PRAISE FOR *THE DR. SEARS T5 WELLNESS PLAN*

"In this powerful and informative book, Dr. Bill Sears shares how lifestyle changes transformed his life and how these can help transform yours. He continues to inspire me and millions of others. Highly recommended!"
—DEAN ORNISH, MD, AUTHOR, *THE SPECTRUM* AND *DR. DEAN ORNISH'S PROGRAM FOR REVERSING HEART DISEASE*

"Dr. Sears offers advice that is not only holistic and truly empowering, but suitable for the entire family. This is a rare invitation to find and share vitality with the people you love most, and I love that!"
—DAVID L. KATZ, MD, MPH, FOUNDER OF TRUE HEALTH INITIATIVE AND AUTHOR OF *THE TRUTH ABOUT FOOD*

"Dr. Sears's book takes you deep inside your body and helps you discover clear directions to a better looking and feeling you. Once you start reading, you'll be unable to put it down."
—VINCE FORTANASCE, MD, AUTHOR OF *THE ANTI-ALZHEIMER'S PRESCRIPTION*

"Dr. Sears has an amazing ability to take science-based information and present it in a simplified way. Transform 5 adds a whole new perspective to making healthy living simple and fun."
—DOMINIQUE HODGIN, MA, NE, NBC-HWC, EXECUTIVE DIRECTOR OF EDUCATION, DR. SEARS WELLNESS INSTITUTE

The
Dr. Sears T5
Wellness
Plan

The
Dr. Sears T5
Wellness
Plan

**FIVE CHANGES
IN FIVE WEEKS**

TRANSFORM YOUR MIND AND BODY

William Sears, MD
and Erin Sears Basile

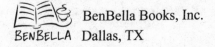 BenBella Books, Inc.
Dallas, TX

Copyright © 2017 by William Sears and Erin Sears Basile
First trade paperback edition 2019

Illustrations by Deborah Maze
Drawing on page 227 courtesy AnnaBelle Crain
Fitness photography by They Call Me Lolo Photography

BenBella Books, Inc.
10440 N. Central Expressway, Suite 800
Dallas, TX 75231
www.benbellabooks.com
Send feedback to feedback@benbellabooks.com

Printed in the United States of America
10 9 8 7 6 5 4 3 2 1

Library of Congress Control Number: 2017040930
ISBN 9781944648701 (trade cloth)
ISBN 9781946885777 (trade paper)
ISBN 9781944648718 (electronic)

Editing by Leah Wilson and David Bessmer
Copyediting by James Fraleigh and Jennifer Greenstein
Proofreading by Cape Cod Compositors, Inc. and Kim Broderick
Indexing by Debra J. Bowman
Text design and composition by Aaron Edmiston
Cover design by Ty Nowicki
Cover photo © iStock / Zocha_K, BrianAJackson, barcin, herreid, villagemoon
Printed by Lake Book Manufacturing

Distributed to the trade by Two Rivers Distribution, an Ingram brand
www.tworiversdistribution.com

Special discounts for bulk sales (minimum of 25 copies) are available.
Please contact Aida Herrera at aida@benbellabooks.com.

To our children, who are the motivation for my transformation:

James
Robert
Peter
Hayden
Erin
Matthew
Stephen
Lauren

To my wife, Martha, may this transformation keep me part of your life for many more years.

Finally, to our fourteen grandchildren, may my example become a legacy for your healthy living.

—WILLIAM SEARS

To all my past, present, and future T5 clients and family members.

—ERIN SEARS BASILE

CONTENTS

Part II: Transform 5 for the "Big Six": Gut Health, Brain Health, Inflammation, Heart Health, Diabetes, and Cancer

CONSULT YOUR DOCTOR FIRST

While T5 is a science-based health transformation plan, you may have special medical needs that merit some modifications. Be sure to consult your healthcare provider before you start, especially if you are taking medications. T5 may affect the dosages you need.

⊕ VISIT US ONLINE

The Dr. Sears T5 Wellness Plan isn't just a book—it's a multimedia health-support program. We will be your extended T5 family, providing a second helping of more topics and a list of over 100 *scientific references* supporting our T5 plan. Go to DrSearsWellness .org/T5 for all this and more:

- Download the ten "T-tips"—colorful, full-page reminders you can post in your kitchen, bedroom, and home workout room to help keep yourself on track.
- Watch video clips of how-to-do-it tips from Dr. Bill and Coach Erin.
- Get updates to the T5 plan.
- See testimonies from happy T5 transformers.
- Visit Dr. Bill's virtual office to learn how to help your body make its own medicines and heal your hurts.
- Enter Coach Erin's workout space to get moving.
- Visit the Sears family kitchen to learn the art of making delicious, healthful smoothies.
- Join our growing family of transformers and interact with them. See our schedule of Facebook parties and webinars.

WHY THIS BOOK IS FOR YOU

Want to feel better, look better, and live healthier? Live every day feeling more energetic, clear-minded, and higher on life?

Are you a young person who wants to *stay* youthful and healthy, even when you're old?

Are you an older person who wants to feel younger?

Do you have medical issues such as brain pains, heart hurts, joint aches, or gut upsets that keep you from enjoying life to the fullest?

Want to lower your pill bill by teaching your body to make its own medicines?

If you answered yes to any of those questions, Transform 5 is for you.

Almost every day, we hear patients and friends saying pretty much the same thing: "I've finally made the decision to take charge of my health. I just need a plan that's easy to understand and fun to follow."

The T5 plan is just what the doctor and health coach ordered. Five steps in five weeks that will transform your health and your life.

By choosing this book, you are well on your way to transforming your health, with a little prescribing and coaching from us.

—DR. BILL AND COACH ERIN

WELCOME TO OUR T5 FAMILY: STARTER TIPS TO A NEW LIFE

A LIFE TRANSFORMED—DR. BILL'S STORY

I'm alive because of Transform 5. My new life started on April 22, 1997, the day I was diagnosed with colon cancer—the disease that had taken the lives of my father and my mother-in-law. A medical crisis that could have ended my life instead transformed it.

On the gloomy afternoon when I came home from the hospital, I wasn't feeling much like Dr. Bill, author, teacher, and lecturer on family health. I was just another patient recovering from a five-hour surgery and looking unhappily ahead to radiation and chemotherapy.

But despite that—or maybe because of it—on that day and in the weeks and months that followed, I began a *transformative* change in my thinking. My life was on the line. If I didn't make some serious adjustments in the way I was living, the quality of my life would slide downhill, and it would be over all too soon. I made a vow to get well and stay well, for the sake of my beloved family and friends, for the many precious patients I cared for, and, yes, for myself.

I made the decision to transform, and made it my mission to help others transform.

I decided to learn everything I could about leading a healthier life. I studied, read, and talked to my friends and colleagues who are doctors and medical scientists. And that is how Transform 5 was born.

The life-saving, life-changing steps I took years ago are the driving force behind this new book. I've spent years developing, field-testing, and fine-tuning my T5 health principles, and now I want to share them with anyone who is ready to feel better, inside and out, for life.

Here is what I accomplished by transforming through our T5 plan, and what you can expect as well:

- *Weight loss*: I dropped 45 pounds and kept it off—and I *love* the way I eat, even more than before.
- *Leaner form*: My waist is seven inches smaller (waist size is a better indicator of your health than weight), and my body is more toned.
- *Stronger bones and muscles*: This happened naturally as I lost waist and weight.
- *Better brain health*: Along with more physical energy, I have more mental energy.
- *Better breathing*: My resting rate decreased from twelve to five breaths per minute. A slower breathing rate boosts energy and helps cardiovascular health.
- *Better vision*: My eyesight improved so much that I tossed out my glasses.
- *Good gut feelings*: I have no digestive issues—and I had colon cancer. If you're feeling good in your gut, you're feeling better all over.
- *Better blood work*: My HDL—the good cholesterol—is up, my blood pressure is down, and my blood sugar is in balance

24/7. My doctor said, "At age seventy-six you have the blood chemistry of a young man."

- *Less of the "shuns"*: I no longer suffer from indigestion, constipation, or inflammation.
- I feel like a "senager," a senior with the health of a teenager.
- In short, everything works and nothing hurts!

⊕ Catch Dr. Bill and Erin's T5 passion: DrSearsWellness.org/T5.

MY BIG MENTAL MAKEOVER

During my transformation, I switched on the *wisdom of my body*, an inner voice that prompts, "Think this, not that!" "Eat this, not that!"

> My wish for you: Everything works and nothing hurts.

Dr. Bill

Next, I changed my habits. I made a list of the things that I had to do. Of course, I didn't *want* to do most of these things. I just knew I *had* to. But over a few months, something astonishing happened in the way I felt about the healthy-living habits on my list. I went from *don't like* to *like* to *crave*. I realized my transformation had begun. I saw the difference. I felt the difference.

You will feel not only healthier but happier. In chapter seven, you will learn—and begin to feel—one of the happiest T5 skills: *how to think-change your brain.*

FEEL IT, CRAVE IT, SHARE IT

Sharing T5 with patients, friends, and family gave me a huge dose of what I call the "helper's high," that priceless feeling a doctor gets from helping others transform their lives. "Doctor" is Latin for "teacher," and I couldn't wait to begin teaching my patients the self-help skills that transformed my own health. But first, I wanted to simplify and streamline my program. Healthcare begins with self-care. Or as the proverb goes, "Physician, heal thyself."

Dad, we not only want you to be at the weddings of your grandkids, we want you to dance with them.
—HAYDEN SEARS

> ▶ View Hayden's story at DrSearsWellness.org/T5/Testimonies.

MORE SKILLS, FEWER PILLS

Patients often ask me, "Doctor, what can I take?" Wrong question. The right one is, "Doctor, what can I *do*?" Transform 5 gives people the skills to take charge of their health and lower their pill bills.

Ready to take charge of *your* health? To feel better, look better, and live better? You're ready for Transform 5—just five steps in five weeks for a lifetime of:

- **Immune system health:** T5 targets inflammation, the number-one trigger of disease and disability. Chapter eight shows how to reduce the -*itis* illnesses and prevent and beat cancer.
- **Brain health:** T5 can help protect against conditions like depression and anxiety, as well as neurodegenerative diseases like Alzheimer's.
- **Heart health:** T5 helps protect cardiac health in people of all ages.
- **Gut health:** Good gut health equals good health overall. When you get your gut in order, you'll feel great.
- **Hormonal health:** Learn how to conduct your inner hormonal symphony.

In figuring out how I could live longer and healthier, and as a show-me-the-science doctor, I concluded that there are *five science-based changes* that have the quickest, greatest, and most lasting effects on wellness:

1. Eat more **plant-based foods**, more **safe seafood**, and much less animal-based food.
2. Be more satisfied with **smaller meals**.
3. **Move** more.
4. Think **happy thoughts**.
5. **Share** more.

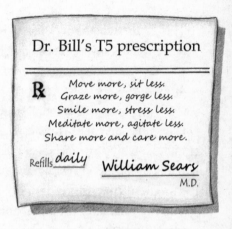

Dr. Bill's T5 prescription

℞ Move more, sit less.
    Graze more, gorge less.
    Smile more, stress less.
    Meditate more, agitate less.
    Share more and care more.

Refills *daily*   **William Sears**
                                    M.D.

T5 does all five.

5 STEPS IN 5 WEEKS: YOUR JUMPSTART TO A MIND AND BODY MAKEOVER

These five changes translate to five simple steps that are the core of Transform 5:

1. **Enjoy the "5-S" Diet:** Eat delicious foods that are simple to prepare and leave you feeling full and satisfied.
2. **Graze on five daily mini-meals:** Forget the "three squares a day" routine. The T5 approach is far more satisfying and healthier, too.
3. **Move more:** Five categories of exercises you can do for the rest of your life that benefit your body and your brain, too. Plenty of options here, so there's something for everyone.
4. **Stress less with five daily stressbusters:** They take only a few minutes a day, so you can stay mellowed out no matter how busy you are.
5. **Share T5 five times:** Transforming with others reinforces your new, good habits, so recruit a team of five from your family and friends to transform with you. You'll stick to it better, and you'll feel great about sharing something this good.

MAKE YOUR OWN MEDICINES—NATURALLY—WITH T5

This is the real "wow" factor of T5—the reason it works so well—the reason T5ers say, "I feel so much better!"

T5 greatly enhances your ability *to make your own medicines internally.*

Yes, you read that right. As of this writing, no other health or fitness plan takes this approach. Transformers "make their own medicines" by tapping into the body's two personal pharmacies: (1) the endothelium—that is, the lining of the blood vessels; and (2) the microbiome lining of the intestines.

These two "silver linings" dispense your own personal medicines. The endothelium is a natural pharmacy that contains trillions of endocrine glands, which I think of as microscopic medicine bottles that release the right dose of "medicine" at the right time, without the side effects of prescription drugs. Exercise and eating real foods like fruits, vegetables, and omega-3-rich fish helps your blood flow freely through your blood vessels. This opens your personal pharmacy so that it dispenses the right amounts of hormones and other natural biochemicals—your internal "medicines"—to keep your body and your brain in tip-top shape. This discovery was such a "wow" moment that it won the Nobel Prize. (You'll learn more about it in chapter three, and about the microbiome in chapter six.)

Are your personal pharmacies open or closed? Your endothelial pharmacy is easily damaged by eating what we call "the sticky stuff"—bad sugars and bad fats—the stuff that literally sticks to the endothelium and closes off those endocrine glands. When this occurs, the "pharmacy" is all but out of business, its shelves barely stocked. The results are disease and disability. Transformers know that keeping their natural internal pharmacy open is easy when they follow the T5 plan.

> Download a full-color illustration of your endothelial pharmacy at DrSearsWellness.org/T5/Endothelial-Pharmacy.

> ▶ View a three-minute, Telly Award-winning animated video on opening your personal endothelial pharmacy at DrSearsWellness .org/T5/Endothelial-Pharmacy-Video.

MEET TRANSFORMED COAUTHOR AND CERTIFIED HEALTH COACH ERIN

Hello, everyone! Welcome home!

As your health coach, and as Dr. Bill's Transform 5 colleague and daughter, I can't wait to share the experience, strength, and knowledge I've gained from T5—and from 15 years of dealing with my own health challenges. Whether you're dealing with depression, stress and anxiety, or chemical dependency, or simply want more energy and a healthier life, you're not alone. Believe me, my journey has not been easy, but I have found a sense of peace and serenity that I wouldn't trade for the world.

One day in 2011, I woke up and stepped onto the scale, and it read 204 pounds. I felt awful about myself, and I knew something had to change. This was where years of crash diets had brought me. Each time, I'd lose 20 or 30 pounds, then gain it all back and more. I felt lost. My self-worth was below zero. I had hit rock bottom.

But, slowly, I began making progress on my inner issues and came to love myself just enough to realize how much I am really worth. That helped me to climb out of depression enough to make better overall health choices. My outer appearance started to match my newfound self-respect. As the number on the scale went down, the passion inside me grew. I was living and feeling the Transform 5 plan. Here's how that worked, on an emotional level, for me:

1. I got my emotional health in balance and looked at past patterns that had gotten me into the dark place.
2. I set my body up for success by fueling it with nutritionally dense food and a meal plan of five small meals throughout the day.

3. Consistent exercise. A very wise friend, my dad, told me, "The best exercise is the one you *do*." I started with Zumba, because I love to dance and it didn't feel like work. I added strength training and yoga, and the fat really began to melt.

4. I changed my relationship with food. Don't get me wrong—I still love to eat. But I'm so much happier and healthier now that I'm putting quality food into my body. For example, I enjoy my Juice Plus+ smoothie every day.

5. I got a tribe of people into my life who lift me and support me and vice versa. And I stay engaged with things that give me joy and motivation, like music and coaching.

This new chapter in my life has fulfilled me more than I could have imagined. I call it Erin 2.0. I'm down 65 pounds, with eight inches off my waist. And I'm living life every day to the fullest.

I am now a Dr. Sears Wellness Institute Certified Health Coach, a yoga teacher, and a fitness instructor. And I am honored to have the chance, through this book, to help others find their best selves. Thank you for that. My role as health coach is to help you make this program part of *your* new, healthy, transformed life. Here is my hope for you:

Focus on health from the inside out, and take back your life!

🌐 GET A COACH

You may need a coach to get you off the couch—a Certified Health Coach to help you *personalize your plan.*

BECOME A CERTIFIED HEALTH COACH

Many of our top transformers have taken this online training to learn more about the science behind Lifestyle, Exercise, Attitude, and Nutrition (or LEAN) and the psychology of coaching.

Find a coach in your area or learn about becoming a coach yourself by visiting DrSearsWellnessInstitute.org.

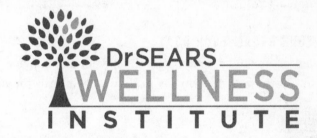

FIVE TIPS FOR GETTING STARTED

Get your head ready to go and you can't fail. Here are five great ways to get your mind into a T5 groove.

1. GO TEAM!

Put together your own T5 team—you and several other transformers—so you can keep each other motivated and accountable. Team transformers have synergy; they feed off each other's enthusiasm. Our team goals:

- *Do it!* Start the five-week transformation plan together.
- *Feel it!* Record your results and cheer each other on.
- *Share it!* You'll find new ways to make T5 work for you. Share these tips with your team and others. (See how to share T5 on page 161.)

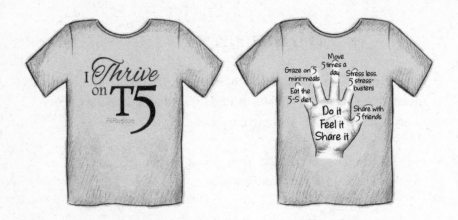

2. MAKE YOUR DREAM YOUR GOAL

A goal is a dream with an action plan. T5 is your action plan. You'll go quickly from *dream it*, to *do it*, to *feel it*. Here are our goals for you during these five weeks:

- *Feel better* mentally and physically.
- Feel such a *complete inner transformation* that you won't want to lapse back into unhealthful habits again—a lifetime transformation!
- Feel empowered to *share your transformation* program with your loved ones.

Are these *your* goals? If they are, you're sure to succeed.

You will think-change your brain. Even if you're not a naturally goal-driven person, you can become one. One of the most exciting medical discoveries over the past decade is how you can *think-change* your brain. In chapter seven, we will give you tools to help you get the willpower to rewire your brain.

Think-change your brain!

Your thoughts may be full of *what if*, *I can't*, or *I don't want to*. We will literally help you grow your brain's *I can do it* center. PET scans (as you will see on page 124) reveal that you can literally grow transformation centers, such as positive-thinking centers, that you never had before. We will show you how. All you have to do is follow the plan. Soon, your brain will convince your body to do it and feel it.

3. TAKE A HEALTH RETREAT

Here's a tip we got from some "fast transformers." They took a weekend off and spent that time thinking about and planning what they would do and imagining how that would make them feel. During that retreat, they made a commitment to *make health their hobby*. They read this whole guide and made lists of the changes they wanted to achieve, based on their personal needs, level of commitment, medical and financial situations, and so on.

On your retreat, read a little at a time, pausing to meditate on what you've read. Let one T5 tip sink in at a time. Think how you would tailor that tip just for you. Read some more. Take a walk and think about it. Throughout your retreat, keep saying to yourself, "I will do it," and, "I want to feel it" until those phrases are stuck in your mind. Picture yourself enjoying more physical energy and greater mental clarity.

We promised you T5 would be easy to follow and fun to do. So we've divided this book into two sections. In Part I, as each of the Transform 5 tips is discussed, we simply tell you what to do, with a bit of why you should do it. In Part II, and in the endnotes, we explore the science underlying the T5 steps. (Wherever you see the 🌿 in the main text, flip to the endnotes section to learn more!)

Throughout your retreat weekend, imagine having the health to live your dreams and achieve your goals. *Picture the new you.*

I'm transforming!

4. JOURNAL YOUR PLAN AND YOUR PROGRESS

List your specific transformation desires and record your progress. Certain changes have different feel-better effects on different people. Keep tabs of what changes worked best for the new you. If you write it, you're more likely to do it—and enjoy it.

YOUR DESIRES:	YOUR RESULTS AFTER FIVE WEEKS:
• More energy • Feel better physically • Feel better mentally • Look leaner • Enjoy more friends	
YOUR MEDICAL ISSUES: • Medical tests, such as inflammatory markers and cardiovascular profile • Medications, hurts, intestinal upsets, illnesses	
I DID THIS: Drank a smoothie a day	I FELT THIS: More energy, good gut feelings

Over the five weeks, your progress might chart something like this:

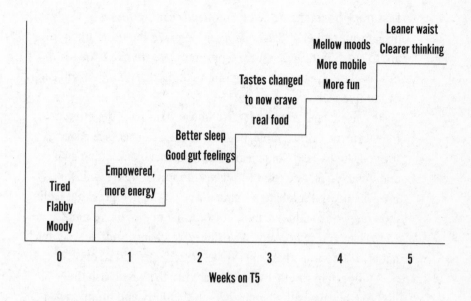

5. CHOOSE YOUR OWN TRACK—PERSONALIZE YOUR PROGRAM SO IT WORKS BEST FOR YOU

T5 is a *personal growth plan*. Identify where you need to grow and T5 will help you get there. *How* fast do you want to feel better? You can choose the *fast track*, and do everything the way we've laid it out. Or you can choose where to start and how to proceed. The important thing is to get on board! *Choose the track that suits your personal train and gets you to the destination you want.* If one part of T5 makes you feel *I just can't* . . . then skip it. (You can always come back to it.) Use as many of these keys as you can to unlock your health potential. What transformation plan is best for *you*? One you will *do*—and *stick to.*

> Set up sustainable habits.

1. **Fast-track transforming.** We've noticed that the *sooner* transformers feel at least *one healthy result*, the more likely they are to stay on the Transform 5 program. *Do all five changes for five weeks.* Or, start your program making *one change* from each of the five steps.

2. **Make one change per week for five weeks.** This pace fits *gradual* transformers. For example, begin with the 5-S Diet (see page 5) for your first week. Some team members make one eating change and quickly feel one result: "When I stopped gorging and started *grazing*, my gut felt better within a week." Let that good gut feeling motivate you to add one more transformation tip: move more, ache less. Then you're hooked. "I've done two changes and feel so much better! If I do four changes, I'll feel better yet," and so on.

    Will going too fast with T5 backfire the way crash diets do? No, because all changes benefit the body and brain. Fast weight-losers on fad diets become fast regainers, because these changes are neither natural nor healthful for the body. All the T5 changes are healthy. They don't shock your body or leave you feeling deprived. That's why the brain welcomes your fast T5 track and tells you, "Finally you are doing it right. Keep it up!"

3. **Fastest track.** If you are absolutely jazzed about getting there as soon as possible, go completely clean and green and do all five steps at once for *two weeks*:

    - Stick to the 5-S way of eating 100 percent (page 5).
    - Graze according to the rule of twos (page 56).
    - Move: Do isometrics for five minutes, five times daily; strength-building twice a week; and cardio three times a week. Also consider stretching and/or yoga once a week (see page 87).
    - Meditate daily (page 139), do deep breathing five times a day (page 132), practice the five stressbusters (page 128), and go outside and play (page 114).
    - If you can, do all of these with at least one other person.

If there were a T5 Health Ranch you could visit for a two-week intensive program, this is pretty much what it would look like.

In short, before you start, have an honest chat with yourself about what track will lead you to success. Most people start with the 5-S diet, but the right way is the one that works for *you*.

I'm not following the prescribed weekly plan of meals first. I'm shooting for mental health first. I always eat better when I'm feeling stronger mentally.
—SUSAN PHINNEY

I'm so terrified of failing like I have with every diet I've tried. I really want to tackle the stress part and look at what is holding me back. I'm dedicated to making this stick! The powerful thing about T5 is that this is *my* program to be lived as I need it.
—SUZANNE LUNAK

YOUR T5 SYNERGY

For optimal health, each T5 component has to work in synchrony with the other four. Eating the diet described in this book won't do as much good if you aren't grazing and moving. Too much stress can sabotage everything. And if you don't share, you will likely soon not care. When you do your best at all five components of T5—eating, grazing, moving, thinking, and sharing—each boosts the effect of the others. That's synergy.

WHAT T5 TRANSFORMATION FEELS LIKE

Think of your body as a symphony orchestra. Hormones are the instruments, and when each plays in tune and perfect harmony, you have the beautiful music of wellness. You can feel this! The T5 program brings your body into harmony. The more you do, the more effects you will feel in terms of these eight "Re-" words:

RESULTS

The time-tested T5 program gives every transformer a quick mental and physical "feel better" result. That's your motivation to keep progressing through the five stages of change: *learn it, do it, feel it, crave it, share it.* Make one simple change, feel one healthful result, and you're hooked!

I feel so good, I'll never go back!

REFRESHED

You know those doorknob tags in hotel rooms that say "Do not disturb" on one side and "Please make up room" on the other? We once saw one that said "Please refresh room." We were charmed. And it's what we want for you. Makeup is superficial. Get refreshed from the inside out.

RESET

T5 resets the inner workings of your body so that it can enjoy hormonal harmony. Your endocrine system is like a system of hundreds of dials interconnected by biochemical signals. As you transform, your body will turn up some dials and turn down others, getting your hormones in harmonious balance.

Three of the main dials are stress, appetite, and energy. Resetting means you will be dialing into a hundred-year-old concept called *the wisdom of the body.* When someone says, "I feel transformed!" they are feeling this hormonal harmony reset. As you will learn on page 243, *hormonal balance* is the current buzz phrase in treating the root cause of many diseases.

REENERGIZED, REJUVENATED, AND REPAIRED

Get ready to feel and look healthier and younger. Enjoy greater physical stamina and mental clarity. And if you suffer from *-itis* illnesses, your body is likely to heal those hurts.

REVEALED

"Wow, you look great! What are you doing?" When it shows, it's time to tell. Share your story. It's amazing how every time you share your story, you get the "helper's high" and a big new dose of motivation.

RESHAPED

First you reshape your brain. Then you reshape your belly as your tastes gravitate toward the good gut feelings of real food. This is *metabolic programming*; the cells in the lining of your gut change. You will almost hear your gut speak: "You're finally feeding me real food. Thanks! Please keep it up." Good gut feelings will cause you to crave this new, healthful way of eating and living.

T5 BOOSTS SEX DRIVE

Sexual desire and performance go up with T5, especially for men. Besides enjoying more energy, there are two more reasons men get more manly. Endothelial function improves with T5, and that makes for better blood flow *everywhere*. (See "Getting Husband on T5" page 267, and "The Case Against Colas," page 84.)

Also, T5 helps you stay lean. Belly-fat cells become estrogen producers and lower testosterone levels—guys, this ain't good! Alcohol also suppresses testosterone; cutting back on alcohol helps you stay lean. (See "Drink Smart," page 268).

A TOP TRANSFORMER'S TESTIMONY

We feel so passionate about sharing T5 because it gives us a big dose of what we call the *helper's high*. (More on this in chapter five.) Meet Gerry, an investment banker who made his smartest investment ever—*investing in his future.*

I had been going to my general practitioner for years, being treated for hiatal hernia, acid reflux, and abdominal pain under my diaphragm. I had also been diagnosed with high cholesterol, liver dysfunction, hypothyroid, gout, sinus and ear infections, difficulty swallowing, and hoarseness, and I was prediabetic. I was taking three medications daily to curb my reflux, gout, and thyroid disorder. My systems were breaking down. I was a mess—stressed out and convinced I had throat cancer.

I visited my general practitioner one day as I was recovering from walking pneumonia and influenza. He scheduled an appointment for me with a gastrointestinal endocrinologist who ordered a battery of tests: esophagram with barium swallow, abdominal ultrasound, endoscopy, biopsies, EKG, and blood analysis.

Soon after, I had a meeting with one of my clients, Dr. William Sears. He could tell I was distraught, and I shared with him my situation. He said my doctor was right in ordering the tests. Then he stepped out to his car and returned with a copy of his book The Inflammation Solution *to help me understand why I hurt. He also prescribed his T5 program, a draft copy of the new book he was working on. He said, "Gerry, just read it and do it." I began reading T5 over the weekend. I couldn't set it down. It described my symptoms to a T. It was a science-made-simple-and-fun approach to tackling confusing medical problems. It described why you hurt, how you heal, and how to help your body make its own medicines.*

I immediately went shopping for my food supply, ordered my supplements, and began the T5 program. I began eating in accordance with the T5 recommendations, and started my new twice-a-day exercise program. I felt a drop in my stress level. I was ready to deal with whatever life would throw at me. And while this isn't recommended, I chose to wean myself from all my medications. I had been on my new T5 regimen for thirty-one days and then I underwent the testing my doctor had recommended. On the day I met with him to review the results, I felt terrific, better than I had in years. I hardly cared what the results would show. My doctor asked me how I felt, and I explained I was pain-free and off all medication. He told me all of my tests had come back negative, and all systems were functioning the way they should. My throat and stomach biopsies were clear and showed no sign of corrosion or irritation. He was amazed. He wanted to know what I had been doing. I told him about Dr. Sears's T5 program. Of course, he suggested I continue doing whatever I had been doing, as it was working.

Over a year later, I am without pain, reflux, gout, and sinus infections. I no longer have any difficulty swallowing, hoarseness, or pain from my hiatal hernia.

My new lifetime avocation is wellness and coaching. I have become a Certified Health Coach with the Dr. Sears Wellness Institute, and have begun helping others achieve their health and wellness goals by providing science-based, trusted information, positive encouragement, and continued motivation. I am sharing and making a difference in others' lives by helping them make changes in their lifestyle, exercise, attitude, and nutrition.

Those are the letters on my new license plate: L E A N.
—GERRY ROSENFELD, CERTIFIED HEALTH COACH

T5—TRANSFORMATION FOR ALL AGES

Naturally, people of different ages will see the value of the T5 differently. If you begin and end each day tired and hurting, you know you're ready for a transformation. But what if you feel great all the time, just because you're young?

"BUT I FEEL FINE!"

T5 is preventive medicine. You may not realize prevention until years later when you continue to "feel fine," yet your friends feel sick.

MESSAGE TO YOUNG READERS: WHY WAIT FOR A WAKE-UP CALL?

The sad fact is, sometimes the wake-up call comes too late. It shouldn't take health crises like we had to scare people into taking better care of themselves. And not everyone is lucky enough to recover as we did. All too often it's extremely hard to reverse years of damage done to bodies and minds.

So when you read in this book about "older people's" issues like Alzheimer's, type 2 diabetes, or the various chronic *-itis* diseases, don't skip that page. We're talking about you. Now.

First, new insights reveal that these preventable diseases are happening at younger ages. The increase in autoimmune *-itis* illnesses is *highest* among millennials. Moreover, the groundwork for many diseases of later years is laid during childhood and early adulthood. In the words of University of California professor Vincent Fortanasce, author of *The Anti-Alzheimer's Prescription,* "Alzheimer's begins in adolescence."

No matter how young and healthy you are, *transform now*. It's never too early to take charge of your health. That's the greatest gift you can give your older self. Look how your parents' and grandparents' generations have messed up:

- 25 percent of women over 40 take prescription antidepressants (even though they often don't work and have risky side effects).
- 33 percent of Americans are prediabetic. (Nearly every one of them would remain "pre" if they did T5.)
- Most Americans over age 65 take seven or more pills for their ills. (Many of these pills are proving to be unsafe when taken too strong for too long.)
- Our generation is sick and tired of being sick and tired. That doesn't have to be your future.
- It's far easier to *prevent* an illness by doing T5 at your age than it is to reverse that illness when you are older. The younger you are, the faster you heal.

BIOHACKING AND TRANSFORMING

Biohacking is a new buzzword that I love and use in my medical practice. It perfectly describes the way T5 teaches you to "hack" into your inner pharmacy to help it work better for you. I recently recorded a podcast with Dave Asprey, author of *The Bulletproof Diet* and one of the pioneers of biohacking. Enjoy Dave's talk on his website, Bulletproof.com.

OUR WISH FOR PARENTS

You have a golden opportunity to transform your lives *and* transform your children's lives by instilling lifelong healthy habits. One evening I was giving a health talk to a large group of parents at a grade school. This was in the wealthy community of Newport Beach, California, and many of the parents held jobs such as investment banker. I opened with this: "Tonight you are going to learn about the absolutely best long-term investment you can give your children." That got their attention. "Give your children the inheritance of healthy living habits, and be there for them as long as you can."

At her wedding, our daughter Hayden toasted us with this: "Thanks, Mom and Dad, for giving us kids the gift of health."

What could be better than that?

T5 TESTIMONIES

Before we get into the specifics of Transform 5, we thought you should hear from some people who have already made it part of their lives.

SIMPLE CHANGES, BIG RESULTS

I needed something simple that I could stick with and that would fit my lifestyle. T5 just made sense! I started making small changes

*and was amazed at how my energy levels began to increase. I was
so inspired by feeling awesome that I've been able to stay motivated and make healthy choices in my food. I'm also much more
educated on what motivates my eating, like not turning to comfort
food when I had a hard day at work. I'm down thirteen pounds in
my first month, and feel like I can conquer the world.*

—SUSAN PHINNEY

PAIN—A GREAT MOTIVATOR

Over the years, we have found that pain relief is the biggest reason why
people start T5 and stay on it. Feeling better—physically and mentally—is
an even greater motivator than weight loss, although the two often go
together.

*As an avid runner for the last few years, I found myself stressed,
tired, and still using food to cope. I hadn't lost a pound, and I
had been diagnosed with plantar fasciitis. With Coach Erin's help
and the T5 program, I gained a new perspective on health that I
would have never received had I not been injured. I was forced to
focus on my inward health and unhealthy patterns. I developed
more-sustainable low-impact training habits, like yoga, as well as
taking control of my portion size through mini-meals.*

—ESTHER ALVA

A BALANCED APPROACH FOR LIFE

*What drew me to T5 was the balance. It didn't feel extreme. I've
tried so many diets that did help for several months, but when I
strayed, it was hard to get back on them. They were expensive and
very restrictive.*

*I focused on the one big change at first. I printed out my T5
shopping and recipe lists and I picked out the recipes I knew I
would enjoy. I stuck to shopping in the outer ring of the grocery*

store and went home and prepped for my week. I did have some headaches, but I knew they came from my severe decrease of sugar and caffeine. That was okay with me, because I knew my body needed to detox.

In a few days, I could feel the difference! My whole family has gotten on board. I make an effort now to take regular bike rides with my kids on the trails behind our house. I've lost 17 pounds, three inches from my waist, and two sizes in jeans!

I have tried many diets, but T5 helped me to know that this is a life change. Yes, the weight is coming off slowly, but I also have more energy, and I feel better. When I'm done with a meal I am totally satisfied and full, because the carbs I've had are healthy! I am so thankful for T5! The scale had not moved since I had my son nearly three years ago. Now I'm hitting lower and lower numbers! Nothing tastes as good as eating "clean" feels!

—TINA EATON

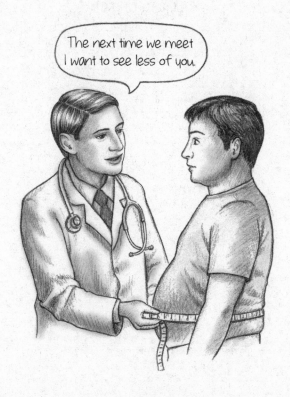

GETTING RID OF POUNDS AND PILLS

I needed a complete transformation. I was taking twelve prescriptions for all my highs: high blood pressure, high blood sugar, and high cholesterol. I was sixty pounds overweight and six inches too big in the belly. I was tired, had foggy thinking, and I was what Dr. Bill scientifically termed a "metabolic mess." He looked at my waistline and said, "Next time we meet I want to see less of you."

Dr. Bill put me on his Transform 5 program, and to learn more, I became a certified Health Coach through the Dr. Sears Wellness Institute. Within five weeks, I began feeling the health effects. I now am off eleven of the twelve medicines. I shed the sixty pounds and six inches, and I've kept it off for eight years. Before my transformation, I was a yo-yo dieter. In August of 2016, my cardiologist, after viewing my test results, said, "Bill, at age seventy-six, you have the heart of a thirty-year-old."

—BILL BRIDEGROOM

PART I

FIVE CHANGES IN FIVE WEEKS

✐ You hold the five keys to your transformation in the palm of your hand. Download this visual reminder from DrSearsWellness.org/T5/Hand. Hang it all over your home and workplace, and display it as your cellphone wallpaper.

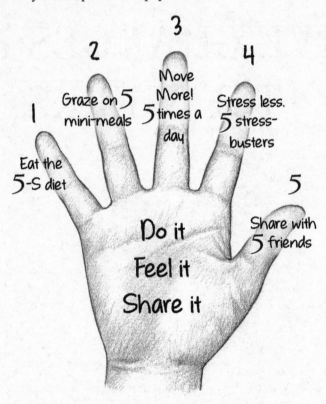

Now that you are fired up about investing in a new you, it's time to walk you through each of the five changes. You will learn *what* to do and *why* you should do it. If you're interested in the science behind each T5 change, you'll find a second helping of motivating information in endnotes and suggested reading at the end of the book.

The first two changes (and chapters) have to do with nutrition—what, how, and when to eat. But first, we want you to understand the biggest reason *why* we eat this way.

Three simple words: *avoid sugar spikes*.

Increased blood sugar triggers the release of insulin. Insulin is the hormone that, among other things, regulates blood sugar levels. The standard American diet (SAD) typically dumps big loads of "sticky stuff"—especially carbs (sugars)—into the bloodstream that have to be knocked down by big jolts of insulin from the pancreas. This is why we use "sugar spikes"—the *cause*—and "insulin spikes"—the *effect*—interchangeably.

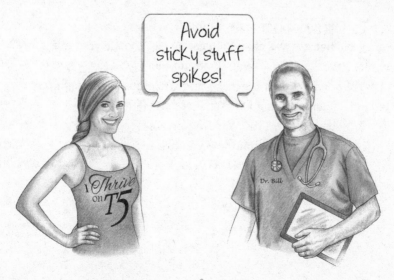

Sugar spike, insulin spike, sugar spike, insulin spike, all day long. That's bad for you in so many ways!

Constant insulin spikes are why we get sick and tired and fat.

T5 blunts spikes. It levels out blood sugar throughout the day.

Beginning on page 39 we'll show you *why* preventing spikes is the T5 key to health. But all you really need to remember is this: "Why am I making this change? I'm avoiding spikes." If someone says, "You look so good. What are you doing?" tell them, "I'm lowering my spikes!" Then show them pages 41 and 86 to explain the *what* and *why* of sugar spikes.

T5 GOES DEEPER THAN DIETS

T5 is a mind-body *transformation,* an inside job, not a superficial and temporary eating change. And the deeper inside your body the T5 effect goes, the better you will feel and the longer it will last.

Every organ of your body is only as healthy as the blood vessels supplying it. T5 grows more and healthier blood vessels to all your vital organs. But let's go even deeper.

Every tissue in your body, from a fiber of muscle to a bit of your skin, is only as healthy as each cell in it. T5 *energizes* your cells.

Feeling good begins in your gut. The lining of your gut is your quick-change artist; a change in eating can change your gut lining within a week. T5 gives you good-gut feelings.

Your body is your business card. Be prepared for admirers to inquire: "You look so good! What are you doing?"

Proudly answer, "T5! Want to join me?"

Let the journey to your new you begin.

CHAPTER 1

ENJOY THE 5-S DIET

W hat is the perfect diet?

It's a way of eating that is science based, delicious, nutritious, and time tested—a way of eating that you love because it makes you feel great mentally and physically. And, of course, it's a diet that will last.

The eating plan for you is the one you will do—and stick to. We want to transform you from reader to doer. Or to put it another way, T5 is not a *diet*, it's a *do-it*. That's exactly what Erin and I wanted when we needed to transform our minds and bodies following life-threatening medical crises, and we did extensive research to discover what that diet would be. Our 5-S way of eating is based on foods that:

- *Taste* good,
- Are *filling* and *feel* good in your gut,
- Are *nutrient dense*—the most nutrition per calorie,
- *Balance* your immune system—the best definition of "health food"—and
- Are proven by *science* to have the greatest health benefits.

After our transformations, people would ask us, "What diet are you on?" Our answer: "The real-food diet," which simply means all the good stuff is left in and no bad stuff is added.

So if someone says to you, "You look so good! What diet are you on?" that's your answer: "The real-food diet." You'll love the look of surprise on their face. This simple, delicious, and nutritious diet is the one I personally eat and have been recommending in my medical practice for over a decade. It is not a low-fat, low-carb, or high-fad diet. It is science-based, real-food eating that will transform your life.

Remember, the best diet for *you* is one you will consistently *do*. Customize this diet to one you will enjoy the most, working in your favorite treats, such as the 90/10 approach: 90 percent the 5-S diet and 10 percent your personal favorites and treats, so you'll never feel deprived.

Why do we call it the 5-S diet? These will be your new *five food groups*, all beginning with the letter S:

THE 5-S DIET

1. **Smoothies.** Enjoy one every day.
2. **Salads and spices.** Go *green* with organic arugula, kale, and spinach. Go *red* with tomatoes and peppers. Add a tablespoon of extra-virgin olive oil to increase the synergy and intestinal absorption of these nutrients. Enjoy turmeric, black pepper, ginger, garlic, rosemary, chilies, and cinnamon.
3. **Seafood.** Our top T5 pick is wild salmon, 12 ounces a week.
4. **Smart snacks,** especially seeds and nuts.
5. **Supplements that are science based.** Fill in your nutritional gaps with supplements like concentrates of fruits, berries, and vegetables; omega-3s; and probiotics.

COACH ERIN'S KITCHEN MAKEOVER

Start your new 5-S diet by making over your kitchen and you're sure to stick with it. Throw out the really bad stuff, the chemical foods (see page 81)

such as those containing high-fructose corn syrup, hydrogenated oils, any #
color symbol (such as red #40), and flavor enhancers such
as MSG. Refill your fridge and pantry with healthier
choices. (See our Shopping Guide at DrSears
Wellness.org/T5/Shopping-Guide.)

Purge your pantry and fridge!

Next—be honest with yourself. Can
you have ice cream in the house without
overdoing it? I can't! Think about what
your *trigger foods* are, and get rid of
any temptation you can't resist.
Out of sight, out of mind, out
of tummy. (See our "instead
of" chart, page 74.)

5-S isn't about what
you can't eat. It's about all the
wonderful, nutritional food we *get*
to eat. Replacing those trigger foods with
healthier options is key!

COACH ERIN'S 5-S BEGINNER SHOPPING LIST:

- A journal
- A blender (doesn't need to be expensive, just powerful enough to blend leafy greens)
- An insulated bottle to shake up your smoothie when you are on the run
- Pint and quart Mason jars for making salad in a jar (see page 328)
- A cooler or insulated lunch bag, if you need to pack your food for the day
- A fitness tracker (optional; see "Share with Tech-Savvy Transformers," page 176)
- Medium-weight resistance band
- Light (5–10 pound) and medium (12–20 pound) weights
- Yoga mat
- A comfortable workout outfit (optional, but fun)

SMOOTHIES: ENJOY ONE A DAY

This is the quickest, easiest way to reshape your tastes, reset your eating habits, and start feeling better inside. Whether you call your blended bounty a "smoothie" or a "shake" is up to you. We use both interchangeably. Many transformers say they feel the effects within a week of making this one simple change—a smoothie a day. We call it *the sipping solution.*

- Your head feels better—clearer thinking.
- Your body feels better—more energy.
- Your gut feels better.

The sipping solution is a "supergrazing" way of eating. It's the quickest way to put your body into balance. (See "Why Grazing Is Good for You," page 56, for more information on grazing.) During my health crisis in 1997, my body was out of biochemical balance. I needed to see and feel results fast. I came up with the sipping solution and have been doing it for twenty years. As a happy, healthy, leaner doctor, I have prescribed this delicious, nutritious way of eating to hundreds of transformers in my medical practice. I have promoted it on many television and radio programs to audiences all over the world, and it was the subject of a feature article, "The Supergrazer Solution," in *Prevention* magazine's September 2010 issue.

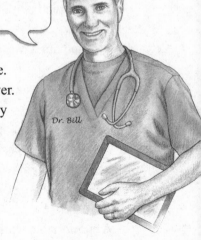

A smoothie a day keeps the doctor away!

Dr. Bill

My sipping solution was literally a lifesaver. After surgery for colon cancer, followed by radiation and chemotherapy, my gut wasn't ready for me to eat—at a time when I needed the best nutrition to help my body heal. Solution: First, choose the best healing foods that are the most gut friendly. Second, blend them into a smoothie and sip on it all day long. That one simple change helped me heal, as it has hundreds of my patients with various ailments. The sipping solution became my top transformation tip for health.

EAT THE FRUIT. DON'T DRINK THE JUICE.

There's a big difference between gulping store-bought orange juice and peeling and eating an orange. An eight-ounce glass of orange juice has maybe three oranges, but without the fiber. You gulp it down fast, and your blood sugar spikes fast. But when you eat an orange, you take time to peel it and chew it, and the natural fiber blunts the sugar spikes.

JUST DRINK IT—OUR T5 SMOOTHIE PRESCRIPTION

Select items from each of the five food categories below. Start with a few ingredients that you already know you like. Gradually add more. Be sure to add *protein* and *healthy fats*—your smoothie will taste better and keep you fuller longer than a carb-only drink. Aim for about 20 to 25 percent proteins, 25 to 30 percent healthy fats, and 45 to 50 percent healthy carbs.

1. Healthy Fluids	2. Healthy Fats
• Kefir, organic, plain	• Avocado
• Coconut milk, unsweetened	• Nut butters
• Almond or cashew milk, unsweetened	• Coconut oil, virgin
• Goat milk, Meyenberg	• Coconut chunks
• Green tea	• Ground flaxseeds, hemp, or chia seeds
• Organic juices: green vegetable, pomegranate	
• Milk, whole, organic, 100% grass fed	

3. Healthy Proteins

- Greek yogurt, organic, plain
- Nut butters
- *Juice Plus+ Complete* or other multinutrient protein powder mix; 13 grams of protein per serving
- *Hawaiian Spirulina Protein*, a plant-based protein powder; 16 grams of protein per serving

4. Healthy Fruits and Greens

(organic whenever possible)
- Blueberries
- Strawberries
- Açai berries
- Pomegranates
- Papaya
- Kiwi
- Banana
- Greens: kale, spinach, chard, celery

5. Special Additions: Flavors and Nutrients

- Figs (for more fiber and sweetness)
- Cinnamon
- Hawaiian spirulina
- Wheat germ
- Cacao powder
- Grated organic orange peel
- Shredded coconut
- Mint
- Ginger root (for a spicy perk-up)
- Half lemon or lime (for a tart taste)

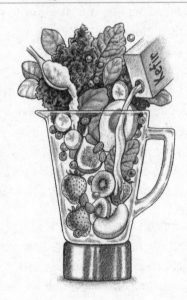

See DrSearsWellness.org/T5/Sipping-Solution for a video of Dr. Bill and Erin making smoothies.

COACH ERIN'S SMOOTHIE TIPS:

- No time to blend up your morning smoothie? Simply shake your Juice Plus+ Complete or other multinutrient mix in a Blender Bottle. (Add your beverage of choice, or even just water.)
- Drink a smoothie before or after your workout. If you exercise first thing in the morning, this is a great way to get fuel for your workout without upsetting your tummy. It is also wonderful for recharging and repairing stress on the body after a workout.
- Sip a smoothie for an afternoon pick-me-up instead of a candy bar.
- If ice cream is your diet downfall (as it is for Dr. Bill and me), enjoy a smoothie instead. My favorite smoothie uses chocolate, banana, and almond butter—as delicious as ice cream and so much healthier!

My smoothie turns me from blah to hallelujah!

WHY IS IT CALLED A SMOOTHIE?

Because it smoothes out your blood sugar spikes.

It's delicious. It fills you up and satisfies your hunger, because it's made with fiber-filled carbs, protein, and healthy fats. It satisfies your craving for a treat and tells your brain to stop begging for more.

After three to five weeks of the sipping solution, you can feel one of the most important effects of T5: you're comfortably satisfied with smaller meals. Another perk of the sipping solution is that you have a sip when you feel *slightly* hungry rather than waiting until you're famished, which prompts overeating.

The sipping solution will make you feel better fast. The sooner you can feel your transformation, the more motivated you will be to continue. You feel better faster because you enjoy the five R's of an inner transformation:

- **Reduced.** No, not just weight. You gradually become satisfied with less food. Taking small, frequent sips programs your gut to be comfortably satisfied. And that translates into less extra fat being stored around your middle.
- **Reshaped.** Not just your belly, but also your tastes. At first, you might not like certain healthful foods, like kale. But you will, I promise! Start with a few leaves and progress to a handful.
- **Relieved.** Because blended food empties faster from the stomach, it relieves reflux (i.e., heartburn), a pain in the esophagus that afflicts millions of people.
- **Regular.** One of the earliest and most gut-friendly feelings you are likely to experience is an increase in the number and softness of your daily stools (more about this at AskDrSears.com/DrPoo). Because blended food travels faster through the intestines, sipping is a solution for constipation. (See why your microbiome loves blended foods on page 206.)
- **Re-immunized.** Want to make your immune system healthier? Eat the T5 way. Fruits and vegetables help support your immune system, at all ages.

BERRY, BERRY GOOD

Berries are one of the best nutrients for all your organs, especially the brain. I call blueberries the "brain berry." See more about berries and the brain on page 222.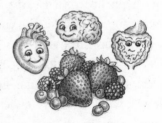

FIVE STARTER TIPS FOR BEGINNING SIPPERS

1. **Start slow.** Some new sippers find it easier to *start low* and *go slow*. In the first week, make a small, simple smoothie just for breakfast. Then gradually add more ingredients to make a smoothie large enough for breakfast and lunch each day (I personally average thirteen ingredients). I suggest this, because drinking Dr. Bill's super smoothie (pages 9–10) right from the start may give some sippers uncomfortable gut feelings instead of good ones. It can help to ease your gut into this new way of eating. Start with a few of the ingredients that you like most and you know from experience will agree with you, then gradually add more.

I made one simple change starting with drinking more water and drinking a daily smoothie with the fruit and veggie capsule supplements. By day three I had so much more energy! I've changed my perception from "diet" to "lifestyle."
—SARAH SLADE BRANHAM

2. **Go BIG.** Want to feel better fast? If you're fast-tracking T5, here's the sipping solution for you. Gradually increase the volume of the smoothie you make from 12 ounces (one glass) to as much as 48–64 ounces—a whole blender full—and sip all day to your gut's content at least five days a week. It's your breakfast, lunch, and morning and afternoon snacks. Then eat a healthy dinner. Within five weeks you are likely to feel so transformed, mentally and physically, that you'll want to continue your new way of eating.

SHAKE IT—AFTER EXERCISE

Drink a 12-ounce smoothie before and after your workout. The increased delivery of protein and healing antioxidants will help repair and grow your muscles.

---

3. **Shake it and share it!** Share your recipes and other sipping tips with your new "health club" of other transformers. Share what's happening with your social media network. "I added this . . . and felt this . . ." The sipping solution for you is the one you will do. Experiment with various on-the-go containers so you can enjoy sipping on your smoothie on the way to work, while traveling, in the gym, or just while you walk.

4. **Make it fit your work schedule.** The sipping solution is easy to do at home. But it can be just as easy at work and on the go. Just put your smoothie in a couple Blender Bottles, sip on the way to work, and refrigerate the rest at your workplace. (See "Transforming While Traveling," page 273.)

DR. BILL'S ENERGY TIP

On work days, I add extra healthy fats (nut butters, avocado, coconut oil) for extra energy, so I'm always satisfied and never hungry.

---

5. **Avoid five mistakes most "shakers" make.** *Don't skimp on the protein.* Of all nutrients, protein has the *highest satiety factor,* meaning it comfortably fills you sooner. As a general guide for your day-long sipping solution, add to your smoothie around *half a gram of protein per pound* of your weight. My daily smoothie averages 60 grams of protein.

- *Don't forget fat.* The biggest mistake that new sippers make is leaving out the fat because they don't want to get fat. Wrong! (A bit more on "Five Fat Facts You Have to Know" on page 16.)
- *Don't forget fiber.* This is also important for blunting sugar and insulin spikes. Fat and fiber are partners in *satiety*. Like proteins, they make you feel full and satisfied sooner, so you don't overeat. The 5-S diet is naturally high in fiber (35–45 grams a day). The fiber in your food paints a layer of gooey stuff on your intestinal lining. The rest of the nutrients you eat, including carbs, have to make it through the goo to enter the bloodstream. That slows down absorption, which *blunts sugar-insulin spikes*—which is good for your health.

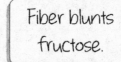

Fiber blunts fructose.

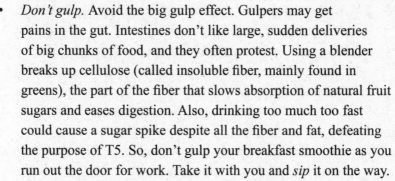

Dr. Bill

- *Don't gulp.* Avoid the big gulp effect. Gulpers may get pains in the gut. Intestines don't like large, sudden deliveries of big chunks of food, and they often protest. Using a blender breaks up cellulose (called insoluble fiber, mainly found in greens), the part of the fiber that slows absorption of natural fruit sugars and eases digestion. Also, drinking too much too fast could cause a sugar spike despite all the fiber and fat, defeating the purpose of T5. So, don't gulp your breakfast smoothie as you run out the door for work. Take it with you and *sip* it on the way.
- *Don't oversweeten.* Remember, a big T5 effect you want to feel, or in this case taste, is to reshape your tastes to enjoy the natural sweetness of real foods. No need to add "sugar" and certainly *not artificial sweeteners* (see why on page 82). After a few weeks, the natural sweetness of fruits should satisfy your sweet tooth. Our favorite natural sweetener: figs!

FIGS: A FABULOUS FRUIT

Besides being full of fiber, figs add a natural sweetness and pleasant texture to your smoothie. Since the fig season is short, load up on fresh organic figs while they're available, then slice and freeze them in small containers. More nutrition-conscious supermarkets often stock frozen figs as well.

FIVE FAT FACTS YOU HAVE TO KNOW

1. *You don't get fat by eating healthy fats.* You get fat by eating *junk carbs.* (See why on page 195.)
2. However, "Eating fat doesn't make you fat" is only true of certain kinds of fats—plant fats and wild seafood fats. Excess animal fats can cause obesity.
3. Fats increase the absorption of fat-soluble nutrients, such as vitamins A, D, E, and K, as well as important antioxidants in plant foods called carotenoids and flavonoids.
4. Adding healthy fats to your smoothie helps you feel comfortably fuller longer. This is especially important for waist watchers. When you eat a healthy-fat breakfast, you tend to eat fewer calories and lose more weight compared to dieters who eat no fat for breakfast.
5. Fat gives your smoothie an enjoyable taste and texture.

How much fat in your smoothie? I suggest one tablespoon of nut butter or coconut oil, or half of a medium avocado.

SALADS AND SPICES: SAVOR THEM

Remember all those times your mother said, "Eat your vegetables"? Maybe you didn't listen, but she was right. Science proves it. The best change you can make in your diet: Eat more vegetables. Consider these scientific veggie facts:

- Veggie eaters outlive meat eaters, and they spend less time in the hospital.

> Eat five servings of veggies a day to keep the doctor away.

Dr. Bill

- The incidence of every illness you don't want to get goes down when you eat more vegetables.

VEGGIES DELIVER AWESOME ANTIOXIDANTS

Want to look younger? Eat more antioxidants.

A smoothie for breakfast and a salad for lunch or dinner is just what the transformation doctor ordered. Just as Dr. Mom preached, "Put more color on your plate," put more color in your smoothie. Antioxidants are natural biochemicals that are among the most important examples of nature's medicines. Some antioxidants give fruits and vegetables their vivid colors. The blue color of blueberries (anthocyanins) and the yellow, orange, and red of vegetables and fruits (carotenoids) are the result of internal medicines these plant foods make to stay healthy. If plants didn't make their own antioxidants for pest and sun protection, they would get sick and die quickly. When we eat these plants, the natural medicines they contain help keep *us* from getting sick and delay aging. The 5-S diet is high in natural antioxidants. Or, as your mother might have put it, 5-S is a *colorful* diet.

Oxidation means combining something with oxygen to form a new chemical. Rust is oxidized iron. When something is on fire, it is being oxidized very fast. When your body burns carbs for energy, that's oxidation at work, too. And that process can leave your body, as it were, rusty.

The 5-S diet is basically an anti-rust program, because it is full of anti-rust nutrients called antioxidants. Like any engine that burns fuel, your body produces exhaust, or what is called oxidants (or oxidative stress). As a tribute to the great Designer, your body both produces and takes in from food those anti-rust chemicals we call antioxidants. When the production of oxidants and antioxidants is in balance, the result is beautiful music, the harmony of health.

The smart avocado. To see how oxidation can damage brain and body tissue, cut an avocado in half. Leave one half unprotected and exposed to the air. On the other half leave the pit in place (it contains the avocado's own protective antioxidants) and sprinkle on it some lemon or lime juice (full of natural antioxidants). After six or eight hours you'll see the difference. The unprotected avocado half looks rusted, oxidized, aged, brown; the protected half looks young and healthy.

This is what you do for your tissues when you eat more antioxidants. So as you sip your smoothie and enjoy your colorful salads and seafood, just say to yourself, "I'm keeping my body and brain from rusting."

FIVE REASONS WHY SALADS ARE SMART

1. **Eat more for less.** Ever wonder why smart eaters begin their meals with a big salad? Salads have a *high satiety factor.* You have to chew them more, which makes you feel satiated sooner and improves digestion. The high fiber content fills you up faster, so you become more satisfied with fewer calories. In fact, being satisfied with fewer calories is one of the underlying reasons your body transforms fast with T5.

   > Big eaters can enjoy a big salad without getting bigger around the middle.

   Dr. Bill

2. **Salads don't spike.** There it is again, the T5 mantra: *avoid spikes.* As with the sipping solution, the high-fiber, slower-eating, and low-glycemic-index (less spikey) carbs in vegetables prompt your body to feel more comfortably full sooner.

As a recovering overeater, I noticed the bigger the salad I ate, the smaller the rest of the meal I wanted. I upsized my salad, downsized the entrée, and downsized my waist.

3. **Salads help you stay lean.** Eat green, stay lean. Later in this book you will learn that there is a strong correlation between a leaner waist and a lasting health transformation. Vegetables help keep you lean for several reasons.

Vegetable-rich salads are free *foods.* You can eat as much as you want as often as you want. A vegetable medley will likely become your favorite all-you-can-eat buffet. Because they're so filling and satisfying, it's almost impossible to overeat vegetables.

Of course, that doesn't mean you can use a lot of salad dressing. One tablespoon of olive oil is best. (See "Give Yourself an Oil Change," page 245.) At any rate, while I don't advocate becoming a strict vegetarian, a high-salad diet is as close as you can get to an all-you-can-eat daily diet and still maintain a healthy weight.

You burn more, and store less. Because you burn so many of the calories in the vegetables just chewing and digesting them, no excess calories are left over to be deposited in belly fat. Also, studies have shown that salad eaters tend to have a higher metabolic rate (i.e., calorie burn) than meat eaters. Perhaps it's all that chewing of high-fiber plant foods at the top end and microbiome action (see page 191) at the other end that accounts for this.

ENJOY SMOOTHIES AND SALADS FOR SYNERGY

The 5-S diet is super-synergistic. Smoothies and salads deliver one of the most transforming principles of nutrition, another S word—synergy. When you team up a whole bunch of colorful foods in your salad or blender, you get synergy—each antioxidant increases the effect of the other. We call it the *rainbow effect*: eat five foods together and get the nutritional benefits of ten or more.

4. **Science says salads are smart.** When you eat more vegetables, diseases go down and health goes up, especially 🖐 :

- Healthier brain
- Healthier heart
- Good gut feelings
- Fewer -*itis* illnesses

5. **Salads satisfy your microbiome.** In chapter six, you will learn why your loveable little gut bugs, your microbiome, thrive best on salads.

LOVE YOUR LEGUMES

Want to eat more and weigh less? Eat more beans, peas, and lentils. I noticed that when I added a half fistful of beans or lentils to my salad, I felt fuller faster. Fat scientists—I mean those who study obesity—have been trying to figure out a better way to lose weight than eating less, because nobody has come up with a good way to get people to eat less. A better strategy for a lifetime diet is one that lets you eat as much as you want and still weigh less. We've already discussed vegetables as one component of a tasty, filling diet. Legumes are another.

Science shows that when people add a lot of lentils, peas, and beans to their diets, they tend to eat more in volume but lose weight and keep it off. This actually has been studied by comparing calorie cutters to legume eaters who didn't cut calories. The legume group came out way ahead in remaining slimmer and had better blood chemistry, especially regarding insulin sensitivity. As we said earlier, it's not so much the quantity as the quality of the food that makes the difference.

TIPS FROM COACH ERIN ON ENJOYING YOUR VEGGIES

Does just thinking about all those high-fiber veggies and legumes make you bloat? Try these tips:

- Aid digestion by sprinkling on fresh lemon juice.
- Lightly steam your veggies.

- Chop them up fine.
- Don't go for too much variety too soon. Start with a few favorites and add variety gradually.
- Eat slowly and chew longer.
- Watch your portion size. Yes, veggies are "free foods," but listen to your body so you don't overload.
- Choose dressing and toppings that don't add extra salt, sugar, and omega-6 oils.

DR. BILL'S TOP FIVE SALAD-EATING TIPS
To make your salads more nutritious and delicious:

1. **Eat your salad first.** A salad will fill you up faster, so you won't want to eat too much of the (likely) less healthy main course. Also, salads may blunt sugar and unhealthy fat spikes caused by the "sticky" entrée.
2. **Enjoy a hot salad.** For taste and variety, once a week I lightly steam my salad for just two minutes. This melts the cheese, warms the hummus, and softens the spinach, kale, and black beans. Yum! While raw vegetables are generally more nutritious, light cooking releases more of the nutrients in vegetables like kale, spinach, and tomatoes. This is called increased *bioavailability*. I love that term. It means that more of the nutrients you put in your mouth are absorbed by your intestines and get into your tissues. (See how steaming brings out flavor, page 66.)
3. **Spice it up.** Spicy salads are savory and healthful. I like to add a teaspoon of turmeric and a half teaspoon of black pepper to my salad. Also, I usually add about a tablespoon of olive oil and one to three teaspoons of vinegar—balsamic or apple cider. Science suggests adding vinegar is smart—it blunts sugar spikes. This is how I justify one of my occasional treats, dipping bread in olive oil and balsamic vinegar.
4. **Make salad a main course.** A salad of dark leafy greens, vegetables, nuts, salmon, olive oil, and eggs will serve as a very tasty, satisfying, and transforming main course. Top your salad with

a four- to six-ounce wild salmon fillet for a delicious lunch or dinner. Mix it up by *adding beans to your greens.*

5.   **Slow your salad eating.** Dr. Bill's slow salad-eating tip: use chopsticks. It's fun, it improves your dexterity, and it slows down your eating. I added chopsticks to my T5 regimen several years ago, and now I prefer them at every salad meal. Need to really slow down your eating? Use your non-dominant hand to grab each bean.

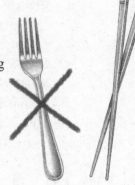

GROW YOUR OWN GARDEN, GROW A SMARTER BRAIN

As I write this I am munching on sweet, delicious tomatoes home-grown in our Tower Garden.

The more antioxidants we eat, the better for our brain. That's because the brain is composed mostly of fat and blood vessels—the two tissues most vulnerable to oxidation (see page 214). Fruits and vegetables are great sources of antioxidants, but the longer and less carefully they are handled from farm to fork, the more natural antioxidants they lose. Best solution? Shorten the farm-to-fork time from weeks to minutes by growing your own.

Imagine you're making a smoothie or a salad. When it's time to add the kale, straw-berries, tomatoes, or parsley, you go out and pick a handful. That's smart, and it helps you stay smart.

Also, it's a great way to get kids involved. Picky eaters often love to eat the veggies they help grow.

(See AskDrSears.com/Tower-Garden and the endnotes.)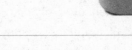

ERIN'S SALAD BAR

Here's a great list of ingredients for making your own delicious salads. As you go down the list, pretending you're at a salad bar, add less food from each category:

Greens: Mixed greens, kale, arugula, spinach

Veggies: Cucumber, tomatoes, bell peppers, carrots, radishes, beets, broccoli, mushrooms, onions, cauliflower, pepperoncini, zucchini, squash, corn, bean sprouts, celery

Beans and legumes: Kidney beans, edamame, chickpeas, black beans, lentils, peas

Lean protein: Salmon, tuna, turkey, chicken (organic, free-range), eggs, feta cheese, goat cheese

Healthy fats: Olives, avocados, olive oil, raw seeds (pumpkin, sesame), raw nuts (almonds, walnuts, cashews, pecans)

Always put dressing on the side to avoid overdoing it. Shoot for one tablespoon. Best is to pour from bottle to tablespoon, then drizzle on the salad. Pouring directly from the bottle encourages overuse. One healthy choice is olive oil with balsamic vinegar. Avoid creamy dressings such as ranch. Keep it fresh and fun with theme salads—Italian, Greek, Mexican, Cobb, fruits and nuts with goat cheese.

Yes, I've turned into my Dad.....
I HAVE to have my salads!

SALAD IN A JAR—FAST FOOD THE T5 WAY

This hip new salad trend is a great way to eat the T5 way when you're on the go. Transformers tell us they love it!

Use a pint-size jar for a regular salad or a quart size jar for an entrée salad.

This is a five-layer salad (our favorite number!) that you can make in any combination of ingredients you like.

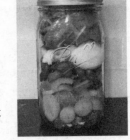

Layer 1: Dressing
Layer 2: Hearty vegetables and legumes
Layer 3: Pasta and grains
Layer 4: Protein and cheese
Layer 5: Lettuce, nuts, seeds, and dried fruit

After you fill the Mason jar with the different layers, just put the top on and close tight.

There's no rule for how much to put in each layer. You can even skip a layer or two. The layer you *always* want to include is the second, the hearty vegetables. Just make sure you have enough other ingredients to keep the dressing and lettuce away from each other until you're ready to enjoy your salad.

For more information on making a T5 salad in a jar, see Appendix C, page 328.

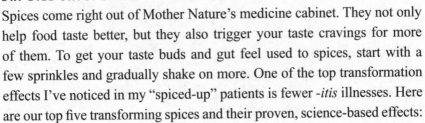

   (▶) Watch Erin's video of how to make salad in a jar at DrSears Wellness.org/T5/Salad-In-A-Jar.

DR. BILL SAYS: SPICE UP YOUR TRANSFORMATION ✌

Spices come right out of Mother Nature's medicine cabinet. They not only help food taste better, but they also trigger your taste cravings for more of them. To get your taste buds and gut feel used to spices, start with a few sprinkles and gradually shake on more. One of the top transformation effects I've noticed in my "spiced-up" patients is fewer *-itis* illnesses. Here are our top five transforming spices and their proven, science-based effects:

1. **Turmeric.** Sprinkle a quarter to a half teaspoon of turmeric on your daily salad. This yellow spice used in curry, a daily staple

in Indian and Asian cuisine, is becoming increasingly popular in America. Science says turmeric has terrific health benefits:

- Anti-inflammatory
- Anti-cancer, especially colon cancer.
- Anti-Alzheimer's—reduces the buildup of "sticky stuff" deposits in the brain.
- Anticoagulant—keeps blood cells from sticking together too much.

Turmeric tip: Partner it with black pepper and extra-virgin olive oil to increase intestinal absorption of the turmeric—a spicy example of food synergy.

At first, I didn't like turmeric on my salads, but after reading about its health benefits, I now have a taste for it. I even pack turmeric in my travel case. Erin, on the other hand, loves turmeric in cooked food, but not on her salads, so she supplements with turmeric capsules.

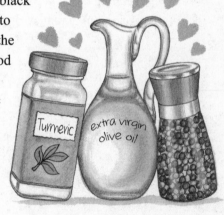

We work better together.

2. **Black pepper.** Like turmeric, black pepper is one of the most researched spices. It eases digestion and arthritis. To retain more of pepper's flavor and health benefits, grind your own in a peppermill and request freshly ground pepper when dining out.

3. **Cinnamon.** Sprinkle a teaspoon of cinnamon into your morning smoothie, oatmeal, or coffee and enjoy both the sweet and spicy flavors. A healthy substitute for sugar, cinnamon is a smart way to gradually reshape your sweet tastes. For an occasional splurge, I sprinkle cinnamon and raw honey into my coffee. The sweet health effects of cinnamon are:

- Blunts sugar spikes
- Lowers blood levels of sticky fats

4. **Ginger.** Along with cinnamon, add a chunk of ginger root about the size of your thumb into your morning smoothie, and occasionally squeeze it into tea, chop into marinades, and add it when cooking or baking. Ginger is good for you. It's an anti-inflammatory and it eases nausea and indigestion.

5. **Garlic.** Yes, foodies, I know. Garlic is an herb, not a spice. But it does spice up your eating *and* boost cardiovascular health by keeping blood cells and blood vessels from getting too "sticky." Also, it may reduce risk of colon cancer.

SEAFOOD: WILD SALMON AND OTHER SAFE SELECTIONS

In our search for the "perfect" food, we looked for these attributes:

- Filling, not fattening
- Tasty
- Just the right amount of healthy fats
- No added sugar
- High protein
- Low salt
- High essential vitamin content
- Inflammation balancing
- Nearly impossible to overeat
- Validated by many scientific studies

And the winner is: wild Pacific salmon (for nutrient profile, see end-notes).

Doctor's orders: Eat two servings (around 12 ounces) of safe seafood weekly. If you're not fond of fish, eat it anyway. Your seafood tastes will naturally go from *don't like* to *like* to *crave.* You'll feel it. All my research has led me to this conclusion: A six-ounce fillet of wild salmon is the most nutrient-dense (i.e., most nutrition per calorie) food you can eat.

FIVE FISH FACTS THAT WILL TRANSFORM YOUR EATING

1. **Fish is filling.** Like salad, seafood has a high satiety factor—less of it leaves you more satisfied. That's because fish is mostly fat and protein, the two highest-satiety nutrients, and contains little or no carbohydrate, the least-filling nutrient. Being satisfied sooner and with less volume helps you to enjoy and stick to T5 eating. That's why we rank a four- to six-ounce fillet of salmon (200–290 calories) and one egg (a measly 75 calories) as two of the best picks for high-satiety foods. 🖌

2. **Fish is full of fat.** And I mean *good fats*. In fact, fish contains the *smartest* fats. The most prevalent fats in seafood, DHA and EPA, are the healthiest fats for the brain and body (see endnotes). 🖌 Also, there's no need to worry about the cholesterol in seafood. As with eggs (see page 284), with rare exceptions, eating cholesterol in healthy foods does not significantly raise blood cholesterol levels. 🖐

3. **Seafood is brain food.** You tell your doctor you want to keep your brain sharp all your life. You want to be able to think clearly and stave off afflictions like depression and Alzheimer's. You ask her what's the best, science-based medicine. Doc scribbles on her prescription pad: "Go fish!"

    Surprised? There are thousands of scientific studies showing that seafood is brain food. During the writing of this book I had the opportunity to "go fishing" with top brain scientists. Science says that seafood can reduce the incidence and severity of brain illnesses and disorders like Alzheimer's, depression, bipolar disorder, and autism. What's more, unlike many prescription medications, it's safe and doesn't have any nasty side effects. (See chapter seven, "Transform Your Brain Health," where we take you inside the brain to learn why seafood is smart food.) 🖌

4. **Seafood is *see* food.** Age-related macular degeneration (ARMD) affects more than two million Americans. It's the leading cause of blindness. We have learned a lot about the effect of omega-3s on the brain by studying the eyes. This makes sense, since the retinas and the maculae within them are really part of the brain. Science

tells us that people who eat more omega-3s suffer less ARMD. No wonder. The retina of the eye is mostly fat and blood vessels, and omega-3s improve the health of fat and blood vessels. Go fish!

When I began my T5 program in 1997, one of the first effects I noticed was better vision, enabling me to retire my glasses. Additionally, children whose mothers ate fish during pregnancy had better eye health, especially premature babies.

5. **Seafood is healing food.** To control inflammation balance, go fish! Many scientific studies show the omega-3 oils in seafood help all *-itis*es, including:

- Cognitivitis (a term I use to describe neurodegenerative diseases such as Alzheimer's)
- Iritis (eye)
- Dermatitis (skin)
- Colitis (colon)
- Carditis (heart)
- Arthritis (joints)

Meet my imaginary partner in medical practice, the multispecialist, Dr. O. Mega III.

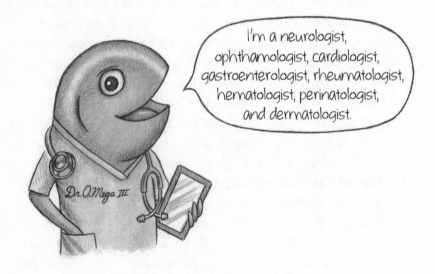

I'm a neurologist, ophthamologist, cardiologist, gastroenterologist, rheumatologist, hematologist, perinatologist, and dermatologist.

DR. BILL'S FISH TIP

"But I don't like fish" is a complaint I hear from some wannabe transformers. Believe it or not, you can transform your tastes to the point that you're hooked on fish. First, look at the head-to-toe health benefits of seafood we've just discussed. Imagine the health benefits! Once your thinking overrules your gut reaction—"Must . . . like . . . fish . . ."—you will come to look forward to your frequent doses of this great natural medicine. Meanwhile, gradually increase the amount of healthy seafood you eat to an average of twelve ounces (two fistfuls) per week. (See endnotes to learn our recommendations for the safest, and most nutritious, delicious seafood.)

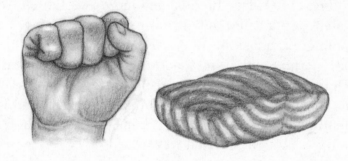

COACH ERIN: LEARNING TO LOVE YOUR SALMON

Don't love fish? Don't fret! Remember, your body and brain are so smart that your taste cravings will change in time. My husband does *not* like salmon, but he will eat it the way I cook it because of the sides and seasonings I use. (See Lemon Dill Salmon in Appendix C, page 333.) Some tips for savoring salmon:

- Choose high-quality wild Pacific salmon (see endnotes for our suggested source).
- Try sushi.
- Mix with your favorite flavors and with foods you like. Make a salmon salad.

- Try sides that complement salmon, like wild rice with onions and almonds, sweet potatoes, and Brussels sprouts. (See Appendix C.)
- Drizzle lots of lemon.
- Try toppings: capers, dill, Dijon mustard, even a honey glaze for a sweet treat.
- Start with a small portion (3–4 ounces).

Because of your recommendation, I have been eating Alaskan salmon for the past year. I eat salmon three or four times a week and love it. I was diagnosed with a rare autoimmune disease a year ago. I changed my eating habits. I am now consuming a Juice Plus+ protein shake every day, gluten-free breads, and more vegetables. What has made a big difference is eating salmon. Today, I am in complete remission. As of January 2017, all my blood tests are normal and all my doctors tell me I am a "walking miracle." I attribute this to my better food choices. My memory has been restored, I'm thinking clearer, and I am not feeling depressed anymore. Salmon is my brain food.

—BARRY SMALL

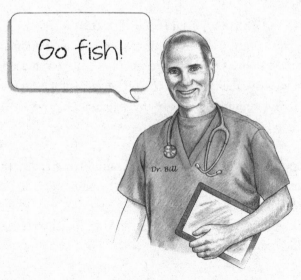

Read more about selecting seafood and the dosage of omega-3 supplements you need for the medical issues you have in *The Omega-3 Effect*, by William Sears and James Sears.

SMART SNACKS: SEEDS AND NUTS

In the next chapter you will learn why grazing is good for you—that is, why most of your eating should be snacking the smart way. But for now, let's focus on what to snack on. Smart snacks have these five features:

1. Filling but not fattening
2. Satisfying but not overfilling
3. Rich in proteins and healthy fats
4. Tasty, with good gut feelings
5. Health benefits, mainly to the brain, gut, and heart

SOLD ON SEEDS AND NUTS!

Seeds and nuts are Mother Nature's perfect blend of proteins, healthy fats, healthy carbs, and fiber—in other words, the perfect snack. I wasn't a big seed-eater until one day the light bulb switched on. If little seeds can grow into apple trees, avocado trees, tomatoes, pumpkins, and all the other plants, there have to be healthy nutrients in them. I am now a daily seed-lover and nut-muncher. Pumpkin and sunflower seeds add great nutrition and flavor to your trail mix. Ground flaxseeds are great in your smoothie. And ground sesame seeds make a savory spread called tahini.

Some tips on how to go nuts in your transformation:

- Make your own trail mix. Because each nut has its own special nutrients, mix five of your favorite *raw* nuts and seeds together.
- Pack a snack baggie of your mix in your purse or pocket. Enjoy a palmful, around a quarter cup, as a snack.
- When you crave carbs, go nuts instead. Eating sweet carbs out of a box when you are hungry usually prompts you to eat still

more unhealthy carbs, and often you're *still* hungry. Instead, slowly munch on a tablespoon of nuts and notice two nut effects: your carb craving dials down, and you feel satisfied sooner (see endnotes). ✋ And when just nuts don't do it, add a *bit* of dried fruit to your medley of nuts.

EAT MORE NUTS, LOSE MORE WEIGHT

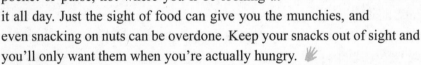

Nuts used to be a no-no because they are "high in fat." That was back when we'd been sold on the idea that fat, any and all fat, was the villain. But in fact, nuts are high in *healthy* fats. Researchers show that nuts are a weight-control food. Why? Because they help you feel fuller faster. Nuts contain all three of the most filling nutrients: protein, healthy fats, and fiber. And yet, *out of sight, out of mouth* is a wise weight-control trick. Put that bag of nuts in your pocket or purse, not where you'll be looking at it all day. Just the sight of food can give you the munchies, and even snacking on nuts can be overdone. Keep your snacks out of sight and you'll only want them when you're actually hungry. ✋

For more T5 snacking guidelines, see "Snacks Are *Good* For You," pages 73 and 361. For a nutritional ranking of nuts and seeds, go to DrSears Wellness.org/T5/Nuts-Seeds.

SUPPLEMENTS: THE TOP FIVE SCIENCE-BASED ONES FOR T5

Because not everyone eats the first four S's every day, we added a fifth S, supplements. Remember that supplement means *in addition to,* not *instead of.* Real, whole foods are always the better option. Supplements fill the nutritional gaps when you don't consistently eat healthfully. ⚡ But before you pop a supplement pill, ask yourself these two questions:

DO I NEED IT?

- Do you eat at least *ten fistfuls* of vegetables and fruits every day? If you don't, **you need a daily fruit and vegetable supplement**.
- Do you eat at least *two fistfuls* of seafood rich in omega-3s weekly? If you don't, **you need a daily omega-3 supplement**.
- Do you live in a sunshine state year round, get at least fifteen minutes of bikini-clad sun exposure daily, and have a healthy vitamin D blood level? If you don't, **you need a daily vitamin D supplement**.
- Are you an amateur or professional athlete, a vigorous exerciser, or have vision and inflammatory issues? **You may need an astaxanthin supplement**.
- Do you eat mostly the standard American diet—processed, fiberless foods? If you do, **you need a daily probiotic**.

HAVE I SEEN THE SCIENCE?

Suppose you go to your local health food store for a supplement a friend recommended. Before you buy it, look at the label to find the maker's website address. Then use your smartphone to go to the website and look for scientific studies done by university researchers that prove two biological facts about this supplement:

- Is it *bioavailable?* Researchers determine bioavailability by drawing blood from people after they've taken the supplement to prove that adequate quantities get into the bloodstream. Many supplements just go in one end and come out the other without being absorbed.
- Is it effective? Is there reliable research showing the supplement does good things for the body?

⊕ Since science continuously reveals new information about supplements, see AskDrSears.com/Supplements for updates on which brand names we continue to recommend.

"Show me the science" is my top advice when patients ask me about nutritional supplements. Companies that are proud of their science show it on their websites.

OUR FAVORITE FIVE

The following are the categories of science-based supplements we most frequently recommend in our medical practice and in our T5 program:

1. Fruit and vegetable supplements. If you came to our medical office for consultation on how you could eat better to feel better, I would ask:

- Do you grow your own fruits and vegetables in a home garden?
- Do you consistently eat ten fistfuls of fruits and vegetables daily? For most people at most ages a fistful is a serving. So, a serving for a baby is a baby fistful, and a serving for a big guy would be a big fistful.

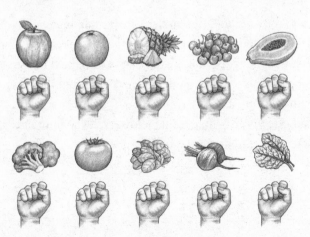

Do You Eat 10 Servings a Day?

Since most patients answer "no" to these two questions, I advise eating a fruit, vegetable, and berry supplement. At this writing there is only one such supplement well-supported by science: Juice Plus+ Garden Blend, Orchard Blend, and Vineyard Blend.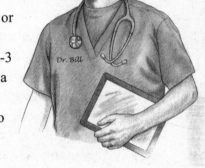

2. Omega-3 seafood oils. You don't like fish? The tips we gave you a few pages back for learning to love salmon didn't work for you? Wild-caught salmon is too expensive or hard to find?

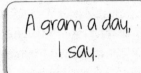

You have only one choice left: an omega-3 supplement, available as fish oil or from a sea-plant algae source.

How much should you take? It's easy to remember: A gram a day, I say.

KNOW YOUR OMEGA NUMBERS

Having the right *balance* of omega-3 and omega-6 oils is one of the most important T5 healthy eating concepts.

A simple fingerstick blood test can measure levels of these fats in your blood (available from www.VitalChoice.com). The two fat numbers you need to know are:

- The percentage of omega-3 fats in your red blood cell membranes.
- Your omega balance—the relative percentage of omega-3 to omega-6 fats.

3. Astaxanthin. Wild Pacific salmon is not only a great source of omega-3 oils; it also gives you a big dose of one of nature's most powerful antioxidants and anti-inflammatories—astaxanthin.

Astaxanthin is the natural carotenoid pigment that makes salmon pink. Mother Nature loads salmon with it to protect and empower their bodies as they swim many miles upstream to spawn. The usual dosage for optimal immune system health is four to eight milligrams a day, which would require you to eat six ounces of wild salmon at least three times a week. If you're like most people, even salmon lovers, you don't eat this much. You need a supplement.

We recommend Hawaiian astaxanthin, because it is natural astaxanthin from sea plants, not synthetic astaxanthin made from petrochemicals. Wild Pacific salmon contains around one milligram per ounce, eight times the amount of astaxanthin found in farmed Atlantic salmon. Also, some farmed salmon uses synthetic astaxanthin mostly as a food coloring, not as a nutrient.

Here's what science says about astaxanthin:

- Supports the *immune system*
- Supports healthy *vision*
- Helps protect against *dementia*
- Helps protect skin from *sun damage*
- Helps control excessive *inflammation*
- Smoothes the *endothelium*—less sticky stuff for better cardiovascular health
- Lessens after-exercise inflammation
- Because it gets into all layers of the skin, it has better dermatitis-easing effects than topical anti-inflammatories
- Crosses the blood-retinal barrier, so it can have vision and possible neuroprotective effects

4. Vitamin D. A top vitamin D researcher, Dr. Michael Holick, calls vitamin D the "D-lightful solution for health."

If you're an indoors person or live in a climate with few sunny days, get your vitamin D blood level measured. If it's above 50 mg/ml, great. If not, you may need to take around 100 IU of vitamin D_3 per day for each

1 mg/ml you need to raise your level to 50. For most people this will amount to 1,000 to 2,000 IU per day. Take this supplement with your fattiest meal of the day, since some fat is necessary for optimal vitamin D absorption.

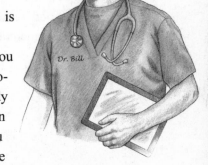

Go outside and play, especially on a sunny day.

Dr. Bill

To make enough vitamin D naturally, you need *fifteen minutes* of unprotected sun exposure (no sunblock) to your almost-naked body around three days a week. Getting fifteen minutes of sunshine in a swimsuit gives you roughly 5,000 to 10,000 IU, depending on the time of year, time of day, latitude, and your personal skin tone.

Six ounces of salmon gives you around 4,000 IU of vitamin D. In T5 we recommend our two favorite natural sources of vitamin D: *salmon and sunshine.* Because everyone is different in their ability to make their own vitamin D, you may still need a supplement.

5. Probiotics: What they can do for you. Probiotic literally means "for life," but it refers to supplements that contain certain bacteria—bugs that are so good for you, you can't live without them. Probiotics have been extremely popular in Europe for decades, and they've finally made it to America. These nutraceuticals proudly reside next to omega-3 oil capsules and fruit and vegetable supplements in many medicine cabinets. (For more about selecting the right probiotic for you, see the "Meet Your Microbiome" section in chapter six.)

T5 EATING MADE SIMPLE

- *Blend it and sip it.* This makes foods easier to digest with lower spikes.

(continued on next page)

- *Color it.* Provide lots of antioxidants (natural healing nutrients in foods).
- *Slow it.* Eat slowly to avoid overwhelming your gut with too many changes too fast.
- *Enjoy it.* Food has to be tasty or you won't stick to it.
- *Feel it.* Feel good during and after eating.

A SECOND HELPING: WHY T5 WORKS, WHY IT LASTS

In this chapter you've learned *what* to eat, and in chapter two you will learn *how* to eat. But as your transformation takes hold, you might naturally wonder, "What's going on inside my body to make me feel so much better?"

So, before we move on from *what* to *how*, let's take a little time to talk about *why*.

Five biochemical changes are going on in your body—at the molecular and cellular level—as you transform into the new you:

1. **You open your inner pharmacy to make your own medicines.** You feel empowered with more skills and fewer pills. (See pages 92 and 93 to discover where in your body these pharmacies are and what medicines your personal pharmacy makes.)
2. **You reset your "appestat" to feel more pleasure while eating less.** Starting on page 161, we take you on trips throughout the bodies of several transformers to show how T5 reprograms your body and brain to enjoy food more while eating less.
3. **You think-change your brain.** In chapters four and seven you will learn self-help skills that will rewire your brain to grow your happy center and shrink your sad center. Yes, you read that right. We will take you inside your brain to show you how.

4. **You lower sticky-stuff spikes.** Enjoy a body in balance. Inflammation imbalance is the root cause of *-itis* illnesses (see page 241). We get sick and tired and fat because of *sugar spikes*. T5 stabilizes blood sugar and insulin levels.

5. **You stay lean.** Your goal is waist loss, not weight loss. (See page 47.)

We'll talk about the first three effects in that list later on in the book. For now, let's look at the science behind the last two: lowering sugar-insulin spikes and staying lean.

T5 LOWERS "STICKY STUFF"

Fellow transformers: The next few pages are some of the most important in the whole T5 plan. Get ready to change what and how you eat.

We came up with our sticky-stuff explanation of illness years ago as an easy-to-grasp explanation to our patients who wanted a deeper understanding of why they hurt, why their thinking was foggy, why they got fat.

I would launch into a long biochemical explanation of these problems and in seconds their eyes would glaze over. As a doctor and author, I've always tried to practice KISMIF—*keep it simple, make it fun.* So I came up with a simple answer to their health questions, especially, "Why am I sick and tired?" My answer: "Too much sticky stuff in your body." I wanted a term that would stick—and it has.

STICKY STUFF MADE SIMPLE

Sticky stuff is the root cause of most ailments. You put too much sticky stuff in your mouth, you get too much sticky stuff throughout your body. For those of you who like real medical terms, sticky stuff causes the three "shuns":

- Oxida*tion*: "rust." T5 is an anti-rust program.
- Inflamma*tion*: wear and tear, *-itis* illnesses. T5 is anti-inflammatory.

- Glyca*tion*: The process of sugars sticking to proteins and fats, which clogs up your blood vessels and damages other tissues. T5 blunts sugar spikes to help prevent glycation.

The medical category of sticky stuff is what your doctor measures as "markers," biochemicals in the blood that go up when there is too much sticky stuff floating around in the bloodstream. For example, a frequently measured marker, hemoglobin A1c (HbA1c)—I call it "frosted hemoglobin"—is elevated when persistently high blood sugar sticks to the hemoglobin in the red cells. If your HbA1c is high, your blood sugar has been too high for too long, indicating you are at risk for type 2 diabetes. The actual biochemical term for sticky stuff is *adhesion molecules,* such as VCAM (vascular cell adhesion molecules) and ICAM (intercellular adhesion molecules). Another memorable term is AGEs (advanced glycation end products). Translation: sticky sugars that *age* tissues.

KIDS LOVE THE STICKY STUFF ANALOGY

You put sticky stuff in your mouth, you get sticky stuff all over your body, especially in your blood vessels. A few years ago, a mother and her seven-year-old attended one of my lectures on sticky stuff. The next evening at dinner, the mother told me that her child had scolded her husband: "Daddy, you shouldn't put that sticky stuff in your mouth. You'll get sticky stuff in your blood." That child gave me confidence to stick with the sticky stuff theme of this book. (See endnotes for another sticky burger story, "SAD from top to bottom," page 373.) ✋

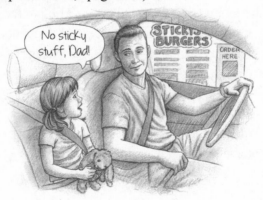

THE TOP BENEFIT OF SPIKE-LOWERING T5

Now you understand what T5 really does inside your body—lowers sticky-stuff spikes. But *where* in your body does T5 exert the greatest effect?

Inside your blood vessels.

Every organ in your body is only as healthy as the blood vessels supplying its cells with nutrients and oxygen and carrying away waste products. Keep your blood vessels healthy and each organ will stay healthier. That's what T5 does, as shown in this tale of two vessels:

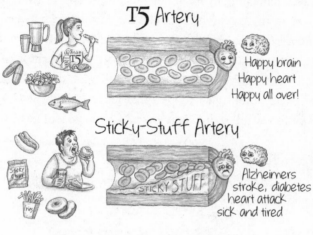

T5 Artery

Happy brain
Happy heart
Happy all over!

Sticky-Stuff Artery

STICKY STUFF

Alzheimers
stroke, diabetes
heart attack
sick and tired

Which artery do you want?

This drawing of two arteries represents the underlying cause of the illnesses most doctors see every day. A baby is born with wide-open, shiny vessels—no sticky stuff. Mother's milk and real foods help keep them that way. But most of the time, the child goes out into the real world of unreal foods and starts accumulating sticky stuff. No problem—yet. It seems that the Great Designer of blood vessels knew that we would put lots of sticky stuff in our mouths beginning at an early age, so he made our bodies with extra-wide blood vessels, so the blood would flow fast enough despite the sticky stuff accumulating. Yet, sticky stuff gradually builds up on the lining of the blood vessels and on the blood cells, causing them to stick together, and the *young adult* has a heart attack or stroke.

Notice the artery of a T5er—smooth linings, less sticky stuff, better blood flow, better health. Which arteries do you want in your body and brain?

YOUNG AND SICK

Once upon a time, when I was in medical school, we took classes on adult-onset diseases, those that only happen to older folks. Those classes no longer have "adult-onset" in the title, because these diseases now occur with increasing frequency in young adults: coronary artery disease, type 2 diabetes, autoimmune diseases, and so on.

Why is this happening to our young people? Simple answer: *they spike when they eat.* In my research, I noticed the correlation between the rise in sugar-processed foods and the rise of these diseases in the young. Eating unreal foods leads to unreal health. Look up the "nutritional" content of fast food chicken nuggets—it reads more like a list of chemical compounds than actual food. Fast foods spike fast and high, leading to fast sickness. Real foods spike slow and low and promote wellness. Got it?

SPIKE-LESS FOODS

Now that you understand how spikes make you sick and fat, naturally you want to know which foods spike and which don't.

Spike-less foods	Spike-more foods
Vegetables	Soda, sweetened beverages
High-fiber fruits	Most cereal in boxes
Proteins	Feed-lot chicken and beef
Healthy fats	(See the "Terrible 5," page 81.)
Wheat-free grains (e.g., quinoa)	
Seafood, wild	
Wild game	

What's more, it's really the whole *meal* rather than the individual *foods* that either blunts or causes spikes. Sometimes you can take a "spikey," say a fruit with a high glycemic index, and partner it with spike-less foods like you do in a smoothie, and the meal becomes spike-less, even though the individual fruits may spike. This is why the low glycemic index (see page

278) has fallen out of favor in preference for the *glycemic load*, which simply means the "spikiness" of the whole meal. Call it the *spike index*. We made up this new word to simplify glycemic confusion. The 5-S diet is a spike-less way of eating.

ENERGIZE ME!

Eliminating spikes isn't the only effect of the 5-S diet. Let's look at another transformation that happens inside your cells.

Organs are made of specialized cells, so every organ in the body is only as healthy as its cells. To transform your organs, you need to first transform your cells. The top feel-good effect that transformers report is more energy. Here's why. Inside your cells are miniature "generators" called *mitochondria* that are genetically programmed to produce energy on demand. In the hardest-working organs, like the brain and heart, each cell has thousands of mitochondria. When you transform your mitochondria to have more energy, you transform your cells, which transforms your organs and your whole body. The T5 way of eating, thinking, and living energizes the mitochondria.

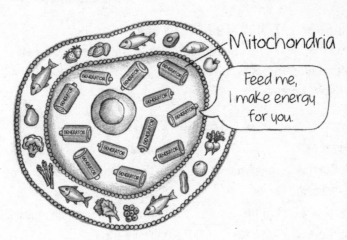

Each cell has a genetic language and communication system that prompt it to work properly. T5 tells the cellular communication centers how to talk. This is the new science called *epigenetics*—the outside influences (mainly how you eat, think, and live) that teach the cell how to behave.

STAY LEAN! WHY "DIETS" DON'T LAST AND T5 DOES

As we like to say, T5 isn't a diet—it's a do-it. Transformations last. Most diets don't. Fad diets seldom last because they're in conflict with the brain. Your brain is designed to oversee and protect your body from dumb decisions by your body's owner. For example, when the brain gets the message that you're on a "grapefruit diet," or some other malnutritional crash diet, it goes on red alert: "Something awful is happening to this body—I better protect it." So it sends countless messages throughout your body that say "Too much, too fast, cool it!" In short, it makes you so miserable that you start eating again, and gain back all the weight you lost and likely more.

On the other hand, the brain *loves* T5, because you're doing what you're genetically programmed to do. The brain and body shout: "We thrive on T5!"

While we don't think of T5 as a "diet," we realize many transformers do T5 because they *need* a diet—a diet for life. Here's the skinny on how T5 helps you stay lean.

HOW YOU GET FAT, HOW YOU STAY LEAN

"Lean" is the medically correct term, not "skinny" or "thin." Having just the right amount of body fat for your body type is lifesaving, health saving, and downright smart.

THE BIG FAT FIVE	
You get fat by:	**You stay lean by:**
Eating fiberless, processed carbs	Eating fiber-filled carbs
Eating "unreal" foods	Eating real foods
Eating too much too fast	Eating smaller meals more slowly
Sitting too much	Moving more
Stressing too much	Worrying less

Which of the "big three" nutrients is most to blame for the obesity epidemic? Don't blame fats; the portion of daily calories from fat in Americans' diets has declined in recent years. And we can't blame protein; it's the lean nutrient, is hard to overeat, and usually accounts for only about 20 percent of daily calories. That leaves only one macronutrient to blame: *carbohydrates*, which have increased from 40 percent to 55 percent of the daily diet over the last couple of decades. Not only is the increased sugar making us fat, we are consuming more of the worst processed sugar, fructose. As Americans have doubled the daily fructose they consume, the incidence of obesity has doubled. Any correlation? We believe so.

HOW UNHEALTHY CARBS MAKE YOU FAT

Yes, we've talked about this. Now we're going to discuss it in a little more detail, because eating chemical carbs is the worst sabotage to your transformation. Let's follow the sugar into the fat.

You gulp down a big soda. This triggers a sky-high blood-sugar spike. The spike causes the brain to send a biochemical message to the pancreas to release a lot of sugar's buddy, insulin, whose job is to escort sugar into the cells, where it can be burned for energy. This causes insulin levels to spike, too, often overshooting the needed amount. (Too much insulin in the blood makes you hungry for carbs to balance it out. That makes for a vicious cycle.)

Next, insulin delivers the sugar to the "door" of a cell, a structure on the cell membrane called a receptor, and finds a sign on the door that reads, "We're full of sugar already, no vacancy, go away." Foiled by this resistance ("insulin resistance" is another term for type 2 diabetes, now an epidemic) the insulin has to unload its sugar somewhere else. If the sugar can't be used, it has to be stored, which was a good thing through all the prior ages of human history when carbs were hard to come by. The body doesn't like to waste calories, so it *waists* them—that is, insulin deposits the excess sugar in the body's energy bank, the belly. Fat cells, especially belly-fat cells, exist to store sugar in the form of fat. And that's how *you* get fat!

Over time, insulin resistance leads to low energy. Cells won't let in enough fuel for sufficient energy production. The blood sugar gets sticky, the belly gets bigger, and you get a bad case of the highs—high blood sugar, high blood pressure, and so on. This is called *metabolic syndrome.* Simply put: *You get sick and tired and fat.*

Ten percent of diabetes patients have type 1 diabetes, a genetic condition in which the pancreas doesn't produce enough insulin to process sugar. The other 90 percent have type 2 diabetes, in which insulin becomes *ineffective*, even when there's way too much of it in the bloodstream.

How your liver gets fat. The sugar story gets even more sour. Insulin isn't needed to process the fiberless fructose in processed foods and drinks. (The chemical names of various kinds of sugars end with *-ose.*) Fructose is a stored sugar. It goes from the gut through a shortcut called the portal vein directly into the liver to be piled up in storage boxes called glycogen. Again, this is a naturally good thing—this stored sugar gets released into the blood when blood sugar gets low, as after an overnight fast.

However, too much fructose makes the liver *fat.* When more fructose arrives than the liver can package for fast delivery, it stores it as fat, hence the epidemic of *fatty liver disease*, which is now happening at younger ages.

Organ by organ, high levels of sticky stuff in the blood make you sick. Even Alzheimer's is now called by some "type 3 diabetes."

Ready to cut back on your carbs?

Fantastic fat cells. T5 is one of the few wellness plans that praises fat, both the fat in real foods and the real healthy fat where it belongs in your body. Inside fat cells is a peptide hormone called leptin, from the Greek word for slender. Think of leptin as the biochemical signal fat cells send to the brain, saying, "We're satisfied. Time to stop storing energy as fat and start burning it." In short, leptin makes you stop feeling hungry. Think: "Leptin helps me eat *less* and stay *lean.*

When leptin behaves as it's supposed to, you are more likely to stay lean. When it misbehaves, you are more likely to get sick, tired, and fat. When you ignore your leptin prompts, your body and brain start ignoring these appetite-regulating signals. This is called *leptin resistance.* Obesity follows. So listen to your leptin. When you're not hungry, don't eat. Let leptin do its job of helping you stay lean.

FAT NEWS! WAIST CONTROL, NOT WEIGHT CONTROL

This may be the only wellness book you'll ever read that doesn't try to make you feel ashamed of your weight. We don't even want to talk about weight. *Waist control* is much more important than weight control. New insights show that body composition—your body fat percentage—is more important than scale weight. In fact, some of our transformers have actually *gained* weight (but lost waist) on the 5-S diet, because they needed to. They gained muscle and lost fat. Their body-fat percentage actually went down even though their weight went up. (Muscle weighs more than fat.) Just what the doctor ordered.

The two science-based rules of weight loss:

- Body *composition* (percent of muscle tissue) is more relevant to your health than body *weight.*
- *Waist size* is more meaningful than what the scale says.

WHY RAPID WEIGHT LOSS CAN BE BAD FOR YOUR HEALTH

"What?! I bought this book to lose weight!" Take a deep breath and read on. When you subject yourself to the malnutrition of a fad diet, you tend to lose both fat and muscle tissue. That's not good. Your diet should make you strong, not weak. The T5 effect gives you more muscle and less belly fat.

Don't do dumb diets. There are even more reasons to avoid crash diets. Healthy people have some fat on their bodies. When you lose too much good fat too fast, your body panics and erroneously concludes, "There must be a famine out there, so I'd better switch into body-fat conservation mode and eat more while I can." Biochemically, that means the good fat cells dial down their leptin production, cutting back the "eat less" signals to your brain. Just when you're trying to get rid of excess belly fat, your body starts telling you to eat more. Lower leptin levels are a curse for dieters. You're likely to regain what you lost and more, and feel sick and tired the whole time.

ERIN'S DIET CRASH

Before T5, I tried and failed at many quick-fix solutions to my health crises, but this one takes the cake.

I was to be the maid of honor in my best friend's wedding. I *knew* my dress was too small, but I didn't do anything about it until two weeks before the wedding. I searched for quick weight-loss "solutions" and landed on—*ta da!*—the cabbage soup diet! Well—the dress fit. But I was miserable during a time that should have been joyful. Instead of celebrating my friend and enjoying a beautiful moment, I was obsessing about my weight. And you *know* how this story ends. I went back to my old eating habits and gained back all the weight and more—and a new dose of shame along with it.

IN SEARCH OF THE PERFECT DIET

The perfect way of eating would be one that:

- Does not cause blood sugar and insulin levels to spike,
- Puts the body in both omega and inflammation balance (see "Know Your Omega Numbers," page 350, and "Inflammation Balance," page 243),
- Tastes good and changes cravings, and
- Doesn't need you to count grams and calories.

Slow carb, not low carb. T5ers don't bother counting carbs or calories. (See why, page 282.) What counts is where the calories come from—real food or fake. If you *have* to know, here is how the calorie distribution shakes out in the 5-S diet:

- Fat: 35–40 percent
- Protein: 20–25 percent
- Carbs: 35–45 percent

T5 isn't a low-calorie or low-fat or low-carb or a low-anything diet. Those diets don't last. The best way to describe it is to say, "I'm on a *slow*-carb diet."

Scientifically, if slowly, all the "low" diets are losing credibility. You will lose weight with a severely low-carb diet, but because our taste buds love carbs, two problems may result. First, you may get tired of the tasteless low-carb diet, not stick to it, and regain the weight you lost. Second, your energy declines, because carbs are still the fuel your muscles and brain prefer.

The ideal diet is a slow-carb diet, in which the carbs come from fiber-filled real foods, especially vegetables, legumes, fruits, and whole, unprocessed grains. Because slow carbs are always partnered with fiber, and sometimes with a bit of protein and fat, they are absorbed into the bloodstream slowly, which prevents spikes.

Our bodies are designed to run on these real, nature-made carbs. The body needs to dispense glucose as an energy source *slowly* over the course of the day as needed. That's why we need to snack on small, frequent feedings of slow carbs during the day: "Eat as you burn." Any excess gets stored as fat.

NO ADDED SUGARS!

One simple change you can make to feel the quickest effect: avoid foods and drinks with "added sugars" on the label. Instead, eat sugar that is naturally partnered with fat, protein, and fiber.

THE T5 RIGHT-CARB DIET

Suppose you eliminated all "added sugars" from your diet and ate only carbs that *naturally occur in real foods,* which would translate to around 35 to 45 percent of your total daily calories. Here's what would happen in your body, and the effects you would likely feel:

- Reshaping of tastes
- Stable blood sugar and insulin levels
- Less fat stored in belly-fat cells
- Less inflammation and -*itis* illnesses

- Steadier moods
- Less fat in the liver
- Less excess cortisol (stress hormone) production

Protein power. Proteins can protect you against carb spikes. Naturally, as you decrease carbs, you would need to increase your fuel intake from proteins and fat. What's good about that?

- You feel fuller and more satisfied faster.
- Protein triggers the release of glucagon. This hormone, like insulin, is made in the pancreas, but it has the opposite effect. Insulin stores carbs as fat, but glucagon *releases* carbs stored in fat cells. So when you eat proteins, you don't get a carb crash as you do with a meal full of junk carbs. Also, unlike carbs, a high-protein meal reduces the hunger hormone, ghrelin.

Enjoy an egg a day. Eggs have the highest *biological value* of any protein, meaning you absorb and utilize more of the protein from an egg than from any other food.

- An easy figure that I have used in my medical practice is *a gram of protein per pound of your ideal body weight a day.* ✺ This may sound like a lot of protein. But increasing your protein intake like this will cause you to naturally eat fewer carbs—another of the T5 goals. The protein-rich 5-S food choices listed in the endnotes are likely to provide this amount. For example, a six-ounce salmon fillet provides 40 grams of protein. ✺
- A question I sometimes get is: "Can I eat *too much* protein, and how much is too much?" First of all, it's hard to overeat proteins. Refined carbs stimulate overeating by keeping you hungry all the time, but proteins do the opposite. Because proteins enjoy a *high satiety* perk, the more you eat, the fuller you get, so it's

hard work to eat too much protein. Second, you would have to eat half of your calories in the form of protein each day to cause problems for your liver, which is highly unlikely as long as you're not on one of those super-high-protein fad diets.

A few months after we gave her some carb counseling, one T5er, a twenty-nine-year-old trial lawyer named Giovanna, reported a natural transformation in her food cravings toward real-carb eating: "When I eliminated meat and junk carbs from my eating, I started craving more vegetables to fill me up—otherwise I was hungry."

So that's another great T5 effect. Rather than having to cut carbs, *you'll start craving healthier carbs.*

BIGGEST LOSERS BECOME BIGGEST REGAINERS

Ever wonder what happens to most of the fat-shedders from the TV show *The Biggest Loser*? Their skinny stardom is short-lived. A 2016 survey published in the *New York Times* showed that most regain the weight they lost, and some gain even more. No wonder!

Sudden, dramatic weight loss causes your body to think something is wrong—it can't tell the difference between a crash diet and starvation. A rapid fifty-pound weight loss sends your body into survival mode, which means conserving fat. Your metabolism gets dialed down to burn fewer calories.

Also, the biggest regainers suffer from hormonal confusion, causing them to battle cravings and go on binges. They've lost weight, but many also lost their ability to regulate leptin, the hormone that stops you from feeling hungry. Because they lost so much weight so fast, their leptin levels dipped so low that they were hungry all the time. When scientists explained to the biggest regainers what was happening to their bodies, they realized it was not their weak willpower that caused them to regain the weight, but rather something bad that had happened to their biology. To explain how T5 keeps you lean and prevents you from becoming a regainer, let's follow two people who wanted to lose lots of weight.

Regina regained. *Regina dropped 100 pounds just like those contestants on* The Biggest Loser. *But because she lost too much too fast, she didn't transform into a healthier self. Instead, her body naturally reacted as if threatened with starvation.*

Lois lasted. *Lois did T5, which meant taking things at the right pace. Slow, gradual changes prompted the wisdom of her body to feel, "I like what you're doing—please keep it up." Her metabolism didn't overreact. Better yet, Lois added a hefty dose of daily exercise to keep her metabolism in the "burn calories" mode. Lois lost her excess weight the right way—a slow, gradual transformation of body and mind. She got lean and stayed lean.*

In our next chapter, we'll move on from *what* to eat to *how* to eat. But first, a word from Coach Erin . . .

DETOXING WITH T5

Since you are likely to urinate more (because you drink more water) and have more bowel movements (because the 5-S diet is so intestine-friendly), you will be naturally detoxing your body. But as you transform from your "old normal" to your "new normal," you may also experience withdrawal symptoms from quitting processed food, sugar, and too much caffeine. Some transformers think they have the flu. That was my own experience and that of fellow transformers I've coached.

Years and years of eating processed sugars and added chemicals train the brain to "need" these foods. Those addicting foods hijack the brain's reward pathway, making us dependent on them—this is a lot like dependency on nicotine, cocaine, or heroin. Our brains become greedy and unsatisfied. We crave more and more of the stuff that's bad for us.

This is precisely why we need to transform our eating. And there's a kind of paradox here. You'd think that giving up unhealthy foods and chemicals would make us feel better, not worse. And, with time, it will. But the problem is that your body builds up a tolerance, just as with a drug addiction. It's like that old junk-food advertising slogan: "You can't eat just one." One leaves you wanting another and another and another. Sugar addiction is real. I know it definitely played a part in my depression, anxiety, and weight gain. Today I still feel much more clearheaded after a day of really healthful eating, versus those days when I have a few too many added treats. (See the endnotes to learn about "a big, fat, sweet lie.")

HOW FOOD ADDICTION HAPPENS

Sugar spikes cause a release in the brain of the chemical messenger dopamine—the same reward response that happens when we take addictive drugs. Over time, more sugar is needed to attain the same "sugar high." Detox symptoms are most commonly experienced as headaches, fatigue, irritability, spinning mind, inability to focus, increased stress, hunger, cravings, insomnia, and muscle aches. But the good news is this only lasts for a few days.

I would love to tell you that my cravings for sweets have completely gone away, but that would be a lie. I have a huge sweet tooth. The difference today is that I can find balance. Identify your *trigger foods* and don't keep them in the house. Transform 5 does not say that you can never have a treat. We simply want you to understand how powerful the processed-sugar/junk-food addiction can become. As you work through the T5 changes, you will learn what balance works for your body.

WAYS TO EASE WITHDRAWAL:

- Keep your blood sugar levels stable by eating five meals a day the T5 way, and eat enough fat and protein.
- Spice it up with ginger and cinnamon, which sweeten your food naturally.
- Reach for an apple when the sweet tooth attacks, and add almond or peanut butter.
- Don't use artificial sweeteners. They cause you to crave more sweet things. If you must use something, use Stevia or a little bit of raw honey (see why, page 361).
- Consume foods high in B vitamins such as dark leafy greens, beans, fish, eggs, and plant-based milks.

- Find healthy ways to trigger the dopamine response in your brain, like dancing, fun activities with friends, and nonfood treats like a pedicure or massage.
- Stock your house with healthy food choices, and get rid of the unhealthy ones, especially your trigger foods.
- Drink extra water.

In the next chapter, you will learn about a tale of two eaters: Gracie the grazer and George the gorger.

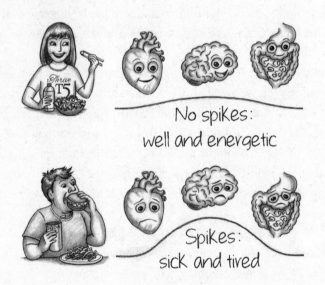

No spikes: well and energetic

Spikes: sick and tired

George spikes; Gracie doesn't. George barely survives; Gracie thrives. Graze for good living!

CHAPTER 2

GRAZE ON FIVE MINI-MEALS

This one simple word is key to transforming your health: *graze*.
Over a decade of noting how people eat, I've observed that slow and mini-meal eaters—grazers—are generally healthier than fast and big-meal eaters—gorgers. Doctor's promise: if you read and heed this chapter, your bites and meals will get smaller and your gut will feel healthier.

Grazing is usually defined as eating small, frequent meals throughout the day. Our T5 way uses grazing to mean:

- Downsizing breakfast, lunch, and dinner.
- Eating two or three palm-sized snacks between meals.
- Ensuring each meal and snack contains nutrient-dense real foods, such as:
  - Fruit and/or vegetables
  - High-protein foods
  - Fiber-filled real carbs
  - Healthy fats

CHEW-CHEW, TIMES TWO

You've heard the wisdom "chew on it a while," meaning to take time to mull something over so you can make a smart decision. This applies literally to smart eating.

"Chew-chew, times two" isn't only about enjoying your food more. It aids digestion two ways: (1) chewing makes more saliva, which contains enzymes that break down carbohydrates; and (2) chewing sends biochemical signals to the stomach, small intestines, and pancreas, saying, "Incoming food! Start secreting your digestive juices." The more digestive work you do in your mouth, the easier it is at the lower end of your intestinal tract. Chewing each bite at least twenty to thirty times stimulates more flow of saliva, giving the whole digestive process a jumpstart.

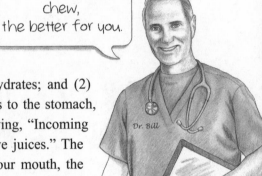

DR. BILL'S RULE OF TWOS

- Eat *half* as much.
- Eat *twice* as often.
- Chew *twice* as long.

You will feel good in your gut!

WHY GRAZING IS GOOD FOR YOU

Grazing makes you feel so much better, you'll soon be hooked on this transforming way of eating. Grazing is the healthy way to eat, because it changes you from the inside out via three transformation effects:

- Lowering sticky-stuff spikes—the top T5 health effect
- Feeling full faster—good gut feelings
- Transforming your tastes—eat less, but enjoy it more

Remember, T5 does an *inside* job on your body. Nearly everyone on our T5 team has felt some or all of its effects. You can, too!

GRAZERS ARE HEALTHIER THAN GORGERS

Grazing is one of the simplest and most health-enhancing eating changes you can make. Here are some of the advantages of grazing over gorging. Grazers are:

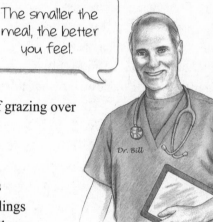

The smaller the meal, the better you feel.

Dr. Bill

- More energetic
- More alert, clearer thinkers
- Able to enjoy good gut feelings
- Likely to have fewer *-itis* illnesses
- More likely to be lean
- Less hungry, more satisfied
- Less moody

Grazing lowers spikes. *Avoid spikes* are the two most important words in preventive medicine, and they are the underlying physiological effect of grazing. T5ers avoid spikes of "sticky stuff," as you read on page 3. The Standard American Diet (SAD) way of eating releases sticky stuff into the bloodstream shortly after eating. This is the root cause of most cardiovascular, neurodegenerative, and *-itis* illnesses. The first step is transforming *what* you eat. The second is *how* you eat. The smaller your bites and the longer you chew, the less you spike.

If someone asks what you are doing to look so good, surprise them with "I'm lowering my sticky stuff."

See DrSearsWellness.org/T5/Grazing to download visual grazing reminders. Paste these transformation tips on your fridge and share them with your team.

GRAZERS NATURALLY EAT LESS AND FEEL BETTER

There's growing neuroscience that proves eating less translates to living longer, healthier, and smarter. Almost all T5ers tell us, "I'm eating less but enjoying it more and feeling better." The reason for this T5 effect is you are changing your body's eating-pleasure signals from the inside. The real-food 5-S diet is naturally full of fiber, rich in healthy fats, and devoid of artificial chemical additives. When you eat slowly, grazing and chewing more, you take more pleasure in eating and feel better inside.

Smaller bites, smaller spikes.

Dr. Bill

Eating less gives you more health benefits. Perhaps you've heard the medical buzzword for eating less: caloric restriction. T5 isn't about depriving you of the pleasure of eating or about being hungry all the time. We prefer to call it "smart selection." We cut empty calories, not nutrients. But the point is that by eating less and smarter, we increase our chances of living longer and healthier lives.

In fact, the list of healthful effects of eating less but more healthfully keeps getting longer. The science-based benefits thus far proven include:

- Less type 2 diabetes
- Less -*itis* (inflammation-related) illnesses
- Live longer, age slower
- Fewer neurodegenerative diseases, such as dementia

Here's my simple explanation for the correlation between eating less and better health:

- Illness and unhealthy aging are due to accumulation of sticky stuff in tissues and clogging arteries.
- Eating less promotes less buildup of sticky stuff.

It could be that simple!

We believe eating less makes the brain and body become *more fuel efficient*, like getting your car engine to last longer and run more efficiently by putting in a more-efficient fuel. Smart selection of food *increases insulin sensitivity*, which means that we become more fuel efficient; increased insulin sensitivity is like getting more miles per gallon from your fuel. Your "engine" idles quietly when stopped at an intersection, but responds promptly and appropriately when the light changes and you step on the gas. You want your insulin level to be low when blood sugar is low, or idling, and then respond promptly to clear the blood sugar after eating so you don't get those dreaded sugar spikes.

GRAZERS ARE LEANER

In my medical practice, I use the more scientific term "prediabetic," rather than focusing on obesity or overweight. Over many years I have observed that *wolfers*—high-speed gorgers—have larger waists than people who eat slowly. When my prediabetic patients transform from gorgers to grazers, they usually enjoy better *weight* and *waist* control for two reasons. Grazing perks up your metabolism and turns you into a calorie burner instead of a calorie storer. And because grazers are more satisfied with less food, they are less likely to overeat. (See related section on appetite control and loving your leptin, page 46.)

Why fast eaters get fat. Your brain has an appestat (actually a bunch of interconnected hormonal dials) that tells you, as you eat, when your fuel tank is getting full. However, these satiety signals take a little time to kick in, so fast eaters speed right through them. They overeat and get overfilled. When you feel stuffed, that means you've filled your gut with too much food, too fast, before your brain had time to register your fullness feelings. Being more satisfied with less food is one of the most lasting T5 effects.

While lecturing in Okinawa, a culture noted for enjoying leanness and the longest lifespan, I learned this slogan: "Eat until you are 80 percent full." The idea is to stop eating before you feel full. Wait at least twenty minutes before eating more; by that time you are likely to feel full.

When you slow down your eating, chew longer, take more time between bites, and take smaller bites, your fuel tank gauge registers "full" well before you've stuffed yourself. So, slow down and take time to enjoy what you're eating. Your body will tell you when it's time to stop.

GRAZERS ENJOY GOOD GUT FEELINGS

Besides inflammation balance, which you will learn about in chapter eight, the T5 way of eating eases two other "shuns": indigestion and constipation. Sipped, blended food empties faster from your stomach, so that less food remains to trigger acid reflux (heartburn). Smaller amounts of sipped, blended food are digested faster, which makes for easier elimination. One of the earliest gut signs transformers notice is that the *number of bowel movements per day doubles*. That's good for the gut. The softer it goes through, the better for you.

Eat real food. Poop real often. Feel real good.
—TRANSFORMER KATHY BEE

TASTES TRANSFORM, CRAVINGS CHANGE

"But I don't like broccoli," you insist. I do insist, and science agrees: adopt the 5-S diet, and you will eventually like broccoli. Taste laboratories at the University of Pennsylvania Monell Chemical Senses Center in Philadelphia have proven that after ten to twenty tries, children, especially toddlers, upgrade their tastes from *don't like* to *like*.

This is your brain on broccoli. We think that works for adults, too. Try broccoli enough, and you'll like it. Your brain *loves* broccoli, because it knows you need it. So, your brain keeps badgering your taste buds until you like and even crave broccoli.

A transformation you are likely to feel early on is the reshaping of your tastes and increased cravings for food that is good for you. That's the T5 strategy—change your mind to change your body. You decide to eat the transformation foods in the 5-S diet that are best for you, whether you like them or not. Your brain and your body reach an agreement. The brain says, "Kale is good for you. We're going to like it." The body says, "Okay, I'll develop a taste for it if you get some good recipes that make it taste good and make me feel good after I've eaten it." That's the deal that moves you from *don't like* to *like* to *crave*. When you choose a transforming food, you turn on an inner switch. The wisdom of your body reinforces your choice: "Keep eating this way. It's good for you." ✋

What your intestines tell you. Your gut also tells you what to eat. The medical term is "metabolic programming." The exact biochemical mechanism behind the relationship between good food and good gut feelings is not known, but it works something like this. Your gut is lined with trillions of cells that are genetically programmed to remember which foods are good or bad for you. They "memorize" the standards for good health, and they continually send signals to the brain, saying, "This food is good for me. Feed me more." But problems arise when these craving cells are confused by years of exposure to unreal foods. Decades of eating fake food leads to fake gut responses. T5 real-food eating retrains this gut lining to crave healthy foods.

Confessions of a chocolate-lover. When I was going through my transformation, the treat I hated to give up most was my daily dose of chocolate. To reshape my tastes and recondition my cravings, I went through this five-step process to ease into increasing my taste for tartness:

1. I convinced myself that the higher the percentage of cocoa, the healthier the chocolate was, because it was higher in antioxidants. Yet, I had to overcome the bittersweet reality of a chocolate-lover's life: the higher the percentage of cocoa, the

more bitter the taste. My only choice was to make bitter taste better. So . . .

2. I ate 60 percent cocoa for a couple weeks, then increased the cocoa content in 5-point increments until I got to the healthful 80 percent.

3. At this writing, I am now stuck at 85 percent—and loving it. What's fascinating is that the 85 percent cocoa that once tasted bitter now tastes sweet. This is a great example of how our tastes change. Once you get away from oversugared treats for awhile, you'll find them distastefully sweet.

4. Choose dark chocolate that has the least processing, because it contains more of the antioxidants called flavonoids.

5. Ditch "Dutched" chocolate. "Dutching" is a chemical process that removes some of the antioxidants.

Because I started shopping the perimeter of the grocery store and buying fewer processed items, my kids and I had to experiment with the kinds of snacks we reached for. We began training our bodies and brains to crave the good stuff, which was easier than we thought because of how good we felt. My kids now love whole-wheat bread, eat more veggies, and ask for air-popped popcorn instead of chips. If you don't buy it, they won't eat it!
—TINA EATON, TRANSFORMED MOM

A tale of two tastes, one tricked, the other transformed. Scenario: The president of Chips Inc. calls in her head chemist and says, "We've got to sell more chips, so we need to get more people to crave our chips. Go to your laboratory and make this happen." The food chemist designs a cheap chemical additive that triggers the pleasure centers in the brain.

I don't know if that conversation ever really took place, but it might as well have. After a few servings of these chemically enhanced chips, you are madly, hopelessly in love with them. Just seeing a bag of them lights up the pleasure center in your brain and prompts you to eat one. Of course, one good chip demands another, and so on. That ad slogan, "Bet you can't eat just one" might have been born on Madison Avenue, but it was conceived in a test tube in a food-additive lab. Your body is chemically changed, for the worse.

"Can't have just one" is pretty much the definition of addiction.

I used to crave chips. Now they taste chemical.
—ERIN

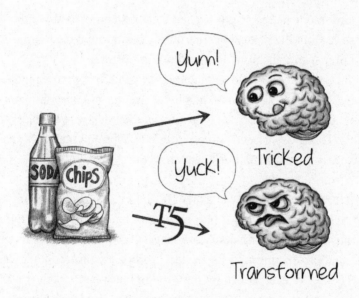

Look how that scenario plays out in two different brains, one tricked, the other transformed. The artificially flavor-enhanced chip registers "Yum!" on the taste buds, which signal the brain's pleasure center to eat every fake-food snack it sees. The owner of the tricked brain gets sick and fat. But after you've spent some time on T5, those taste buds signal "Yuck!" Your transformed brain knows that fake food is going to give you a pain in the gut. Once you're good and transformed, you won't even think about junk food very much. With T5, you instinctively learn to crave what's good for you.

Confessions of a stubborn transformer. One of the earliest transformations I had to make was changing how the *sight* of junk food triggered the "gotta eat it" impulse in my brain. I had to learn to head those impulses off at the pass. I started by convincing my conscious mind that these snacks were bad for me by thinking of all the studies that showed how chemical additives and artificial sweeteners harm my brain and my health:

1. See soda.
2. Visualize the soda sticking on the lining of my blood vessels, piling up in belly fat, and dumbing down my brain.

It took four months of this mental taste reshaping to move the image of the soda from the pleasure center in my brain to the trash bin—so that instead of resisting the urge, I honestly didn't want it.

In fact, the thought of a soda and a bag of chips became repulsive; it triggered "feel bad" signals. What's more, when I did drop my guard and eat some chips, they tasted bad, artificially chemical. *And* they upset my stomach. That was the end of chips for me. My cravings had changed. That's the taste transformation I wish for you.

My transformation trip to a supermarket. Once I had transformed my thinking about what to eat, I put it into practice. I made a list of the top foods that I must eat to feel the quickest, deepest, and most lasting total body transformation. I imprinted those, like a doctor's prescription, into my brain. Then I noticed, as I browsed through the supermarket, it was as if I was magnetically drawn toward the foods that were best for me. I still remember walking past a display of pomegranates one day. It was love at first sight. I had read so much about how good pomegranates were that eventually they made my wish list. Without thinking, I started grabbing them and stuffing them into a bag until it was half full. My body was talking to me, and it was speaking wisely.

THE WISDOM OF THE BODY

I first heard the phrase "the wisdom of the body" in medical school. It means that somewhere deep inside is an inner voice that prompts you to do what's good for your body and avoid what's bad for it. Sadly, as the years go by, many of us stop paying attention to that voice, and eventually can no longer hear it. During your transformation you will start listening again. And the more you listen, the louder the wisdom of the body becomes. "Eat this, not that. Do this, not that." You're being transformed!

"Bill, you're addicted!" One day I was describing my transformation turn-on and how my wisdom of the body was now back in full bloom. My psychologist friend told me that I had developed a "positive addiction." That sounded half nice. Then I realized that's actually a very good addiction to have. I felt it. This is why some of our top transformers, especially those who are in recovery from a negative addiction, such as drugs and alcohol, can be more easily transformed by giving them something to "recover into"—the T5 program.

UMAMI: ENJOYING HEALTHFUL FOOD

Most Westerners were taught that there are four basic tastes: sweet, sour, salt, and bitter. Now a fifth one is being accepted: *umami.* This Japanese word might be translated as "delicious," but it means more than that. More literal translations might be "savory mouthfeel" or "lingering nice taste."

We're hearing the word more in North America as Asian cuisines become more a part of our own. But while *umami* is an actual flavor, the concept of savoring got me thinking about the way we enjoy food here as opposed to other cultures.

My China story. In 2012, I was an invited speaker at the Chinese Nutrition Society, a meeting of healthcare professionals concerned about the trend of Chinese people eating like Americans and getting sick, tired, and fat like Americans. To educate and entertain my audience, I told a tale of two eaters, George the gorger and Gracie the grazer. At the end of one of my lectures a Chinese physician politely asked, "Dr. Sears, why do Americans eat so much so fast?" I said, "It's because we gobble our food with forks instead of pick at it slowly with chopsticks." They liked my answer, but I began thinking that there is more to it than that. Yes, we eat too much too fast. But that is not only bad for our health—it sabotages our enjoyment of eating.

Here are three things we need to do to get the greatest pleasure from eating:

- Chew our food longer.
- Eat our meals more slowly.
- Choose foods that naturally contain nutrients that slowly release more delicious flavors. As we take our time chewing these foods, their aromas ascend from the back of the mouth into the nasopharynx, an area that is very sensitive to the flavor of the food. This area sends biochemical messages to the pleasure centers in the brain that register "delicious."

Get ready to enjoy eating better than you ever have before. The T5 way of eating and the top T5 foods just happen to produce the most *umami* and the best overall eating enjoyment.

TWO WAYS TO SAVOR YOUR MEALS MORE

1. **Favor fermented and chewy foods.** Certain foods release more *umami*, or more flavor in general, because of the way they are prepared. My three fermented favorites are yogurt, kefir, and cheese. Fermentation lowers lactose (lactose-intolerant folks will love this), giving yogurt and kefir a tart taste that wakes up your taste buds and lingers awhile. Because they require thirty to sixty chews, chewy foods often give you the most pleasure: calamari, broccoli, celery, figs, high-fiber foods like artichokes, and my favorite—nuts. (See "go nuts!" page 32.)

2. **Steaming brings out flavor—my hot salad story.** After a few years into my T5 way of eating, I decided I needed to put more variety into my nightly dinner salad. Now, once or twice a week, instead of eating my salad raw, I lightly steam it, just until the greens are warm and soft but not wilted. I scoop the steamed salad into a small baking dish instead of a salad bowl and put a lid on it to keep it warm as I slowly graze on it

throughout the meal—using chopsticks. My first few hot salads blew me away! When I took off the lid, the aroma piqued the pleasure center of my brain even before I took the first bite. The flavors of the spices, the softened cheese, and the olive-oiled vegetables linger longer and have a more savory mouthfeel. I am enjoying the same salad more. Also, I found a completely unexpected perk of the hot salad—not only do I enjoy it more, I am satisfied with less. Two-thirds of the way through, I am full and satisfied.

Why am I more satisfied with less of the hot salad than the raw salad? All the sensations, all the messages between the taste buds on my tongue, the pleasure center in the brain, and, of course, the microbiome in my gut brain are all signaling "like," "pleasure," and "slow down, you've eaten enough." Yet another perk of my hot salad is that I make more saliva, even before the first bite, as my taste buds prepare to welcome the savory salad. This is the *olfactory effect*—you can smell it before you taste it—a mouth-watering experience.

Taste and smell, the pleasure twins. One of the pleasant benefits of our rule of twos is that eating more slowly, chewing longer, and pausing to take a deep breath between bites trigger both the taste and the smell centers in the brain to register a double pleasure. Taste and smell play well together. The tongue is equipped with taste buds and the nose with flavor buds, called olfactory receptors.

For example, it used to be assumed that if you placed a bit of sugar on the tongue and compared it with the sugar in, say, a berry, the brain would register them the same because they are both "sugars." However, sweetness is a function of signals from taste buds registering in the brain. Why does the brain prefer the berry?

Flavor researchers discovered that taste is boosted by the aromas released during chewing. These aromas, called volatiles (airborne molecules), float up into the nasal cavity and trigger the olfactory receptors, located under the mucus lining of the nasal tract. These cells then signal the taste center of the brain, registering "like berry."

Knowing that, let's take a close, scientific look at the relationships between taste and smell and the pleasure center of the brain, so we can better understand how the T5 way of eating moves your reaction to healthy foods from "don't like, but must eat" all the way to *craving*. Specifically, let's swim up that river with a key 5-S food—salmon.

Think salmon. When you're getting ready to make (or order) dinner, think about those five nutrients you get from salmon that are so good for you: omega-3s, astaxanthin, vitamin D, calcium, and vitamin B_{12}. Your brain sends a biochemical text message (scientifically known as neuropeptide crosstalk) to the pleasure center that registers "smart choice, delicious choice—especially with all that tangy honey-mustard sauce." All this anticipation may cause your brain's happy center to release some dopamine, one of the "pleasure hormones." The salmon is still in the fridge, and already your brain chemistry has you licking your chops.

See salmon. Next, you take the delicious, nutrient-dense smart food out of the fridge and begin preparing it. Just seeing it, handling it, smearing it with lemon juice, a drizzle of honey, and a dab of mustard piques your anticipation even more. The "likes" just keep piling up, and you still haven't taken your first bite.

Smell salmon. Upon taking your delectable dish out of the oven, you take a deep whiff of your creation. The flavor buds, those cellular antennae in the back of your nasal cavity, send a "like" message to the pleasure center of the brain.

Chew salmon. Chewing slowly for a long time allows the time-sensitive taste and flavor enhancers in your tongue and nasal cavity to send more "like" messages to the brain. These signals from the tongue and the nose merge into what we call the flavor center of the brain, registering a really big "like." The brain's pleasure center doesn't want to be rushed. When you take time to smell the salmon, chew it slowly, and pause and think or talk between bites, you give the part of your brain that signals "I'm full, stop eating" time to get into the action. Sometimes you will get so comfortably full that you will eat only three-quarters of the fillet and save the rest for your next meal or snack. Smart and satisfied. Again, you *eat less while enjoying it more,* which is the point of T5 eating.

This is how we make every meal a "fine dining" experience involving not only the food but the preparation, the ambiance, the social atmosphere, and the whole interaction of taste and smell. They all work together to play beautiful music as long as we take time to smell the food.

GOOD-GRAZING TIPS

I wrote much of this book while eating. Surprised? During our writing retreats, I enjoy a two-hour breakfast: eat a few bites, write a few lines, walk a minute, go back to grazing. I realized what Mom meant when she preached, "Take time to smell the roses." I take time to savor the chewing and sipping.

USE SMALLER PLATES

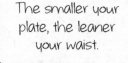

Reduce your plate by a couple of inches and you're likely to reduce your waist by a couple of inches. Also, use the smaller salad fork instead of the big "shovel" fork. Or . . .

USE CHOPSTICKS INSTEAD OF A FORK

As you learned during "Slow Your Salad Eating" (page 22), grazing with chopsticks has a double benefit: it slows down your pace of eating, enabling you to enjoy and digest your food better and feel full sooner. *And,* learning to use chopsticks, developing dexterity, helps grow new brain cells. To *really* grow new brain cells, grab beans or blueberries with chopsticks in your *non-dominant* hand. Your kids will love this one.

TAKE TWICE THE TIME TO DINE

Let's add another "two" to the rule of twos: slow down your eating. The lag time between your stomach filling up and your brain registering the "full" message is about twenty minutes. When you slow down your eating, your brain is more in sync with your gut, so you are less likely to overeat. Remember, if you feel stuffed, you are likely to have spikes. (See the endnotes for a second helping of information about how to regulate your appetite-control hormones, leptin and ghrelin.)

> I'm shrinking my waist and growing my brain.

I have noticed that fast eaters tend to have more health problems, mental and physical. I can often tell how stressed a person is by how fast they eat. At a recent meal, I watched a friend gorge, and respectfully asked, "How long have you been feeling troubled?" Surprised, he opened up about his depression and the antidepressant medication he is trying.

> Fast eaters become fat eaters.

WALK AWAY FROM TEMPTATION

When more food becomes too tempting, take a bathroom break or just get up from your eating place and take a walk around the house. Another of my good-grazing strategies is to put small helpings on your plate and leave the bowl or pan in the kitchen. Out of sight, out of stomach. Just the brief walk from table to kitchen may be enough time off to think, "Do I really need the extra helping?"

Avoid mindless munching. If your eyes, but not your brain, are focused on the food, you are likely to overeat and feel stuffed. That's why you don't want to put a huge bowlful of nuts next to you while watching TV. Instead, leave your favorite munchies in another room, so you have to get up and grab some. If you must snack in front of a screen, better to munch on high-fiber chewy snacks that are hard to overeat, such as celery sticks.

THINK BEFORE YOU EAT

The T5 plan reprograms your body and brain toward making informed decisions that translate into healthful habits. All day long you are faced with choices: what to eat, what to do, and what to think. When you are faced with one of these decisions, ask yourself, "Will this habit or food *help my health*?" If the answer is yes, then do it!

You've heard the term "habit forming." In the same vein that we talked about positive addiction, let's upgrade that to "habit transforming." Habits begin with *patterns of association,* nerve pathways stored in your brain that set off a chain of thoughts that quickly prompt you to an action: see donut, imagine taste of donut, eat donut. Like!

The T5 plan reprograms your brain toward: see donut, imagine how it harms your body, don't like, say no to donut! This reprogramming begins in your conscious mind. Eventually, when you give in and eat the donut—which you probably will—your gut brain, your automatic response, which you have been transforming toward food-refusal messages, will shout, "Don't do that again!" And you'll pay for eating that donut with a pain in the gut. Next time you'll *think* before you eat the donut, and that will bring on a reflexive thought: "I'll get a pain in the gut." You're transformed!

DON'T GO HUNGRY

Being too hungry prompts you to eat too much. A few weeks into T5 eating, you are likely to notice your natural hunger prompts are gentler: "I need a little something to eat." That's because you have been grazing on real foods and have transformed your gut brain and conscious brain never to feel too full or too hungry. Intense hunger, on the other hand, intensely pushes you into mindless eating—too much, too fast—with too little eating pleasure.

EAT EARLY

Late eaters are often restless sleepers, because undigested food may cause reflux or heartburn. Try to finish your

The earlier the meal, the better you feel!

Dr. Bill

meal at least *three hours* before bedtime. ✋ If you become too hungry and find you sleep better with a healthy bedtime snack, see our favorite snooze foods, page 291.

ERIN'S THOUGHTS ON GRAZING

Grazing can seem like a challenge at first, but I promise you will love how you feel and the results you will see. Our American culture says, "Go big or go home," but that saying is not our friend. Our "supersize me" portions are out of control and making us sick. Here is how switching to mini-meals transformed me.

Since college, I have struggled with eating a healthy amount, stopping when I'm full, and not eating out of boredom or stress. But once I started eating five mini-meals, my relationship with food changed drastically. I have steady energy, a clear mind, and emotional stability, and I work more productively.

FIVE GUIDELINES FOR GRAZING:

1. Have breakfast within an hour of waking up to kick-start your metabolism.
2. Eat about every two to three hours (or enjoy the "Sipping Solution," page 8).
3. Have a vegetable at every meal.
4. Watch portions and food quality instead of counting calories.
5. Balance each meal with healthy fats, lean protein, and healthy carbs.

That last guideline may seem like a challenge, but don't worry! Most of us are on the go, so think of the five-meal plan as an adjustment to the traditional three meals a day. You can keep the traditional breakfast-lunch-dinner model and insert two small snacks a day. Spacing out your food will automatically cut down on the size of your lunch and dinner, because you won't be starving when it comes time for that meal. When you have a five- to seven-hour gap between meals, the hunger monster takes over, prompting you to overeat.

A TYPICAL DAY'S MENU OF FIVE MINI-MEALS:

Meal 1: Power-packed smoothie (see suggested ingredients, page 9)

Meal 2: Apple with one tablespoon of nut butter

Meal 3: Green salad with mixed vegetables, a hard-boiled egg, and beans

Meal 4: Carrots, bell peppers, and celery with hummus—or a second smoothie

Meal 5: Salmon with steamed vegetables and wild rice

DR. BILL SAYS: SNACKS ARE *GOOD* FOR YOU

Snacking has gotten a bad rap among obesity counselors, because snacks are perceived as boxes and bags of sticky stuff and fake food—cereal, chips, crackers, cookies, candy, and so on. Healthy snacks seldom come in a bag or a box.

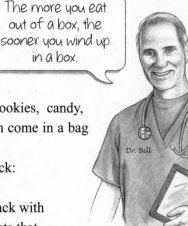

The more you eat out of a box, the sooner you wind up in a box.

Dr. Bill

Five features of a healthy snack:

1. Always partner a carb snack with two or three of the nutrients that blunt sugar spikes: fiber, protein, and healthy fats. Carb-only snacks are not good for you.
2. The *naturally crunchier,* the healthier: nuts, raw veggies like celery.

3. Snack only when your body prompts, when you're just starting to be slightly hungry.
4. A special kitchen KISMIF: keep it small, make it filling.
5. Avoid mindless munching while watching TV or video screens.

Our favorite healthy snacks:

- Palmful of nuts
- An egg
- Celery stick with peanut butter
- Blueberries in yogurt
- Cherry tomatoes with a cheese cube
- Red pepper slices dipped in hummus
- Apple slices dipped in nut butter
- Guacamole dip

COACH ERIN'S "INSTEAD OF" LIST FOR SATISFYING CRAVINGS	
When you crave this ...	Eat this ...
Chips	Air-popped popcorn with a little olive oil or Kerrygold Irish butter Dried edamame, Snapea Crisps Celery sticks
Ice cream	Greek yogurt with frozen fruit drizzled with a little raw honey Frozen grapes
Chocolate cake	One ounce of organic dark chocolate (at least 70% cocoa) Cocoa nibs Chocolate Juice+ Complete shake Chocolate Avocado Pudding (see recipe guide)
Processed dry cereal with added sugar	Steel-cut oatmeal with a palmful of nuts and fruit, sprinkled with cinnamon and a little honey

Soda, including diet soda, sweetened juices	Sparkling water with lemon or lime juice, coconut water, warm lemon water
French fries	Baked Sweet Potato Fries (see recipe guide)
Pasta	Organic brown rice, quinoa, or whole wheat pasta (even better, spiralizer zucchini)
White bread	Whole-grain or pumpernickel bread with nut butter
Cookies	Granola bar (choose the one with the least amount of added sugar, or make your own granola or low-carb cookies)
Something sweet	An apple with 1 tbsp. nut butter or fig paste Unsweetened dried fruit, fresh figs
Pizza	Grilled zucchini pizza bites (see recipe guide)
Hamburger	Salmon or black bean burger (see recipe guide)
Salty snacks	Palm full of raw nuts
Dips	Hummus Guacamole Plain organic Greek yogurt with nut butter
Salad dressing	Hummus, olive oil, and balsamic vinegar
Mashed potatoes with gravy	Steamed broccoli or cauliflower with homemade cheese sauce (or experiment making a "mock-mash" with riced cauliflower)
Sweets before bed	One egg

COACH ERIN'S TIME-SAVING TIPS
FOR SNACKING SUCCESS

1. **Make a "healthy snack" grab box.** Plan your snacks just as you do your other meals when you make your weekly shopping list. That way, you know you have healthy snacks in easy reach. Suggestions for your shopping list:

   - Fruits and veggies (put single snack servings in baggies)
   - Trail mix (also in baggies, ¼ cup each)
   - Whole piece of fruit
   - Hard-boiled eggs (two per bag)
   - Cherry tomatoes with cheese cubes
   - Hummus with whole-wheat pita chips
   - Edamame
   - Celery sticks

2. **Always have a quick and healthy snack visible in the fridge.**

3. **Cook three days' worth of lean protein** (e.g., ground turkey). Here is an example of how a one-pound batch of lean ground turkey can work for multiple meals (3–4 oz. serving size). Cook it all at once, seasoned with spices (salt, pepper, garlic, red pepper), and then use it in several meals, such as the following:

   Meal 1: Lettuce "tacos" on romaine
   Meal 2: Zucchini or rice pasta with meat sauce
   Meal 3: Bowl with brown rice and black beans
   Meal 4: Taco salad with grilled peppers and onions
   Meal 5: Stuffed zucchini with marinara sauce and a little
   mozzarella

For more on snacking and its differences from grazing, see the endnotes. 🖐

A TALE OF TWO EATERS: MR. SPIKEY AND MS. STEADY

Let us summarize what we've learned in these first two steps—what to eat and how to eat—by comparing two friends: one who needs T5 and one who's got it.

Mr. Spikey is hungry. He has driven to the all-you-can-eat restaurant and now stands before the buffet contemplating the huge expanse of food. He has forgotten what his mother told him long ago: "Your eyes are bigger than your stomach." Because he let himself get too hungry, his gut brain and head brain already have him fired up to eat too much too fast. And of course, he heads straight for the sticky food: the mashed potatoes and gravy, two desserts, and the huge slab of roast beef that's being carved to order at the "inflammation station" at the front of the buffet line.

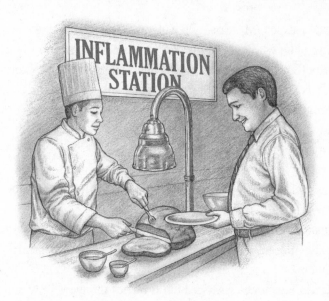

By the end of his first trip down the feeding trough, you can't see his plate due to the pile of food on it. Then Mr. Spikey sits down and goes to work *scarfing* down his food, because that is what his too-hungry body is begging him to do. To add insult to intestinal injury, he washes it all down with a super-size cola—a double no-no. Does he enjoy his feast? He'll tell you he does, but he'd enjoy it far more if he took his time to chew and savor each bite. Instead, he's wolfing it down so fast he hardly tastes it.

Stuffed gut, stressed heart. Over the next couple of hours, all that sticky stuff that Mr. Spikey put in his mouth works its way through his intestines and into his bloodstream, and here's where the big problems begin. When all that sticky stuff floods into Mr. Spikey's blood vessels, they get stressed and actually start quivering, a pre-stroke or pre-heart-attack sign called *vasospasm*. The vessels get too narrow to deliver enough blood, and the level of sticky stuff is so high that it can clog the vessels. Next, all of Mr. Spikey's major organs begin to protest. And because of the constricted vessels, the blood flow slows down like a river filled with sludge. This in turn slows down the function of all the organs. This includes the brain, and Mr. Spikey begins to feel foggy.

Pancreas not pleased. Mr. Spikey's pancreas responds to the sugar spikes by pumping out a whole lot of insulin in a desperate attempt to mop up all that sugar before sugar molecules and other sticky stuff stick to the walls of the vessels. Mr. Spikey's blood flow goes into a hyper sticky state—in medical language, his blood is full of *adhesion molecules*.

Meanwhile, since the body does not like to waste food, it reacts in several ways:

- Instead of wasting those extra carbs, it *waists* them—storing them in belly fat.
- Insulin level *spikes,* causing Mr. Spikey to feel hungry again and crave more carbs to offset the excess, potentially harmful insulin level.
- Stress hormones *spike*, which is one of the ways in which the ups and downs of blood sugar cause mood swings and diminish mental clarity.
- Spikey's body *stores* excess sugars as fat in the liver; this contributes to diabetes and fatty liver disease, which are becoming epidemic.

Remember, the less you spike, the longer and healthier you live.

Mr. Spikey's last spike. As his blood flow slows down, Mr. Spikey suffers what we call "the spike effect." His diet sets up Mr. Spikey for a sad life. Standard American diet = SAD = sick all day. This sticky-stuff effect, if too high for too long, can cause a vascular traffic jam—blood clots, coronary thrombosis, or stroke.

Ms. Steady doesn't spike. She never gets more than slightly hungry—just enough to know it's time to eat. Because she's not too hungry, her body is not prompted to overeat. She picks at her salad with her chopsticks, which immediately gets the brain and body on the right biochemical track. She chews the crunchy salad slowly, savors it, and enjoys each bite. She eats a big salad first because it takes her longer to eat it, it's chewier, and the blood vessels love it because she fills her bloodstream with lots of antioxidants, which will help blunt the effect of any sticky spikes that may come later in the meal. She chews each bite twenty to forty times, and sometimes munches on a bite of shrimp, which may take as many as sixty chews. She takes time to enjoy conversation between bites.

Her second course consists of a four-ounce salmon fillet, grilled asparagus, and some wild rice. Only her plate is in front of her. There are no serving bowls on the table. Out of sight, out of stomach.

Tummy talk. Ms. Steady's tummy feels comfortably full, neither bloated nor stuffed. Her gut brain loves what's going on, because the long chewing has stimulated so much saliva that the food slides down more easily and arrives at the stomach already partially digested to make the gut's job easier. Ms. Steady's blood vessels are pleased. Blood is flowing smoothly during the after-meal rush hour.

Her choice of salmon rather than sirloin is good for her gut and her blood vessels. The omega-3s in the salmon increase production of the enzyme lipoprotein lipase, which helps clear sticky fats—triglycerides—from her bloodstream. After a salmon meal, you don't get the fatty sticky-stuff effect (postprandial lipemia) that happens after scarfing down a steak. Steak fats stick to the blood cells and slow them down, but the smooth fats in the salmon ride along on the surface of the blood cells and make them less sticky, so the traffic doesn't slow after the meal.

When Ms. Steady bypasses the meat counter in favor of seafood and salad, she likely avoids a coronary bypass. Also, a seafood-rich meal causes greater postprandial satiety. Ms. Steady's diet of real food helps her feel great and live longer.

Vessels illustrated. Remember the drawing of healthy and diseased arteries back on page 41 in chapter one? That's what Ms. Steady's and Mr. Spikey's arteries look like. Which ones do you want?

A SECOND HELPING: MORE TIPS ON HEALTHY T5 EATING

Before we move on to the benefits of moving more, a few more random thoughts about eating less and eating more healthfully.

TOO YOUNG TO WORRY?

When we counsel young adults about their sticky-stuff diets, they often say, "But I feel fine. Why should I change?" Here's the math: three sticky meals a day, 365 days a year, for over thirty years. That's over 30,000 meals of sticky-stuff assaults on your tissues. Most people who begin to transform in their forties and after are motivated by the fact that they are already sick—with something like diabetes, heart disease, or cancer. If you're young and healthy, you have a great opportunity *not* to get sick. Prevention is smarter than repair, especially when you consider that some sickness can't be completely repaired. You can't always feel prevention, in the same way you can't always feel disease. The powerful part of the T5 lifestyle is that we get to feel empowered, knowing we are honoring our body through nutrition the best we can each day.

JOURNAL YOUR "INSTEAD OF" CHOICES

Remember Erin's "instead of" list a few pages back? Whenever you make one of those choices, enter it in your T5 journal. "Instead of pasta, I enjoyed salmon." Little changes add up to a lot of health benefits. You are trying to reshape your tastes to enjoy the flavor, health benefits, and good gut feelings of healthier alternatives. Within a few months, you will literally change your gut to crave the healthier choices. Your journal is your motivational record of this transformation. Your gut is called the "second brain" for a reason. When you feed it right, it will tell you so.

After eating the 5-S diet for five weeks, you will notice a transformation in your tastes. Junk foods you previously craved you will now shun. That's because of the transformation that occurred in the lining of your intestines, or "gut feel" of food. Your head brain sends biochemical signals to your gut brain: "Thanks for eating this way. I feel good. Keep it up!"

The longer you can stay on T5, the more persistent and permanent will be your body's *health point*, your personal ideal weight for optimal health. While I was working on this chapter, Martha and I celebrated our fiftieth wedding anniversary on a two-week cruise to Tahiti. You know what a cruise means. Too much food and too many big meals. My habitual T5 eating fell overboard. On day twelve my gut yelled, "You were thriving on T5, but now you're not doing it. We're hurting down here." I suffered the "shuns": indigestion, constipation, and inflammation.

During the first week home, my gut prompts switched back into T5 eating. My good gut feelings returned within five days, the average time it takes to regrow an upset intestinal lining.

BUNS OUT!

My favorite breakfast treat while traveling is eggs Florentine. One day as I was sliding the eggs, spinach, and tomato off the English muffin, the restaurant manager commented, "No wonder you look so healthy. More and more customers are ordering burgers without the bun." This simple change can greatly reduce your carbs.

SKIP THE TERRIBLE FIVE: THE CHEMICALLY PROCESSED "FOODS" THAT CAUSE SPIKES

I call them the terrible five, but *terminal* five might be even better. According to one of the world's largest studies, the Global Burden of Disease

Study, the more of these five foods you eat, the sicker you will get and the sooner you will die:

1. Artificially and sugar-sweetened beverages
2. Processed meats: bologna, hot dogs, bacon, and ham
3. Feedlot-raised meat (see "meat out," page 207)
4. Fiberless foods (e.g., packaged foods that have most of the fiber processed out. See why on page 203.)
5. Hydrogenated oils (one of the fakest and stickiest artificial fats)

ARTIFICIAL SWEETENERS SOUR YOUR TRANSFORMATION

"Added" sugar and artificial sweeteners, in our opinion, are the top causes of our pandemic of obesity, type 2 diabetes, and related illnesses. Here's a crash course on why sweeteners sour your health.

No-calorie and low-calorie sweeteners can cause big health problems. Artificial sweeteners artificially affect your tastes. Aspartame, sucralose, acesulfame, and others stimulate the taste receptors for sweetness many times more strongly than do table sugars or even the natural sugars in fruits. Your taste buds get used to this high-potency artificial taste to the extent that the natural sweetness of a bowl of berries may not seem sweet enough. And since most vegetables are naturally but more subtly sweet, programming your tongue with artificial sweeteners is even more likely to lessen your love for them.

In short, artificial sweeteners reshape your tastes for the worse. T5 reshapes your tastes for the better, to enjoy a more "real" sweet taste. After you spend a few months eating real food, fake-sweetened, processed food will taste yucky. I noticed this after six months of T5 eating. One morning before a lecture I found myself craving a high-protein breakfast. Good! The hotel breakfast only had artificially sweetened yogurt, which I ate anyway. Yuck! What used to taste sweet to me now tasted "chemical"— because it *is* chemical. "Yucky yogurt" is now forever on my red-light, no-eat list.

"Added sugar" leads to added weight. Ever wonder why food processors add sweeteners to foods and drinks? Because the sweetener-eater tends to eat and drink more and buy more. Sweeteners, artificial or added sugar, stimulate the reward centers of the brain, increasing hunger and prompting you to crave more.

Why artificial sweeteners—I call them fakies—cause sour health and increase sugar cravings has been the subject of intense study. Researchers summarize that the more fakies you eat, the more food you eat, the more weight you gain. A probable reason is that the taste buds and the brain get chemically confused, leading to overeating. Basically, fakies trigger binging, just the behavior you don't want when trying to get lean.

One of the hottest topics in neuroscience in the last few years is the startling discovery that artificial sweeteners in "diet" or "lite" foods and drinks may actually make you fat. Dr. Jason Fung, in his provocative book *The Obesity Code*, makes the point that artificial sweeteners can trigger insulin spikes just as sugar does, which we have repeatedly stressed is the root cause of obesity and type 2 diabetes.

Moreover, statisticians have noted that the steadily rising incidence of obesity in America has run parallel to the increasing use of artificial sweeteners in foods and drinks. (For a further exposé of how "big chem" has contributed to our fatness, see the endnotes.) As the sales of fake sweeteners went up, our health got more sour. In summary, artificial sweeteners can mess up your brain, your gut, and your waistline. (See the endnotes for more ways artificial sweeteners sour your health.)

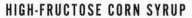

HIGH-FRUCTOSE CORN SYRUP

Despite what you might read, eating lots of fruit, which contains fructose, is good for the body. On the other hand, eating a lot of high-fructose corn syrup (HFCS) is bad for the body. The fructose in fruit and the fructose that is processed in the factory, like HFCS, behave differently in the body. Fruit fructose behaves healthfully; HFCS does not.

Real sugars in fruit are absorbed more slowly, so they don't spike. Also, real fruit contains fiber, which keeps the fructose from rushing too quickly into the bloodstream. HFCS, on the other hand, flows quickly and directly into the bloodstream, causing big, sharp spikes. It's as simple as that.

ARTIFICIAL SWEETENERS—NOT FOR KIDS

Fakies shape children's tastes in the wrong direction, and when growing brains are most vulnerable to taste-shaping. The biggest, baddest fakie: *corn syrup* added to infant formula! Feeding fakies to infants and children is bad for three reasons:

1. They are more likely to be used in fake foods, so children's tastes are being shaped not only toward the artificial sweeteners, but toward fake foods in general.
2. They confuse the gut and head brains, so they are likely to stimulate overeating.
3. They promote obesity.

THE CASE AGAINST COLAS

Sweetened beverages will sabotage your transformation in three ways:

1. *Most fattening.* Sodas are the epitome of the term "empty calories." Full of sugar and transformation-tricking chemicals. Zero nutrients.
2. *Most sickening.* The sugar cravings they trigger and the chemical tricks they play on your brain make you sick and tired.
3. *Most artery-stiffening.* According to Dr. Michael Greger, author of the riveting book *How Not to Die*, phosphates found in meats, colas, and processed foods are medically considered "vascular toxins." This means endothelial

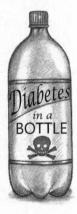

dysfunction can occur within hours following a high-phosphate meal. So look for "phosphate" on the label; it's a bad word. And men, if "tonight is the night," stick to a salad and skip the soda and meat.

A sad soda story. Besides inflammation, there is another "shun" that forms sticky stuff in your blood and in your tissues. *Glycation* is a tissue-damaging chemical reaction caused by excess sugars becoming sticky, building up on arterial walls, and slowing blood flow. What's one of the biggest sources of glycation for young people? You guessed it. Soda.

COACH ERIN: HOW TO BREAK YOUR SODA ADDICTION

- Start by reducing your intake for a few days to soften withdrawal.
- Substitute sparkling water (not club soda) with a splash of fruit juice or fresh-squeezed lemon or lime.
- Mix up a big pitcher of water infused with fresh fruit and rosemary.
- Don't use artificial sweeteners, as this will trigger your cravings.
- Kick the soda habit with a friend. Check in every night to see how you're doing. Accountability helps!
- Don't think about what you're "giving up." Think about what you're gaining—a longer, healthier life.
- Give yourself a healthy reward at the end of each week or month you've been soda-free. Choose something not food related, like a pedicure or a fun new outfit.
- If you're a spiritual person, then every morning turn your cravings over to God and ask for help.
- Supplement with unsweetened green tea if you need the caffeine fix.

Try this taste-reshaping test:

- Eat mostly *real foods*, those that have no added sweeteners or flavor enhancers on the label. (In fact, real foods are less likely to require a label. They're the fruits and vegetables around the perimeter of the supermarket.) Wean yourself gradually, until your diet is 90 percent real foods, 10 percent treats.
- Within five weeks, sweetened foods that you previously liked and even craved will taste artificially chemical (because they are.)

Voila! You're transformed!

CHAPTER 3

MOVE MORE!

FIVE WAYS TO ENJOY IT

Move more to make your own medicines. Yes, you read that right. Inside your body is your own personal pharmacy, and movement opens it. How I learned this involved reading a lot of obscure medical journals, a friendship, a Nobel Prize, and a salmon dinner. And it became one of the two fundamental principles of Transform 5: *avoid sticky stuff* and *make your own medicines*.

HOW TO MAKE YOUR OWN MEDICINES

As a sick doctor who wanted to get well, I formulated, followed, and still follow the T5 program. In those early years of searching for the keys to regaining my health, I kept thinking that somewhere in our bodies there must be a kind of natural pharmacy that makes most of the medicines we need. How else would the human race have survived all those years before the advent of neighborhood pharmacies? If you were designing the human body and wanted it to last long and stay healthy, you would put a pharmacy in there, right? But where? The people who run Walgreens and CVS know location is everything. Where would you put that internal pharmacy to quickly and easily dispense its medicines? As close as possible to the bloodstream, of course. And that's exactly where it is. My pharmacy-finding search led me to an organ that is most important to health and longevity, but which we know little about—the *endothelium*, the lining of the blood vessels.

Only one cell layer thick, the endothelium, or what I call the "silver lining," is where our internal pharmacy resides. No health books mentioned the endothelium as the site of the internal pharmacy. I found the fascinating, life-changing research about the endothelial pharmacy buried in obscure medical journals that only an inquisitive doctor with a bit of ADHD would study.

Our illustration shows, in a whimsical way, how your internal pharmacy consists of trillions of microscopic squirt bottles that inject medicines custom-made for you into your bloodstream at the right time, at the right dosage. Unlike the medicines you buy, the medicines you make have no harmful side effects, only healthful effects.

Sam the sitter and sticky-stuff eater

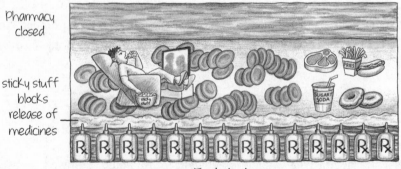

Pharmacy closed

sticky stuff blocks release of medicines

Endothelium

Mandi the mover and real-food eater

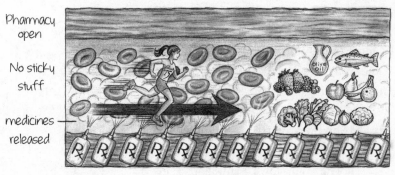

Pharmacy open

No sticky stuff

medicines released

Endothelium

IS YOUR INTERNAL PHARMACY OPEN FOR BUSINESS?

My childlike concept of the endothelial pharmacy produced a revelation. What if the difference between chronic good health and chronic illness depended on whether your endothelial pharmacy was open 24/7 or closed?

By this time, I had formulated my simple explanation of illness: *we put too much sticky stuff in our mouths, and we get sticky stuff all over our organs.* Then the light bulb went on: people who follow the T5 way of eating don't have sticky stuff lining their endothelia and clogging the openings of all those little medicine bottles.

So for the past fifteen years of my medical practice I have used "make your own medicines" as a motivator for patients to do T5. Naturally, the better you care for the "silver lining" of your blood vessels, the more medicine it makes for you.

SICKNESS AND WELLNESS MADE SIMPLE

When you put sticky stuff in your mouth, you get sticky stuff in your blood and sticky stuff clogging the openings of your medicine bottles, and you get sick. Keep sticky stuff out of your mouth, and you stay well.

WHAT MEDICINES DOES YOUR INTERNAL PHARMACY MAKE?

Over twenty "medicines" have been discovered, and undoubtedly more are still to come. You make five main types of medicines that:

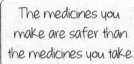

The medicines you make are safer than the medicines you take.

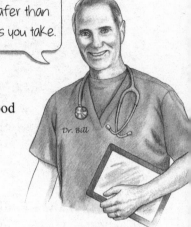

Dr. Bill

- lower your "highs": blood pressure, blood sugar, and blood cholesterol
- elevate your "lows": antidepressants
- mellow your moods: anti-anxiety neurochemicals
- heal your hurts: anti-inflammatories
- keep your blood from clotting too fast: anticoagulants

THE LAST PIECE OF THE PUZZLE: A NOBEL NIGHT TO REMEMBER

Dr. Lou Ignarro, who worked at UCLA, a short distance away from me, won the Nobel Prize for a discovery that transformed my life and will help change yours. Lou and his wife, Sharon, invited Martha and me to their home for dinner. We spent several hours talking about Lou's research, and Martha amused us by donning Lou's Nobel medal.

Soon after, Lou and Sharon were guests at our home for our traditional salmon-at-sunset dinner. I was eager and grateful for the opportunity to learn from this great scientist. While Lou was expounding on biochemistry and biophysics, he noticed that I was not only scribbling notes, but drawing a childish picture. After raising eight children and fifty years as a pediatrician, one naturally begins to think and even draw like a child. (Martha would add, "And act like a child.")

What I was drawing was a crude version of the illustration you saw just above—the one with the medicine bottles lining the blood vessels, showing how they can get shut off by sticky stuff. Lou loved it. Then he filled in the last piece of my puzzle—*how movement opens the medicine bottles.*

MOVE MORE—OPEN YOUR INTERNAL PHARMACY

Brisk movement, exercise, causes blood to flow faster over the surface of the endothelium. Lou Ignarro discovered that faster-moving blood over the surface of the silver lining creates a *shear force* that releases nitric oxide (NO). Think of NO as the pharmacist who opens your medicine bottles to dispense the medicines you need. The more you move, the better job your internal pharmacy does of dispensing medicines.

From that evening on, I referred to Lou as Dr. NO. We started trading NO jokes.

"To make more NO, get up and go!"

"Say yes to NO!"

"NO good nutrition, NO good heart!"

"Sit more, NO less!"

This discovery provides the simple, scientific basis of our Transform 5 program for health and longevity. Keep sticky stuff off your medicine bottles. Move more to get the medicines flowing.

It's a simple, beautiful formula for health:

$$\frac{\text{DON'T EAT STICKY STUFF} + \text{MOVE MORE}}{= \text{MAKE YOUR OWN MEDICINES}}$$

> Go to our website DrSearsWellness.org/T5/Pharmacy on your smartphone or computer to download a full-page, full color "wow!" reminder of how to make your own medicines. Paste this colorful page on your fridge or treadmill. File it in your memory photo library and revisit it frequently. It is the most motivational illustration in this whole book.

WHAT SCIENCE SAYS ABOUT MOVERS AND SITTERS	
Movers	Sitters
Brain grows	Brain shrinks
Live longer	Die sooner
Less diabetes	More diabetes
Fall less	Fall and fracture more
Stay lean	Get fat
Stay happy	Get depressed

A LOOK INSIDE YOUR ENDOTHELIAL PHARMACY

Take another look at the illustration of the endothelium on page 88. Sam suffers from "sitting disease." He puts sticky stuff in his mouth, and it coats the linings of his blood vessels. His internal pharmacy is closed. His blood flow is slower, and his vessels narrower. He is sick and tired and headed for a life of disease, disabilities, and doctors. ✺

Mandi moves a lot and eats according to T5. Her blood vessels are wider and her blood flows faster. Her pharmacy is always open. She has taken charge of her health.

MORE INSIDE DOPE ON BLOOD VESSELS

The pressure is on. When vessels get stiff and sticky, the heart has to pump harder and faster. This increases blood pressure, which further damages the silver lining, which makes the pressure go even higher—a vicious cycle. Eventually, the heart pump wears out, because it had to work too hard for too long to force blood through the damaged arteries.

Sugar-coated vessels. When blood sugar is too high for too long, sticky stuff called advanced glycation end products (AGEs) bind to the elastic fibers in the arterial wall and make them stiffer, as well as blocking NO production. The lining of the blood vessels gets stiff and sticky, and the blood vessels get narrower. The effect is like a lane closure on a congested highway during rush hour, slowing traffic to a crawl. This can contribute to coronary artery clogging and subsequent heart attack. 🖐

This is also why diabetes leads to vascular disease, but you don't have to be diagnosed with diabetes before high blood sugar hurts your blood vessels.

Healthy vessels. When your endothelium is healthy and uncoated, all those little medicine bottles, regulated by nitric oxide (NO), squirt, among many other things, anti-sticky-stuff medicines that coat the red blood cells to keep them from clotting together. Also, during rush hour, when you're exercising, NO automatically widens the highway by relaxing the elastic walls of the arteries, so traffic can flow more smoothly with less congestion.

Get more NO when you get up and go. When you go from being a sitter to a mover, the endothelial cells actually get upgraded and perform better. The more you exercise, the more your blood vessels get used to the extra flow. Exercise increases *cardiovascular reactivity,* meaning that well-toned vessels of regular exercisers widen more easily and with less effort during exercise. That's why I love the term "fit"—that three-letter word that so economically describes the cardiovascular system of a mover. The internal medicine pharmacy of a mover *fits* their emotional and physical needs, sort of like the family doctor prescribing the right medicines.

A WALK IN THE GARDEN—A WAKE-UP CALL

One day shortly after my visit with the Nobel laureate Dr. NO, I was watering my garden when I had a transformative thought: OMG! That's what movement does! It waters the gardens of my body and brain. Now, when I'm teaching kids about health, they love my garden analogy:

- Every organ in your body is like a garden: the better you feed, fertilize, and irrigate it, the better it thrives.
- An organ is only as healthy as the blood flow to it.

- Movement widens blood vessels. Like using a larger garden hose, it increases the volume of blood flow.
- The more you move, the more personal medicines you make, and the more nutrients you deliver. It's like feeding your garden more water and fertilizer. 🖐

This is why the more you move, the lower your chances of getting all those illnesses you hope to avoid:

- Cancer
- Heart disease
- Pains in the gut
- *-itis* illnesses
- Depression and anxiety
- Alzheimer's
- Diabetes

Wow! One simple change that everyone can do—move—has all these preventive-medicine effects.

Which organ of the body is most improved by movement? Most people think it's the heart, but in fact it's the brain.

The brain gets bigger. When you move more, you start making more NO, your blood vessels widen, and blood flows faster and delivers more nutrients to nourish all the organs. This particularly benefits the brain, because it is one of the most vascular organs. As the blood flow increases, more happy hormones flood the brain, in particular NGF—nerve growth factor. So increasing blood flow to the brain is like fertilizing the garden. It's why movers have larger, smarter, happier brains than sitters. 🖐

The heart is happy. Because the NO relaxes the blood vessels, the heart doesn't have to work as hard. Not only does heart rate slow down by a few beats per minute, but reduced blood pressure means that each beat requires less work and your heart will likely last longer. (See more about movement making heart medicines, page 91).

By increasing neurotransmitter activity, improving blood flow, and producing Brain Growth Factors—Miracle Grow or Brain Fertilizers—exercise readies our nerve cells to bind more easily and stronger. Exercise does this better than any other factor that we are aware of at the present time.
—JOHN RATEY, MD, ASSOCIATE CLINICAL PROFESSOR OF PSYCHIATRY, HARVARD MEDICAL SCHOOL

The gut feels good. Moving your body helps keep stuff moving through your digestive tract. Also, your gut bugs, your microbiome, thrives on movement. When blood flow is better, the kidneys filter waste better, so all that toxic stuff doesn't build up to make you feel tired and sick.

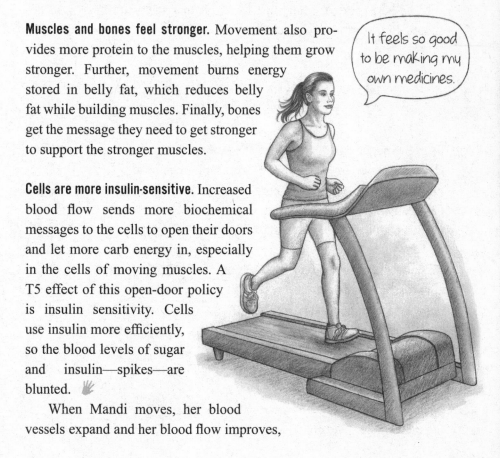

Muscles and bones feel stronger. Movement also provides more protein to the muscles, helping them grow stronger. Further, movement burns energy stored in belly fat, which reduces belly fat while building muscles. Finally, bones get the message they need to get stronger to support the stronger muscles.

It feels so good to be making my own medicines.

Cells are more insulin-sensitive. Increased blood flow sends more biochemical messages to the cells to open their doors and let more carb energy in, especially in the cells of moving muscles. A T5 effect of this open-door policy is insulin sensitivity. Cells use insulin more efficiently, so the blood levels of sugar and insulin—spikes—are blunted.

When Mandi moves, her blood vessels expand and her blood flow improves, delivering to her muscles and organs more nutrients, energy, and oxygen and more of the medicines her body makes. Her insulin and blood sugar levels don't spike. She's healthier, sharper, feels better, and is less at risk for things like heart attacks and strokes.

Because Sam sits incessantly, his blood flow is sluggish. He doesn't feed and fertilize the gardens of his body. Instead of using energy from food for strengthening muscle, Sam stores it as fat. When Sam is sluggish, so are most of his organs. He suffers from brain fog, an overworked heart, lazy gut, and unhappy hormones that cause unhappy moods. Because Sam is sluggish, so is his blood flow, causing Sam to always be on the verge of getting a life-threatening clot in his brain, heart, or legs. Sam's cells become insulin insensitive, and he joins the thirty percent of other Americans with the three D's: disabilities, dementia, and diabetes.

The best perk for Mandi the Mover is that sticky stuff stays off her endothelium, so the medicine bottles remain open.

COACH ERIN SAYS: MOVE YOUR BODY FOR YOUR MIND

In my experience, movement is the safest antidepressant you will find. If I don't move my body every day, I get a chemical imbalance in my brain. In high school, I loved being physically active in cheerleading and musical theater, but in college I found myself stressing out more and moving less. I took to Zumba and swing dancing for stress relief, and, lo and behold, my test scores and homework productivity improved because my mind was calmer.

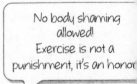

No body shaming allowed! Exercise is not a punishment, it's an honor

Movement calms what I call "the monkey mind." I recently had another reminder of the importance of morning movement. We got a dog who naturally needs to be taken for a walk every morning. At first, I dreaded this routine. But after a couple weeks, it became a vital part of sanely getting ready for the day. Fifteen or twenty minutes of being "where my feet are" every morning helps my entire day go better.

THE FIVE BEST MOVEMENTS YOU CAN DO

To have the butt you want, move the butt you have!
—TRANSFORMER WILL BICKFORD

Now that you are motivated to move more, here's how to make the most out of your movements, have the most fun doing them, and feel the most effects the soonest.

What's the best T5 exercise program? It's the one you will do and stick to. That said, the T5 program is based on, you guessed it, *five* basic kinds of exercise, chosen for their effectiveness, for your enjoyment, and for how easy they are to fit into your life:

1. Isometrics
2. Aerobics
3. Strength building
4. Rhythmic
5. Yoga and Pilates—movement for the mind

IMPROVE THE WAY YOU MOVE

If you're thinking, "But I don't have time to exercise," then you'd better set aside some time to spend in the hospital. As we've said: the T5 program is not a *diet*, it's a *do-it*. One of the reasons so many diets fail is they focus only on the scale. The T5 fitness program works because it focuses on what matters: *waist size* and *body composition*.

In the T5 exercise program you will trade excess body fat for more muscle and enjoy a leaner waist. Making this healthy transformation means you will have just the right amount of body fat for your gender and body type. Science says that those who build more muscle and lean out their waists enjoy:

- Lower incidence of type 2 diabetes;
- Lower blood pressure, blood sugar, and triglycerides;
- Lower risk of cardiovascular disease;
- Lower risk of neurodegenerative diseases;
- Fewer falls and fractures, and stronger bones;
- Fewer inflammatory illnesses; and
- Longer-lasting weight control.

One simple metabolic mechanism explains why all these health benefits happen: Muscle stabilizes blood sugar, even while you sleep.

THE DANGER OF DIETING WITHOUT EXERCISE

When you go on a typical fad diet—the kind that's basically temporary malnutrition—you lose both fat and muscle. Then when you go back to your SAD diet and regain the weight, you typically gain mostly fat. In other words, after you rebound from your "diet," you end up with a body that has a greater proportion of body fat than when you first started. This is another reason why we don't like to call our T5 program a diet. It's a lifestyle.

We realize you're going to make note of your weight before you start the T5 program. But, as you progress, we really want you to emphasize

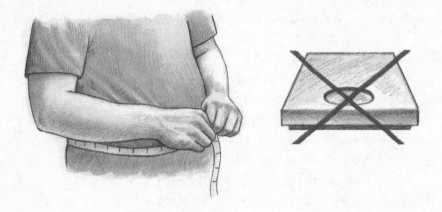

waist control rather than weight control. Your tape measure, belt size, skirt size, and pants size are more meaningful than mere weight change. (See more about *waist management*, page 47.)

We just listed the five different types of exercise we recommend and the overall health benefits they provide. Next, we'll discuss each of them in detail. Each of the five exercises yields its own set of health benefits—mental and physical. Try to fit all five into your life, as there is real synergy between all five types of movements. Your transformation will be greater than the sum of these five parts.

1. ISOMETRICS: THE TOP EXERCISE FOR ANYONE, ANYTIME, ANYWHERE

Isometrics are awesome. My fascination with isometrics as the easiest muscle-toning feature of T5 began with a walk on a golf course with my aforementioned friend, the neurologist Dr. Vincent Fortanasce, who was an alternate on the 1964 U.S. Olympic weightlifting team. "Vince, you guys used to spend many hours just sitting on airplanes during international travel. How did you keep your muscles from getting flabby?"

"Isometrics," he responded. "Here, I'll show you."

Wow! Within one minute I felt as if I'd done a total-body workout. My heart rate was up a bit, I was breathing faster, and I felt better.

Isometrics (so called because muscle fibers don't change length during movement) are exercises in which you "flex and hold" for as long as you can—until you can feel the "burn" of muscle fatigue. You know you're making progress when you find you can flex and hold longer before fatigue sets in. *Time under tension* (TUT) is the principle that gives you the greatest bang for your workout buck. (See TUT, page 108.)

A great thing about isometrics is that you're using your body itself as weight-training equipment—pitting one muscle against another or

Hold me TUT

a set of muscles against gravity. Anyone can do isometrics anytime, anywhere, and you don't need to go to a gym or buy equipment. That's why these must-do, must-feel exercises get top billing in the T5 program.

> Anyone can do isometrics anytime, anywhere.

Dr. Bill

TURN WASTED TIME INTO WAIST TIME

How much time do you spend each day standing in lines and sitting in waiting rooms? You could use that time transforming. Isometrics are especially helpful for professional sitters who spend a lot of time in "bored" meetings. You can lift and hold your legs for a minute or two under the table or flex your biceps and pectorals, and no one will know. You'd be surprised at the end of an hour-long meeting that your body feels like it's had a good workout. Better yet, doing isometrics for two minutes before eating can stimulate production of leptin, the "eat less" hormone that controls your appetite.

One day while standing in line for an international flight, I thought, "Instead of fretting about the long line, I'll enjoy my time doing isometrics." I began *standing strong,* holding my legs and arms tense for a minute (see next section). This kind of exercise is subtle but not invisible. A flight attendant came up to me and said, "Sir, you seem tense. May I help you?" My TUT workout ended with a laugh.

Let's look at some great basic isometric exercises you can do anywhere, anytime.

> ⊙ See videos of Dr. Bill doing isometric exercises at DrSears Wellness.org/T5/Isometrics.

Stand strong. Lean against a post or wall and flex all the major muscle groups from your feet to your chest: flex quads, squeeze glutes, pull in abs, flex and squeeze pecs, and press one fist against the opposite palm while flexing biceps and triceps. Hold these muscles flexed for 30 to 60 seconds, or until you feel the burn in all of them. At first, 30 seconds may be the best you can do. Eventually, you'll be toned enough to hold longer than a minute. The burn (the biochemical fatigue signal that means you are starting to burn calories and build muscle) usually occurs shortly after you feel your heart beating faster and begin breathing more heavily.

Belly suck-ins. You can do these anytime, anywhere, and no one will notice. Suck in your belly button toward your backbone. Also tense your glutes. Hold 30 seconds and release. After a few reps you may naturally feel the need to take a few deep belly breaths.

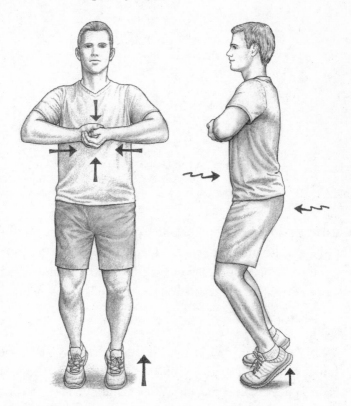

Standing at work. In our Dr. Sears Wellness Institute office in Denver, Colorado, we transform sitters into standers by providing standing desks. Just standing instead of sitting can burn an extra fifty calories an hour. Add periodic isometrics, and you'll burn more.

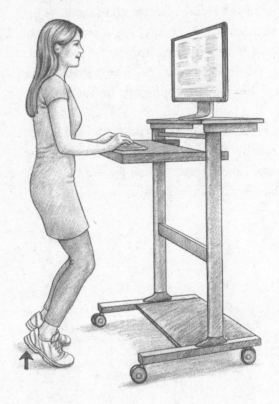

Sit strong. Here's how an on-the-job sitter can become a mover. Lift your legs four to six inches off the floor and hold until you feel the burn in the muscles on top of your thighs, the quadriceps. Add the same upper-body isometrics you flexed in the stand-strong exercise. Try these variations:

Sitting leg lift
- While sitting, lift knees above horizontal. Hold 30 to 60 seconds. Initially, you may need to stabilize your torso by grabbing your chair or desk with both hands. Repeat until you feel the burn.
- *Leg-against-leg.* Lift your legs as shown on next page, then cross them at the ankles, pointing your right toes left and your left toes

to the right. Press the upper leg down and the lower leg up. Then switch legs and do it again.

To strengthen all your leg muscles, especially quads, hamstrings, and lower leg muscles, try leg-against-leg isometrics, illustrated below. I call these my "bored meeting" or "under the table" exercises.

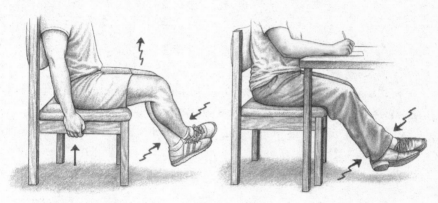

FIST TO PALM PUSH

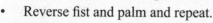

- Flex your arms at the elbows, place one fist against opposite palm, and push one against the other. Hold 30 to 60 seconds.
- After getting used to this basic isometric, try it while also holding your biceps flexed.
- Next, push your fist *down* against your cupped palm. This will tense the biceps on the down arm and the triceps on the up arm.
- Reverse fist and palm and repeat.
- Repeat these isometrics 8 to 12 times.
- Add a *pec squeeze*. While doing the above biceps and triceps tensions, bring your elbows in against your chest and flex your pecs; hold 30 to 60 seconds. Repeat 8 to 12 times.

HEEL RAISES

Lift your heels off the floor. Doing this freestanding will improve your balance, but if that's a problem, hold onto a chair with one hand.

After you have mastered isometrics with individual muscles and muscle groups, do what I call TBT—*total body tension.* Flex, tense, and hold all major muscle groups while balancing on your toes.

DON'T LOCK YOUR KNEES

While doing standing isometrics, slightly flex your knees. This decreases wear and tear on your knee joints and increases tension in the calf and thigh muscles.

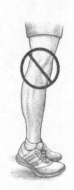

---

2. AEROBICS

Aerobics, cardio, whatever you call it, we're talking about sustained movement that causes your heart to beat faster and your breathing to become faster and heavier. This is a T5 must-do because, as you learned in the last chapter, making blood flow faster through your blood vessels opens your internal-medicine pharmacy so you can make your own medicines. The second reason is the more you move your muscles, the more tiny blood vessels your body makes to improve the blood supply to those muscles (and to other tissues, such as the brain; see pages 225–226). And the better the blood supply, the better those muscles and organs work.

Cardiologists aren't the only doctors who recommend cardio. It is the "medicine" most prescribed by clinical psychologists and psychiatrists, mainly because "making your own medicine" and delivering more of it nourishes your brain better. Fascinating new studies have shown that vigorous daily aerobic exercise can have better and safer mood-mellowing effects than prescription antidepressants, which are increasingly being found to be unsafe, especially if taken for long periods. (Also see: Yes, exercise goes to your head, page 225.)

STEP IT UP

Shoot for at least 20 minutes of aerobic exercise a day. Get a step counter. Your goal is an average of 10,000 steps a day. Most sitters take fewer than 5,000. Set a realistic goal, such as increasing your steps by 1,000 a week (150 steps a day) for five weeks to reach your goal of 10,000 per day. (See related section: "Walk While You Talk," page 120.)

10,000 steps a day, I say.

Dr. Bill

Our favorite means of aerobic exercise is an elliptical trainer. You move more muscles than on a treadmill with lower impact. I enjoy 20 minutes a day on the reconditioned elliptical in my home gym. Our grandkids call it "Grandpa's playroom." This cardio trainer takes up little space in your home. But if getting one doesn't work for you, just taking a brisk walk for 20 or 30 minutes is good cardio, especially if you use a small pair of weights as you walk.

3. STRENGTH-BUILDING EXERCISES

While isometrics and aerobics will maintain, or "tone," your muscle mass, weight-bearing exercises that stretch and stress your muscles are the ones that *grow* them best. Again, a top goal of exercise is to transform excess belly fat into muscle.

COACH ERIN: DON'T BE AFRAID OF STRENGTH TRAINING WITH WEIGHTS

For many women it can be intimidating to walk into a gym filled with scary-looking machines, burly guys, and perfectly trim young women in Spandex. (Although if you tour enough gyms, you'll see plenty of typical-looking people.)

Just remember this. Don't let undeserved shame keep you from feeling better and living longer. Everybody has to start somewhere, and you're in that gym to transform yourself. That's something to be proud of no matter what you look like or how fit you are the first day you walk in there.

And two things about those machines. First, the gym has trainers who will be happy to show you how to work them. More important, the thing with strength training is to keep it simple. Start out with what you can comfortably do, and add more ambitious moves to your workout as you get stronger.

Body-weight exercises—like push-ups, pull-ups, sit-ups, leg-ups, and knee bends—are great, and you don't need a gym to do them. However, adding resistance using exercise bands, free weights, or machines will help trim fat and tone muscle. How much weight should you lift, push, and pull for an effective but safe workout? A good gauge is that you should feel the burn during the last three reps in a set of 12 to 15. If you don't feel the burn by rep number 12, the weights are probably too light. If you feel the burn before rep number eight, you're probably lifting more weight than you should.

And don't worry about "bulking up" like a body builder. At this level of workout, that's not going to happen. My recommendation is to do two full-body strength-training sessions a week. You'll look better, not bulkier.

I will never forget the day about a year into my transformation when I walked into a weight room feeling strong and confident and noticed the looks I was getting. Talk about empowering!

DR. BILL'S ADVICE: BUILD STRENGTH WITH BANDS

I love my stretch bands for muscle toning. They're especially effective if you simply wish to strengthen your muscles rather than bulking up. They are safer than free weights, since you are unlikely to overuse them. I pack my bands in my suitcase while traveling, so I can enjoy a good workout in my hotel room.

> See Appendix A, page 297, for examples of strength-building exercises.

4. RHYTHMICS: DANCING AND SWIMMING

Rhythmics is our word for aerobic exercises that require a lot of brain exercise.

GOTTA DANCE!

Rhythmics are the most fun you can have working out. *And* this kind of exercise boosts balance and brain function. Studies show that dancing seniors are healthier, in mind and body. A study at Albert Einstein College of Medicine revealed that dancing reduces the risk for dementia more than any other physical exercise. Why? Dancing promotes balance, and new dance steps grow new brain pathways. Your brain likes the variety of dancing more than the boring old treadmill.

> Zumba was the first cardio that I LOVED. It didn't feel like work because we were just dancing.

Work out to songs you love and that you can't resist moving to. My three favorites: "Rock Around the Clock" (Bill Haley and the Comets); "In the Mood" (Glenn Miller); and, for a vigorous workout, "Sing, Sing, Sing" (Benny Goodman). You can feel free to choose something recorded after 1960.

Ballroom dancing is my wife's and my favorite hobby as a couple. During our recent fiftieth wedding anniversary dance party, I sang to Martha:

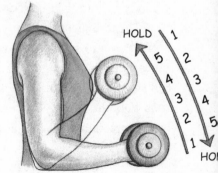

Fifty years ago when you said "I do,"
Did you really think it through?
Then you knew our marriage had a chance,
When your klutzy husband learned to dance.

(See related section: "Swim and Walk Your Worries Away," page 134.)

FIVE T5 TIPS TO GET THE MOST OUT OF YOUR EXERCISE TIME

1. **Think TUT.** *Time under tension* are three magic words for gaining muscle. The longer you can keep your muscles flexed under a weight, the more muscle fibers you will grow. TUT burns more calories and exercises muscles more in a shorter time. Try this test. Take a 10- or 15-pound weight, and flex it up and down fast, the usual way you see untrained people do in the gym. Then take the same weight and move it *slowly,* but without stopping at the top or bottom of your lift, keeping your arm muscles continually under tension. Or, try the 5-5-5-5 technique: lift a weight slowly to the count of five, then hold it at the top for a count of five, then down again to the count of five, and hold again to the count of five. You will feel the burn sooner and stronger than you did while fast-flexing.

2. **Take a HIIT.** High-intensity interval training (HIIT) alternates slow and steady movements (such as running, walking, treadmill, elliptical trainer) with periods when you speed up to your maximum intensity for a minute or two. HIIT burns more calories and builds more muscle tissue.

3. **Cup it up.** While walking, put a smoothie-filled container (such as a Blender Bottle) in each hand. These are your "weights" while you walk. Feel free to make them lighter by drinking the smoothie.

4. **Best time to work out.** "Work out" means (1) moving fat out of your storage banks (the belly is the biggest one) into your bloodstream for burning and (2) working worries out of your brain. The best time to work out to trim that big belly is *before meals*. (When your blood sugar isn't elevated by a recent meal, you start burning body fat sooner.) This is especially true before breakfast, as your body has already been drawing energy from fat for several hours while you slept. It's a wonderful way to begin your day. After a few years on T5, my body, in its wisdom, would give me natural prompts to exercise soon after awakening in the morning and again in late afternoon. Thank you, wisdom of the body!

   (Confession: When I was writing this section, I was speaking at a three-day wellness conference. Most of my talks were scheduled for early morning and late afternoon—the times I habitually exercise. On the third day of missing my exercise "medicine," my body and brain protested: brain fog, fatigue, and worst of all—constipation pains. Departure from my usual 5-S diet and daily exercise routine kept my bowels from moving in their natural rhythm.)

5. **Shake it up.** Enjoy a pre- and postworkout high-protein shake (see recipes, pages 9 and 10) to prefuel and refuel your muscles.

MIGHTY MITOCHONDRIA—ANOTHER REASON WHY EXERCISE GIVES YOU MORE ENERGY, MUSCLE, AND BRAIN POWER

Inside each muscle cell are thousands of microscopic energy generators called mitochondria. The more mitochondria you have, and the more efficient they are, the more energy you have and the more calories you burn. While the T5 way of eating makes for healthier mitochondria, so does movement. T5 movement increases the number of generators. It also increases their insulin sensitivity, so that they need less insulin, which makes the generators run more efficiently.

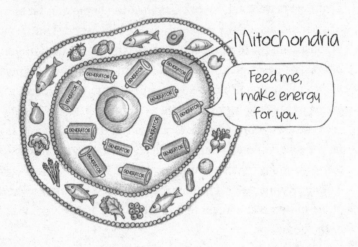

Moreover, when you exercise a muscle to its fatigue point—when you "feel the burn"—you exhaust the mitochondria. The energy-empty mitochondria send a biochemical signal to the brain to tell it to make more human growth hormone (HGH), which reenergizes the mitochondria and builds more muscle. When HGH sends a message to build more muscle, it also sends a message to nourish your brain with more nerve growth factor (NGF). In a biochemical nutshell, *the more muscle tissue you build, the more brain tissue you build.*

5. MOVEMENTS FOR THE BODY AND MIND: COACH ERIN ON YOGA AND PILATES

The complex five-thousand-year-old tradition of yoga is about a very simple thing: happiness. Yoga helps us to remove all obstructing mental clouds, so that we may come to enjoy the sunshine within.
—GEORGE FEUERSTEIN, PhD

My first experience with yoga was in college. I was stressed to the max prepping for finals. After the warmup, which involved a very simple breathing move that anyone can do, my stress and anxiety started to melt away. By the end, I experienced a sense of grounding I was longing for. I was focused and ready for my all-night study session. Today, yoga is a core part of my T5 program, and I am stronger than ever because of it, not just physically, but, more important, mentally and emotionally.

YOGA—STRETCHING AND MEDITATING

In the broadest sense, yoga is a set of Indian spiritual practices, but what we're talking about here are its physical aspects. In ancient Sanskrit, the word means "to yoke" or "to unite" through physical poses (asanas) and breathing (pranayama). These yogic principles align beautifully with T5 and will help you experience one of its main benefits: the balancing of mental and physical strength. The poses offer low-impact muscle strengthening and toning, promote flexibility, and help detoxify internal organs. I recommend a Hatha flow class for beginners. In this format, you move a little more slowly and hold each pose, which helps you learn them and find strength and balance.

Set up sustainable habits. As I write this section, I am working through a hip injury that was ignited by high-impact exercise like kickboxing. For months I refused to do anything differently, because I loved the way those high-intensity classes made me feel. But my stubbornness was dishonoring my body. I had to take an honest look at my workout habits and ask myself, "Is this sustainable?" I had an opportunity to take and teach more yoga classes, and I took it. I have to say that my energy is much more stable, and my physical issues have mostly cleared up. I still enjoy good heart-pumping cardio workouts like Zumba and hiking, but I've reached a healthier balance.

The moral: Choose the movements that are right for you—for your body, your fitness level, and your stage of life.

Yoga helped me shift the self-defeating views on my body and planted seeds of unconditional love for myself. What initially seemed like torture has become one of the most important parts of my adult life. My yoga practice plays an integral role in keeping me happily focused and grounded, peacefully controls my asthma, and prevents my epilepsy from holding me back in life. It has helped me recover from knee surgery and depression.
—PHILIPPE LEVESQUE, YOGA TEACHER

See Appendix B, page 308, where Coach Erin guides you through the most popular yoga poses.

PILATES, THE ART OF CONTROLLED MOVEMENT

Many transformers love Pilates for its low-impact strength-building exercises and focus on building long, lean muscles, flexibility, and core strength and stability. Pilates is more gentle on the joints than weight-bearing exercises and is great for anyone recovering from an injury. As with yoga, breathing is important.

Core is key. Pilates gives a lot of attention to the core muscles—the abdominal muscles and the muscles closest to the spine. (See core moves in strength training, page 297.)

In Appendix B, we demonstrate our T5 version of Pilates-based strength moves using resistance bands.

> Keep your core engaged at all times and use your cleansing breath.

> ▶ See Erin demonstrate and explain favorite yoga poses and Pilates movements at DrSearsWellness.org/T5/Yoga-Pilates.

FITTING IN MORE T5 MOVEMENTS

We've tried to show how all of the T5 modes of movement can fit into your busy life, but there are other ways to add movement as you go about your day. Small changes add up. An extra ten minutes of these "fit ins" each day can result in better muscle tone, a leaner waist, and the loss of a pound every three months.

- Take the stairs instead of the elevator.
- Park farther away when running errands.
- Enjoy a 10-minute power walk on your lunch break.
- When you have a call at home or work, walk and talk.
- Do a five-minute stretching routine to help you wake up.
- When watching TV, do sit-ups or squats during commercials.
- Spend as much of your TV time as possible on your in-home cardio machine.
- Have walking dates with friends instead of sit-down socializing.

- Do calf-raises or other isometric moves while brushing your teeth, doing the dishes, and so on.
- Use a standing desk.
- Play outdoors with your kids.

GO OUTSIDE AND PLAY—THE NEUROSCIENCE OF NATURE

Your mother gave you some of the best medical advice you'll ever get: "Go outside and play!"

As I was healing from colon cancer, I noticed that I felt better—physically and psychologically—when spending more time outdoors, looking out windows, even facing my desk toward the window. As a show-me-the-science doctor, I wanted to study how nature affects what's going on in our brains. So if you're wondering if all this psycho-nature stuff is for real—it is!

Imagine that before taking your therapeutic walk in the park, you stop by your friendly neighborhood neurologist and get wired with sensors that peer inside your brain to see what's going on in there while you walk. Called fMRI (functional magnetic resonance imaging), this technology reveals healthy changes in the brain when you go outside to play—scientific proof of the health effects of the great outdoors. (For a deeper explanation, see the endnotes.)

Our replay theory. T5 exercise is at its best when you're moving *in nature,* and this includes special benefits for the brain. Why? It might be that your brain returns to its natural habitat. We believe that the delightful sights and sounds of nature light up a place deep in your brain that prompts, "This is the environment in which, thousands of years ago, you grew up and where you belong. Welcome back!"

We are wired to walk. For most of human history, people walked. Even riding on the backs of animals is a fairly recent development, not to mention motor vehicles. Our ancestors learned how to use and enjoy nature and how to defend themselves from it. Besides food, nature is the mind's earliest medicine. Most of the diseases of modern living, mental and physical, are due to the fact that we don't fit into the life for which our brains were wired. Our ancestors looked at blue sky, blue sea, blooming fields, rich green forests, and colorful plants. Now we are forced to sit in an unnatural environment of our own creation. We justify this by saying that humans are smart enough to adapt to ever-changing living conditions. This is partly true, yet it also makes us unhealthy. This poor fit is a body, mind, and spirit out of balance.

Longer walks, longer life. Longevity studies reveal that persons who spend more hours in outdoor physical activity tend to live longer. When I lectured recently on longevity at a continuing-care retirement community in Florida, the CEO reminded me of an unsurprising statistic: seniors who live in retirement communities that promote outdoor movement tend to live seven to ten years longer than do solitary, sedentary seniors. We are wired to walk—outside.

At no time in history has nature's therapeutic effect on mental and physical health been more important. While great strides have been made in treating physical ailments, modern medicine still lags pitifully in preventing and treating mental illnesses, which have now reached epidemic proportions at all ages. Ten percent of school-age children are now being drugged for some disorder. Many adults take medications for their minds simply because the doctors don't know what else to do and, quite frankly, don't have the time to do anything but scribble a prescription. Oftentimes when seeing a patient who suffers from some disorder such as ADD, OCD, or depression, I think this person has *MDD and NDD*—movement-deficit and nature-deficit disorders.

Dr. Bill's Rx: go outside and play.

When we're long away from the natural environment we are programmed to be in, we pay a mental price. Of course, few people want to live the difficult life of prehistoric hunter-gatherers who roamed the forests and savannahs, but we *are* wired to walk and to love nature. Even if you work all day before a computer screen, you should be next to a window, preferably open, so you can see and hear the natural world as you work.

An exciting field of research, the neuroscience of nature, validates the health effects of a walk in the woods or playing in a park. This is especially important for children, who now spend far too much time sitting, focused on the artificial light of computer screens. Once upon a time, children ran around outside for exercise and entertainment. They couldn't wait to get outside. Nowadays, they sit indoors and gaze at screens—and they're getting sicker, sadder, and fatter.

That's why I love that studying the neuroscience of nature has finally proved that your mother was right when she said, "Go outside and play." ✋

HEAD-TO-TOE HEALING EFFECTS OF NATURE	
Brain	• Grow more and healthier brain cells • Make more happy hormones • Mellow your moods • Repair damaged tissue • Decrease dementia
Heart	• Lower your blood pressure • Lower your heart rates by reducing stress
Gut	• Less risk of inflammation, indigestion, constipation
Immune system	• Balance stress hormones • Improve infection fighting
Joints	• Lessen arthritis • Improve mobility
Longevity	• Enjoy longer lifespan
For references and additional reading, see the endnotes. ✋	

NATURAL NATALIE AND WIRED WILLIE

Natalie's bed faces a window, so she wakes up to the sights and sounds of nature. Her bedroom is decorated with floral wallpaper, live plants, and pictures showing nature scenes. There are no fluorescent lights in her home. When Natalie's at home, her smartphone rests, the ringer muted, on a table near the door, so she can grab it as she leaves for work. Meals are time for no-tech fun and conversation as Natalie and her family and guests relate to one another face-to-face. At work, she has arranged her office with a window next to her shoulder—so that she can enjoy as much natural eye candy as computer-generated "i-candy."

At night, Natalie gradually darkens her world and dials down her worries to prepare her body and mind for sleep. She does the bright-light tasks long before bedtime. All bright screens are turned off, and mellow music is turned on. Softer sights and sounds are just what the sleep doctor ordered. In the dim light, the eyes send a biochemical message to the brain to reduce neurohormones that stimulate alertness and ramp up sleep hormones such as melatonin. Natalie's brain is in balance.

Willie is wired. He is glued to a screen most of the day. Willie has "tech neck," that hunched-over posture of looking down at his smartphone all the time, even while walking. At dinner, while others are relating to real human faces, Willie is engaged in video games or checking texts. He is learning to relate to machines rather than people. His brain is being rewired in an unnatural way.

Neurons that wire together fire together, so you can see how the brains of Natalie and Willie will wire and fire differently. Some argue that digital activities such as computer games are good for the brain, since the brain thrives on novelty, and to an extent they are right. The point is to grow up with a *balance* between the natural and digital-virtual realms that can equip young adults with the interpersonal and technological skills they'll need in this rapidly changing new world.

EYE FEEL GOOD!

What you see affects your mental health. When you see beauty, you feel beauty. The colors of nature—blue sky, the green trees and grass, sand, rocky cliffs, the colors of birds and flowers—fit the genetic programming of the retinal tissues of our eyes and the nerve pathways that go from our eyes to our brains. The artificial lights of a computer screen do not.

Forty percent of the neocortex, the biggest area of the brain and the part that makes us human, is devoted to processing visual delights.

Neuroscientists call the beauties of nature "visual Valium." Since the eye is actually an extension of the brain, what's pleasing to the eye is pleasing to the brain. When you take a walk in the woods, a stroll in the garden, or just gaze outside the window, the sights you see travel via the retinal-hypothalamic pathway, the nerves that run from the eye to the pleasure and healing centers of the brain. This is the neurological basis for the teaching that sunlight heals.

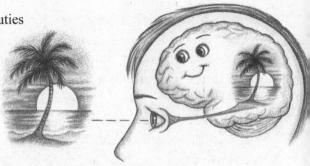

Change my bed, please. Research supports this sunlight solution. Japanese scientists did a brilliant hospital experiment in which they faced the beds of patients healing from surgery toward windows. These patients healed faster than those whose beds faced a wall. Enjoying the sights, sounds, and movements in nature is particularly healing for inflammatory illnesses. Throughout your busy day, try these sunlight solutions:

- To keep yourself from getting bored during a meeting in a boardroom, try to sit facing the window.
- Face a window during your workout at home or in a gym.
- Face your desk toward or alongside a window.
- Choose the window seat on an airplane and enjoy the serenity of sights at 30,000 feet.
- *Enjoy the garden effect.* When possible, look through the window at the sky, trees, or a garden.

LESSONS FROM LEAVES

I wrote part of this neuroscience-of-nature section on a trip to lecture in Singapore, where I visited Gardens by the Bay, the "billion-dollar garden." There I learned how movement benefits the health of plants much as it does in humans.

Even though some of the world's greatest gardeners had constructed this masterpiece and maintained the plants and trees with enough water, sunlight, and natural fertilizer, some plants still withered and died. What plant-growth factor was missing? Movement! In nature, wind moves the leaves and branches, which naturally nourishes the roots. After the gardeners installed fans to move the leaves and branches, the plants, trees, and their roots flourished.

Healthy living lesson: When you move, you flourish; when you don't, you wither.

DON'T WORRY, GO OUTSIDE AND PLAY

Consider the outdoors as not only your personal gym but a trusted therapist. If you have to worry, do it outdoors. Research reveals that woods walkers with the highest stress levels felt the most stress relief when they went outdoors.

Researchers in Japan, a culture that values the healing effects of nature, found a simple way to measure stress hormone levels during a walk in the woods. An enzyme in saliva, salivary amylase, correlates with blood levels of stress hormones. They found that salivary amylase levels were lower following a nature walk and concluded that woods walkers enjoyed less physiological stress during their nature therapy. This aligns with other studies showing physiological benefits such as decreased heart rate, blood pressure, and stress hormone levels following a nature walk. Perhaps this is why some of my most productive moments in writing are while walking on a golf course. (See the endnotes, "Forest bathing.")

WALK WHILE YOU WORK

Want to work your body while working your mind? Smart companies now advise their employees to take a lunchtime walk, because research shows they think and work better afterward.

Walk while you talk. Just because you're at work doesn't mean you can't walk. Get out of the conference room and meet on the move. I frequently schedule "walking meetings." Email less and make more phone calls. Use a voice messaging app like Voxer instead of sending texts. You can walk and talk, even if you're just leaving a voice mail while pacing around your office. I tell my associates who like email, "I think and communicate better by phone. Please call me at . . ." One week I kept a log and realized I could walk an extra half-hour a day by talking instead of typing. That simple upgrade could translate to a loss of ten pounds and several waist inches in a year.

Whiners wear you out. Suppose you need to solve a stressful problem with a stress-promoting caller. Schedule your unavoidable call for a time when you can walk (preferably in nature) while you talk. Movement in nature not only helps you think more clearly about the problem, it also dials down your stress hormones. If the caller turns out to be a whiner who wasted your time, at least you got movement therapy out of the call.

Bring the outdoors indoors. You can't always be outdoors, but you can fill your home and perhaps your office with plants. Researchers at Kansas State University found that surrounding yourself with flowering plants can stimulate calming centers in the brain. And as a last resort, when work, weather, or illness keeps you indoors, watch nature shows on television or computer. Researchers have found that watching scenes of nature has healthful calming and cardiovascular effects.

Nature and ART (attention restoration theory). An interesting study on restoration therapy at the University of Michigan divided participants chosen because they were having problems with sadness or depression into two groups. One was assigned to take a fifty-minute walk in the university's arboretum, the other to walk in busy downtown Ann Arbor on a traffic-heavy street lined with university and commercial buildings. After their walks, the two groups took performance tests. The nature walkers showed better scores. It's not just walking; it's where you walk and what you think about that restores.

Walking in nature is restorative and relaxing. Walking downtown is not, because the brain is continually hyped up, startled by traffic noises, distracted by flashing lights. You have to stay focused, so you don't get hit by a car. Perhaps this is why kids with ADD do better after a walk or run. Such a child's brain is so hyperfocused in the classroom, it gets tired. If these children go outside to dial down—rest, restore, and recharge—they can come back into the classroom better able to refocus. This is not rocket science.

My early nature therapy. I grew up an "underprivileged" child of a single mom in a financially poor but emotionally rich family. Looking back, I had a mentally healthful life. Nature was my playground: the woods, the ballpark, nearby creeks—I spent my days fishing, building, and climbing. The prescription for ADHD in those days was "go outside and play . . . go build a tree house . . . go fishing . . . take a walk in the woods." As a result, my brain has been imprinted with an appreciation of the great outdoors, and I crave going back to these scenes of serenity.

In the schoolroom, I would stare out the window, because I wanted to be out the window. My fourth-grade teacher, Sister Mary Ursula (Latin for "little bear"), had the perfect "medicine" for what would today be labeled ADHD. Every school day around 11 AM and 2 PM, Little Bear would put her hand authoritatively on my shoulder and say, "Billy, you're fidgeting too much. Go outside and run around the schoolyard three times, then come back and sit still." It worked! That brief run was my Ritalin.

IT'S NOT ADD, IT'S MDD—MOVEMENT DEFICIT DISORDER

Neuroimaging studies reveal why persons tagged with ADD are so impulsive. Normally, the brain enjoys a balance of the impulse center and the impulse-inhibiting center. Or, in an automobile analogy, the brakes balance the accelerator.

We believe T5 is like the brakes of the brain. Science agrees in three ways:

1. The smart foods listed on page 222 dial down the overactive accelerator center.

2. Movement mellows the hyperactive center.
3. Neuroimaging studies at New York University's Child Study Center found that meditation improves the attention and impulse-inhibiting centers of the brain.

Suppose your child were diagnosed with ADD or ADHD. You'd want the medicine that is best supported by science and that has no harmful side effects. If I were your doctor, here's what I would likely tell you: "Your child doesn't have ADD or ADHD. Your whole family has NDD (nutrition deficit disorder) and MDD (movement deficit disorder)." My prescription: "Do T5 and you'll thrive."

A friend asked me, "Are you over the hill?"
I said, "Yes, and I'm picking up speed!"
—DR. BILL

CHAPTER 4

STRESS LESS

FIVE TRANSFORMING STRESS-BUSTERS

You want to transform your mind or you wouldn't be reading this book. You've heard it said that you are what you eat. Even more, you are what you *think*. You have already learned how you can transform your brain by changing your eating and exercise habits. Now we'll add the finishing touch: how you can change your brain by changing your thoughts.

My inability to cope with stress and then using food as a drug needed to change. I've been working hard to get in a better place mentally, so I can bring those stress levels down and get back into balance. Tools like taking a walk and breathing help so much! Since living the T5 lifestyle I have switched jobs and I am thriving!

—ESTHER ALVA

THINK-CHANGE YOUR BRAIN: FEEL A MENTAL TRANSFORMATION

You can change your brain by changing your thoughts. We call this process think-changing your brain. *You*, not doctors, can best change *your* brain.

> I feel so much happier after five weeks.
> Even my friends notice my change.
> **—A HAPPY TRANSFORMER**

YOU CAN REWIRE YOUR WORRY CIRCUIT

Your mind is really your thoughts. The best mind medicine is how you manage your own thinking, because thoughts affect the neurochemical pathways in your brain. Transform 5 helps you grow or rewire your happy center and shrink your sad center, helping you become a more joyful person. In your brain, transforming is rewiring. Are you ready to rewire?

We're all control freaks. We want to control our lives socially, medically, financially, and so on. Yet, realistically, our wishes go wrong, and we stress. When Erin and I were going through our transformations, we realized that there is one thing in life that we *can* mostly control:

Our thoughts.

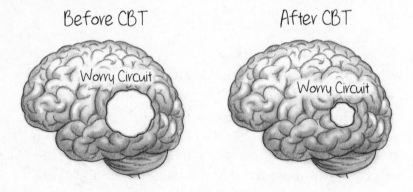

124

Readers, take note: Because stress reduction is near the top of our transformer's wish list, please don't get stressed out by our discussion of stress-management tools. Stay with us as we give you a big helping of stress reducers and take you on a technological tour inside the brains of worrywarts to see how they transformed their minds.

New brain-imaging technology reveals how you really can think-change your brain. The artist's rendering of the PET scan on the previous page shows an overactive area in the brain of a patient with obsessive-compulsive disorder. At right, you can see the decreased activity in the area of the brain, *the worry circuit*, that was previously "infected" with unhappy, addictive, negative thoughts—after ten weeks of using think-changing tools, also called cognitive behavioral therapy (CBT), and with no medication. (See the endnotes for reference.) ✋

These findings showed that when people master thought-switching therapy, which is really mental effort and willpower, they have the power to rewire the circuitry of their brains. This science opens up a whole world of treatment: the personal power of thoughts and how changing your mind can change the structure of your brain.

The more you believe you can think-change your brain, the more you will. As you repeatedly and willfully steer the car down the right road, it becomes more natural, automatic, and requires less effort, less *mental force*, to keep going down the right road. You rewire your brain by shutting down the road to a problem and opening a road to the solution.

MIND OVER MEDICINES

Some of our happiest transformers are those who were able to gradually lower the dose of their pharmacological medications, or even get off them, by learning how to make their own internal physiological medicines. In fact, one of the most frequent reasons people of all ages ask about T5 is, "I want to take less medication, but I don't know how." T5 shows you how.

Of all medications, pills for brain ills are the most challenging for doctors to prescribe correctly and for patients to judge objectively whether or not they work. Because more physicians are empowering their patients to think-change their brains, we hope these doctors will "prescribe" our T5 plan. ✋

Think-changing skills better than pills? In my medical practice, instead of telling a patient, "You need cognitive behavioral therapy," I make it more fun. "We will help you think-change your brain." They like that. Our T5 tools teach you to think differently about your circumstances, repeatedly switching from negative to positive and throwing the negative thoughts in the trash bin. In this book we upgrade cognitive behavioral therapy (CBT) to TCB—**Think-Changing the Brain**.

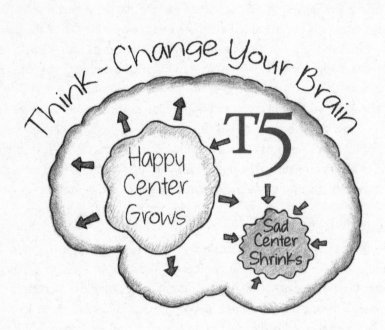

Erin coaches:

Thoughts before TCB	Thoughts after TCB
"I'm so overwhelmed!"	"I am safe. I can get through this one step at a time."
"I have so much to do!"	"What's most important? I'll start there, then do the next right thing."
"I'm so afraid!"	"I am grateful for . . ."
"I feel out of control."	"I will focus on what I can change."

Mental illness has a physical cause. The time has come to downplay the term "mental illness," which has the wrong connotation that "it's all in your head," that it's imaginary. Neuroimaging reveals there is *a physical basis* for mental illness. Actual physical changes occur in the brain.

Suppose you have a physical disability, say a weak muscle in one leg that causes you to walk differently. Naturally, treatment would be to strengthen the muscle and to strengthen the nerves and blood supply to that leg by repeated exercises. The same is true with mental illness. The brain needs to be exercised with physical therapy (such as T5 eating and moving) and mental therapy (T5 stressbusters) to regrow and strengthen the weakened area in the brain.

I was able to decrease my antidepressant dosage after following the prescribed 5-S eating and moving more. I have found more natural ways to boost my happy hormones, like listening to uplifting music, dancing, and helping friends.
—A TRANSFORMED FRIEND

Now you know you can think-change your brain. Next, you will be empowered to build your personal stress-reducing toolbox. Now tell your brain, "Get ready to change!"

FIVE STRESS-BUSTERS TO DIAL DOWN YOUR DIMMER

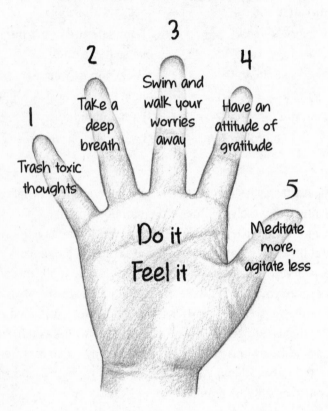

Imagine that you consult a therapist for stress management. After downloading your overload, your therapist says, "Man, you need to dial down your dimmer!"

"My what?"

"Your dimmer is your stress-control center."

The stress-control center resides primarily in the hypothalamus, the area of the brain responsible for peace, happiness, and mental health. It can be thought of as a dimmer switch for mood lighting. There are times you want it really bright, such as when you're working, meeting deadlines, commuting, making quick decisions, and adjusting on the fly to the fast pace of daily life. But when the need for bright lights is over, you want to dial down to mood lighting for romance, meditation, tranquility—whatever mood you need for serenity and peace.

> T5 helps you dial down when you're upset (anxious) and dial up when you're down (depressed).

T5 helps you adjust your dimmer for the right mood at the right time. When you're able to dial down easier, then you're able to dial up better when you need to solve problems and be more creative.

Dr. Bill

1. TRASH TOXIC THOUGHTS

The best stress-management advice we've ever heard: *You can't always control situations, but you can control your reaction to them.* Sounds like something your mom would have said. T5 stress-management steps teach you how to manage your thoughts so that the bad ones don't take over your mind.

Treating your toxic thoughts as junk email is neurologically correct. When a toxic thought enters your mind, it goes to your amygdala, a structure in the brain involved in memory, decision making, and emotions, especially fear. That's the time to say, "Don't go there," and quickly divert that toxic thought into your trash bin. If you dwell on it, the toxic thought can then go into the hippocampus, which is a kind of file cabinet where that negative thought is likely to be stored permanently. Just what you don't want.

> You're not always in charge of your first thought, but you are in charge of your response.

You are what you think, so learn to make good, quick decisions about how you think—and therefore who you want to be.

Your brain photocopies thoughts and stores them in a memory file. You may or may not want to recall and replay various memories, but they are part of your brain. Your thoughts become *you*.

I Thrive on T5

Repel ANTs. "Automatic negative thoughts" (ANTs) cause toxic buildup. The T5 ANT-repellent technique: as soon as a negative thought invades your mind, brush it away as you would a pesky ant. Then immediately think of how to replace that ANT with an anti-ANT. Switch to a positive to reverse the negative. Mentally replay a peaceful, pleasant visual memory from your "happy files," such as your wedding day or your favorite vacation. Remember the movie *Happy Gilmore*? To rescue Happy from his negative mindset, his girlfriend-turned-therapist smilingly advises, "Happy, go to your happy place." Happy then imagines his dream of being a star hockey player scoring the winning goal.

Have a happy hippocampus. The hippocampus, and its partners in emotional reactions, the amygdala and the hypothalamus, are the emotional centers of your brain. The quicker you choose to reroute toxic thoughts into the trash bin, the more likely that these thoughts will be temporary, disappear, and not become part of you. If we instead allow a thought to fester a while, the image or idea will flow into the hippocampus, which acts like a reference library for thoughts. It decides to file thoughts into permanent memories or short-term memories, or quickly trash them, and it does a lot of this work while we sleep. Here is where stress management is important. The hippocampus is one of the most vulnerable sections of the brain to manage unresolved stress because it has a lot of extra stress hormone receptors (microscopic doorways that let in chemical information). The more energy you put into entertaining a thought, the more your brain accommodates it. Imagine that you're asking, do you want the photocopy of your thought to be in regular type or bold? Do you want it to be in indelible ink and be permanent, or easily erasable?

New insight into the neurochemistry of thought shows that the harder you think, the more neurochemicals you produce and the quicker and longer your thoughts are stored in your memory bank. So, if you *quickly trash a toxic thought* as soon as it enters your mind, its neurochemical structures are less dense, less permanent, and more erasable. Isn't that what you want—to quickly and easily erase toxic thoughts? People who have mastered this thought discernment quickly say to a toxic thought: "Go away, that's not me . . . Think this, not that."

Coach Erin's thought changer. Is this thought coming from love or fear?

FIVE THINGS I LIKE ABOUT ME

In our medical practice I use this strategy to lift up down patients: "Paste on your bathroom mirror and on your cell phone wallpaper a list of your top five physical, emotional, and social assets. Replay, refresh, and refill as needed." For example:

1. I like my job.
2. I have pretty hair.
3. I can swim fast.
4. I have two wonderful children.
5. I get up in the morning and nothing hurts.

Quickly replaying what you have dials down your stress about what you don't have.

Put your mind on "mute." Try our favorite mind game. We call it "mind-mute." Whenever your mind is racing or scattered, retreat into a quiet place and think "mind-mute"—your cue to unclutter and clear your mind of difficult thoughts. Partnering this mental clearing with *deep breathing* (see technique below) helps you refocus more quickly. Initially, it might feel as if you are working too hard to clear your mind, which could tend to rev up your mind even more. Eventually, though, your mind will welcome the mind-mute cue to dial down disturbing thoughts.

Dr. Bill's mind-mute tips. As a father of eight, grandfather to fourteen, pediatrician, Special Olympics coach, writer, and lecturer, my mind could be cluttered—if I let it. Turning on mind-mute is my brain-saver.

To master mind-muting:

- Go (literally or in your imagination) to your favorite peaceful place, where you are least distracted—a swimming pool, the woods, or even just a quiet spot in your home or workplace.
- Take a deep breath.
- Do a *five-second* mind-mute. This is usually the longest that brain-cluttered beginners can go before disturbing stuff reinfects their peaceful rest.
- Gradually increase your mind-mute duration to ten seconds, and so on, until mind-mute naturally becomes easier.
- Practice mind-mute at least every hour throughout the day.

Mind-mute and meditation—partners in mental health. Think of this as *advanced mind-mute* because it takes a little more time. First, use your meditation mantra (see page 146) to clear your mind. After a few minutes, once your mind is uncluttered, ease into the mind-mute mode. Think of gradually pouring out sad stuff from a glass. Once it's empty, let it fill up with happy stuff. (See related sections on flotation therapy, page 134, and meditation, page 139.)

2. TAKE A DEEP, CLEANSING BREATH

Deep breathing increases the pleasure hormone dopamine and calms your mind by dialing down blood flow to the worry centers of the brain and dialing up blood flow to the relaxation centers. Do the following at least five times an hour, especially when you are hurting or stressed:

1. Close your eyes. Breathe in deeply, slowly and gently from the belly, through your *nose* for a count of five. Feel your belly expand. Feel, and follow, the air moving in and out of your nose. (Exciting research reveals that nasal breathing triggers the nasal and sinus linings to release a natural healing and anti-inflammatory biochemical called nitric oxide (NO)—we call it a NO-rich nose. See more, page 144, and the endnotes.) 🖐
2. Hold your breath for a count of five.

3. Exhale slowly for a count of five; either through your nose or through pursed lips, which keeps the lungs expanded longer to deliver more healing oxygen.

4. *Humming heals*. Humming while exhaling causes the air in your nasal and sinus cavities to oscillate more, which releases more healing NO from your NO-rich nose. (See the endnotes, "Why cats purr.")

5. Do five deep breathings every hour.

Breathe better to eat better. Do some deep breathing before meals and several times during them. This dials down overactive stress hormones, which are notorious for compelling us to overeat and to eat unhealthful foods. Belly breathing is good for the head brain and the gut brain.

Breathe better to think better. You can change your brain by changing your breathing. Call it self-medicating, if you wish, but deep breathing is one of the most natural ways of calming your mind and uncluttering your brain.

Dr. Bill's breathing tip. Select a two-word mantra: "feeeel" (inhale); "gooood" (exhale).

Erin coaches. I recommend *Pranayama*, a yogic breathing technique using alternative nostril breathing. View the video linked below and breathe along with it. Find a calming, slow-moving visual aid and sync your breathing to it. For example, search "triangle breathing" on YouTube and enjoy a soothing video; inhale while the triangle blooms into different shapes and exhale as it returns to its original shape. My sister-in-law Kristin used this breathing exercise to overcome anxiety while recovering from brain-cancer surgery.

> ▶ See Erin's video on breathing technique at DrSearsWellness .org/T5/Deep-Breathing.

3. SWIM AND WALK YOUR WORRIES AWAY

Need a movement that's easy on your body and benefits your brain? Swimming is one of our top cardio exercises for the following reasons:

- It's the safest exercise you can do, at all ages, especially for muscles and joints.
- It refreshes and just feels good, unlike a sweaty gym workout.
- Swimming is one of the top exercises for the brain.

Swimming heals. If you have an *-itis* illness or a bone or muscle injury that keeps you out of the gym, head for the pool. (See how knee-pumping movements make healing nutrients in the knee joints, page 246.)

NO MORE "TEXT NECK"

In recent years, we've noticed more teens and young adults who have a hunchback posture usually associated with getting old. Just another of the many disorders of the old that are occurring in the young. Try these two neck-friendly exercises: (1) at least ten times a day, for ten seconds, look up at the sky or ceiling; (2) swim the breaststroke, which requires you to flex your neck backward.

Dr. Bill on spiritual swimming. Swimming is a magnificent movement for your mind. It can be more calming than walking, because you can relax your whole body. You can even take a moment to close your eyes and just enjoy the feeling of floating. There's even a name for this: *floatation therapy*. I do not only prayer walks, but prayer swims. While doing the breast stroke, I look at the blue water under the green trees and the blue sky and pray, "Praise God" during one stroke, and "I'm happy" during the next. The rhythm of the body and mind moving and praying together is very calming.

I begin most mornings with my meditation swim. I put my mind in dial-down mode, trying to avoid all clutter in my brain and simply let the sights and sounds of nature sink in. (See related topics, "The Neuroscience of Spirituality," page 231; and "Mind-Mute," page 131.)

Walk in water. In a peaceful pool, immerse yourself shoulder high and enjoy the floaty feelings of a slow, rhythmic walk. Time the touch of each step with a calming word, "Thank (step) God (step) I'm (step) healthy (step)." Or, try: "Walk (step) in (step) wa (step) ter (step)." Synchronizing your mantra with your natural stepping rhythm calms your mind. Focus on giving thanks for what you have: eyes that see, lungs that breathe, and so on.

Make your own mantra. Here's my attitude-of-gratitude mantra during flotation therapy, one word with each breaststroke:

> *Thank you, God, for my life! (Cancer survivor.)*
> *Thank you, God, for my wife! (Of fifty-one years.)*
> *Thank you, God, for my health! (At age seventy-eight, everything*
>   *works and nothing hurts.)*
> *Thank you, God, for my wealth! (Eight kids.)*
> *Thank you, God, for my MD! (Fifty-one years.)*
> *Please make T5 my ministry.*

One day during my flotation therapy session, two friends, one a neurologist and the other a psychotherapist, walked by the pool and saw me "vegging" while floating. I looked up and said, "I'm in therapy." They got the message.

Thank you for encouraging me in a healthy habit that lifts my mood and mindset while exercising my body. Following a nature walk in the hills with my dog, Kona, I follow your prescription for Flotation Therapy with an Attitude of Gratitude! I swim in our warm backyard pool. With each stroke, I speak a phrase of gratitude: "Thank you, God," stroke, "for my loving and devoted husband," stroke, "Thank you, God," stroke, "for my healthy, bright kids," stroke, "Thank you, God," stroke,

"for my community of giving friends," stroke, "Thank you, God," stroke, "for my work that gives purpose, joy, and family income," stroke. The days I focus on an attitude of gratitude while swimming, I feel my spirits and energy level rise! Medicine for my soul!
—KRISTEN SCHULTZ

Tread water to shed worries. This is a relaxing technique that I have mastered. In the deep end of a pool, move your arms just enough to keep yourself afloat while your legs dangle weightlessly, or flutter-kick slightly, or your toes are just barely touching the bottom. Close your eyes and either mind-mute (page 131) or meditate on your mantra. As you enter that almost weightless state, you will notice that your mind sheds the weight of worries.

After having knee surgery and desperately wanting to exercise, I pushed myself too hard too soon trying to go back to my usual cardio routine. Erin suggested swimming, so I had to get over my shame of wearing a bathing suit in public, because my health was worth it. Swimming helped me ease back into cardio safely.
—TRANSFORMER MICHELLE CASEY

Walk your worries away. Just like relaxed breathing, relaxed movement dials down stress-hormone production. (See "We Are Wired to Walk," page 114.) When worry invades your mind, start moving. Go outside and say "hi" to the sky and set out for a brisk walk. Hippocrates recommended, "In a bad mood, go for a walk. If you don't improve, walk more." (See related section, "Go Outside and Play," page 366.)

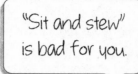

"Sit and stew" is bad for you.

Dr. Bill

4. HAVE AN ATTITUDE OF GRATITUDE

Gratitude is being thankful, appreciating and returning others' kindness. One of the most powerful ways to get out of a stress funk is to focus your thoughts on the gifts that you have at this very moment. Start with simple things: I have a roof over my head, food and water, people who care about me. Slowly, you'll shift from self-pity to serenity. Gratitude starts as an attitude, but the power really comes when you put it into action. Action creates change! You really do have a changeable attitude center in your brain.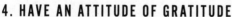

Coach Erin's service story. When I was growing up, Mom and Dad insisted that we kids participate in mission trips. I recall one sobering day in Russia that we spent in an orphanage holding babies, some of whom had never been held much. I returned from the experience with a renewed sense of gratitude and a new perspective on my problem with worrying that had been holding me back. There is power in just one simple act of service. It can . . .

- Make you truly grateful for what you have.
- Light up the compassion-pleasure center in your brain.
- Provide balance to our sometimes self-centered lifestyles.
- Give you the "helper's high."

Erin coaches: serve your worries away. A great way to mellow your mind is to volunteer. Redirecting your focus toward helping someone less fortunate puts you into the helper's high and an attitude of gratitude mode.

HUMOR HEALS

There's a scientific basis for the maxim "Laughter is the best medicine."
Here's a bit of jollyology:

- Laughter raises the blood level of circulating germ-fighting
  soldiers called T-cells.
- Humor boosts cancer-fighting NK (natural killer) cells.
- Laughter lifts spirits, speeds healing, and lowers the blood level
  of stress hormones.
- Laughter increases circulation and helps the heart. That's why
  it's called "inner jogging."
- Humor is contagious. So is sadness. You may stimulate pleasure
  centers in the brains of people who catch your smile. (See related
  section, "Mind Your Mirror Neurons," page 236.)

During a vacation retreat, I wanted to convey
to my kids that dad needed some
downtime. I stretched out in a
hammock and placed a card on
my chest (borrowed from the
bathroom) that said "Out of
Service." They got the picture.

HEALING TEARS

Not surprisingly, crying and laughing are therapeutic partners.
Tears have been found to contain cortisol, the stress hormones, as
if tears are the body's overflow for excess stress. Perhaps there's a
biochemical basis for the phrase "a good cry."

5. MORE MEDITATION, LESS AGITATION

The most successful transformers often become the most mindful meditators. Remember our stress-reduction theme: grow your happy center and shrink your sad center. Meditation does both.

DR. BILL'S MEDITATION STORY

My first personal experience with meditation came between 1957 and 1960 when I was in seminary studying to become a priest. I would begin each day with a walk in the woods, focusing only on spiritual thoughts: "Thank God for . . ." "Praise God for . . ." "Serve God more . . ." No matter how unfortunate your life may seem, everyone has at least a few blessings to dwell on. "I was sad that I had no shoes until I met a man with no feet." After three years I had grown a meditation center in my brain. ✋

My meditation transformation. While doing T5, I realized my meditation center was missing and needed to be restored. Fortunately, it was fairly easy to do, a bit like picking up a musical instrument first learned in childhood. As with muscle, if you don't use it, you lose it. I'm happy to say I have regrown my meditation center. You can grow one, too!

In the beginning, I was somewhat skeptical. I struggled with confusion about meditation—is it real or all in the mind? It's both. All too often we devalue mental exercises because, unlike physical exercises, we can't easily measure their effects. However, brain scan technology has taken the mystery out of meditation by proving we really can change our minds by changing our thoughts. Researchers discovered that meditators have *larger happiness centers* in their brains than nonmeditators. Similarly, the part of the brain that coordinates all the muscles and mindsets involved with running grows larger in people who run. That's exactly what we want to do for stress reduction: grow our happy centers and shrink our sad centers. Meditation is proven to help you do that.

MEDITATE LIKE A MONK

We owe a lot of the scientific findings about how meditation betters the brain to a Nobel Peace Prize winner, the Dalai Lama. He recruited Tibetan monks who had spent much of their lives in meditation into a brain-imaging study that proved what neuroscientists had long suspected: the monks had changed the structure and function of their brains by meditation. The results of this famous "monk study" greatly increased interest in the growing science of neuroplasticity—how the brain changes in response to experience. One of the outcomes of this study was that the more the monks meditated, the less effort was necessary to sustain focused attention. In other words, meditation became easier to do and more automatic. This is just like other exercises. The more you practice, the easier it is to do. Meditation also helps reduce "neural noise," or what we would call brain clutter, that tends to frazzle us.

The biggest misconception about meditation is that it is mainly for monks. On the contrary, this ancient art of mind healing is just what the brain doctor ordered for today's frantic lifestyles. During meditation, the brain doesn't really "shut down." Rather, it blocks out disturbing thoughts and images. Meditation puts you in touch with your inner state and quiets your mind. For those seeking spiritual growth, meditation helps unclutter the mind so you can *talk* to God. Mind-mute and meditation help you *listen*. And that's not all that science says about the stress-reducing effects of daily meditation.

WINDOWS INTO YOUR BRAIN

Suppose you've been meditating for a while and you want to see if it's "all in your mind" or if something good has actually happened in your brain. You stop by your friendly neighborhood neurologist's office to get a picture taken—a brain scan—that will show whether your brain has changed. The doctor gives you a happy report: "Congratulations! Your happy and compassion centers have gotten larger. Keep it up!"

You might be wondering how this works. One method of brain imaging is a PET scan (positron emission tomography), in which a substance such as glucose, carrying a radioactive tag, is injected into the person's bloodstream. The radioactive stuff lights up in color-coded images that show the amount of blood flow to the targeted area of the brain. The more the blood flow, the more they light up. Next, pictures are taken showing how *changes* in blood flow correlate to changes in brain activity, such as when meditating.

When you're meditating, think: "I'm lighting up my happy center in my brain."

COACH ERIN'S FIVE-MINUTE MIRACLE

I had a hard time getting into meditation, because I just could not dim down my spinning thoughts, what I call "monkey mind." Meditation requires us to turn off our thoughts and simply listen. It takes practice, and, as with any new skill, you need to start slow and be patient. Here is what works for me:

1. Refocus your mind. (I read from a book of daily inspirational quotes, *Hope for Today*.)
2. Sit cross-legged on a pillow or chair. Sit up straight, tuck your chin slightly, and rest your palms on your knees, either facing up or down. Relax your muscles.
3. Breathe slowly and steadily in and out through your nose.
4. Be open. Thoughts will come up. Notice them and then let them float away. Return back to the breath.
5. After five minutes, I close by setting an intention of love and service to everyone who will cross my path that day.

MILLENNIALS NEED MEDITATION

While meditation is good for all ages, we believe young adults benefit the most, because their minds are cluttered the most—with busy lives and the barrage of electronic media interaction. This group needs to think more clearly morning to night to make decisions about work, family, personal growth. They need to learn to selectively process those addicting messages that arrive constantly in the age of "i-dependency."

MEDITATION MAKES HAPPY HORMONES

During deep and habitual meditation, serotonin levels may rise, which is why meditation is as or more effective than some medications, not to mention safer. It may even act on the same pathway as some drugs. Other neurochemicals, such as GABA (which is the brain's own natural anti-depressant, anti-anxiety, mood-stabilizing neurochemical), are increased during deep-breathing and stretching exercises like yoga. Meditation increases the release of dopamine, which helps explain the relaxation, happiness, and peacefulness that meditators experience. It also lowers stress hormone levels.

MEDITATION MAKES YOU MORE COMPASSIONATE

Meditation increases blood flow to the compassion areas in your brain. Perhaps shrinking stress hormones and growing more calming hormones in the brain is why meditators are better able to navigate healthfully through stressful situations and often show better decision making and more compassion during stressful situations.

Think good, feel good. Neuroimaging of meditating monks, during what is called "compassion meditation," where the meditator focuses on compassionate thoughts for a person, reveals that the compassion-happiness center lights up a lot. More interesting, even when the compassionate monk was not meditating, the same happy center stayed lit up at a higher level. These studies show that we really can grow our happy centers by feeding them with happy thoughts.

Awful anger. Excessive anger or fear can disrupt your ability to evaluate and respond compassionately in social situations. Anger dials down the compassion center. You act irrationally, make harmful decisions, and are unaware that you are being a jerk, saying things you'll regret later. When the empathy center gets dialed down, you are unable to sense the other person's fears and needs, you become self-centered. The neurochemicals that are released by persistent anger gradually "shrink" the empathy center of the brain. People begin to see you as an angry person.

But the more you meditate on compassion, the more you increase the blood flow and neurochemical stimulation of the compassion centers in your brain, making you less prone to outbursts of anger.

When you get angry, quickly switch gears and let your rational mind apply the brakes on fear and anger. Think through what you're about to do. Take a deep breath and rethink things. This balances your emotions so that you're likely to be more empathetic. This is called *nurturing your inner negotiator*. It's interesting that meditation and spiritual practices strengthen your inner negotiator, making people less anxious and fearful, especially those who are prone to rage. Our conclusion: The more you are prone to rage, fear, and anger, the more you need to meditate.

Erin on the dangers of multitasking. In our culture, many of us feel shamefully unproductive if we're not doing at least three things. Sometimes this seems unavoidable, but is multitasking really productive? I had a moment of insight a couple of years ago. My workload and life responsibilities had tripled. One afternoon my to-do list seemed unmanageable. I just dove in with no real plan and started doing everything at once. Checking an email while waiting for water to boil, going from one task to the next without finishing any. My mind was spinning, all my tasks were half finished, everything was chaos and stress.

When this happens to you, put on the brakes for a moment and think about whether multitasking is helping or hurting. Try dedicating your mental and emotional energy to just one thing a time (okay, two if you really have to) and see if you don't get more things done more efficiently and with less stress.

MEDITATORS LIVE IN THE MOMENT

Much of our mind clutter consists of replaying unpleasant things from the past and worrying about bad things we imagine might happen in the future. But the only time we can actually change is the present, so that's where we need to live. During meditation, the meditator becomes a neutral observer, simply enjoying an enhanced sensation and imagination of the environment without judgment or evaluation—not worrying about past and future, but savoring the present moment. During meditation, blood flow to the judgment and worry center decreases, while it increases in the imagination, sensation, and enjoyment centers. Meditation trains your mind to focus on the here and now.

Meditators put it this way: It's necessary to be silent so you can hear yourself speaking. This is called *centering*. While you can't always control the thoughts that enter your mind, you can keep thoughts about past and future worries from taking over and dominating your mind. That's what meditation does. It mutes negative self-talk, sort of like purging your computer of junk mail.

Or as Coach Erin likes to say, keep your thoughts where your feet are.

MEDITATORS HAVE HAPPIER HEARTS

Meditation dials down your rev-up system and dials up the relax-your-heart center. This enables the heart to relax and recharge. Heart doctors preach, "Relax your brain to relax your heart." In a study of persons with cardiovascular disease, meditators showed a decrease in blood pressure and heart rate and an increase in endothelial function. (Remember that the endothelium is where you *make your own medicines*.) Meditation can lower the blood level of stress hormones and reduce thickening of arterial walls. Meditation calms a "neurotic heart." "Relax!" means both brain and blood vessels. (See "Excess Stress Causes a Neurotic Heart," page 153.)

MEDITATION GROWS YOUR BRAIN GARDEN AS YOU AGE

Meditation increases the blood flow to the areas of the brain devoted to calmness and relaxation. Specifically, meditation increases nitric oxide (NO), the body's own vasodilator. NO also helps release endorphins, the brain-made medicines that relieve pain and increase the feeling of well-being. Long-term meditators also show less age-related "cortical thinning," meaning we lose gray matter and our brains shrink with age.

MEDITATION IMPROVES ATTENTION

Another misconception is that meditation's only purposes are relaxation, bliss, and helping us "zone out." Not so! Meditation benefits the areas in the brain's right hemisphere that promote concentration and sustained attention, which is why it could help teens and adults labeled with ADD and ADHD. I find that periodic meditation breaks, especially swimming meditation (see page 134), are especially necessary when I am writing, to help me relax and refocus. So do frequent mini-meditations throughout the day. Don't think of meditation as wasting time or doing nothing. On the contrary, meditation puts you in control of what's in your mind, or at least helps you deal with it. In fact, science-based therapists now teach meditation to help people with all sorts of disorders. It offers the same kind of mental health benefits as going to the gym does for the body.

Meditate more, fall less. I am a recovering klutz. Martha calls me Dr. Band-Aid. Because I'm usually deep in thought and not watching where I'm walking, my legs are always dinged up. One day, while meditating on what more I could do for the ones I love, I had an "aha!" moment. Falls are a top cause of disabilities in older people. Meditation teaches how to live and think in the present moment. Now, while walking through unfamiliar places, my mantra is:

"Watch where I walk!"

After a week of practice, meditation helped me be more mindful of each step.

Contrary to popular belief, the brain doesn't really shut off when it meditates, but rather becomes more selective in blocking out clutter. Or as Dr. Richard Davidson, a pioneer in brain-imaging during meditation, put it: "The brain on meditation is less 'bothered' by the usual stressors and is more accepting and content."

BEST TIMES TO MEDITATE

For most people, the best times to meditate are shortly after awakening and just before going to bed. Enjoy those two "happy hours" whenever you can.

Dr. Bill's prescription. Also, take frequent mini-meditations throughout the day as needed.

Erin coaches. The two best times to be "unplugged" from your devices are the first hour after awakening and the last hour before retiring.

MEDITATION HELPS SOLVE PROBLEMS

When your mind is dark, meditation can let the sunshine in. When I have writer's block, I take a meditation break. Clearing the mind of clutter and muting the noise helps me downgrade the problem and focus on the solution. During the writing of this chapter, I was invited to the annual NBJ Summit, hosted by *Nutrition Business Journal*, where forward-thinking minds in the field of nutritional healthcare get together to share ideas. In their wisdom, the summit's leaders had arranged a meditation break, led by a monk, in the middle of the information-packed lecture schedule. The message: Cool it, CEOs; you'll be more productive.

Meditating goes to school. Some schools are even replacing detention with meditation. Inattentive and misbehaving kids are encouraged to sit in the room and go through practices like deep breathing or meditation to help them calm down and get centered. They are also asked to talk through what happened. The Holistic Life Foundation offers the after-school program *Holistic Me,* in which kids from pre-K through fifth grade practice mindfulness exercises and yoga. Cofounder Andres Gonzalez quotes parents saying things like, "I came home the other day stressed out, and my daughter said, 'Hey, Mom, you need to sit down. I need to teach you how to breathe.'"

I recently advised a prep school principal to add brief periods of meditation to the curriculum. Children go to school to learn how to succeed in life. The more pressure the school puts on students to achieve, the more they need to learn how to rest and recharge their overworked minds.

MAKE UP YOUR PERSONAL MANTRA

Develop a mantra that works for you. A mantra is a word or phrase that protects your mind from sabotaging thoughts. A mantra can be a simple prayer that helps you quiet the clutter and the chatter of self-talk in your mind. When stress arises, you can open your box of favorite prayer thoughts. Clicking into your prayer is like switching on the relax-and-cool-it center in your brain.

Dr. Bill's mantras. One of my favorites is simply, "Guide me, God." One of my periodic prayers is: *Lord, take my hand. Guide me in your paths. Open* *my mind to know you. Clear my mind to hear you. Guide my eyes to see you in nature. Bless my feet to walk on your land. Quiet my life to feel you. Bless my dear wife. I see You in her. Lead me to serve You. Prompt me to share You. Open my kids to see You in me.*

Coach Erin's daily mantra. I invite gratitude and love into every circumstance I'm faced with daily: "Let my motives be to serve people. Give me patience, and open my ears to hear people's needs and guide them toward discovering their best selves. I am open to what this day has for me. God, align my will with Yours."

ENJOY MUSICAL MEDITATION

We enjoy "M&Ms" for health: not candy, but "music and meditation." Music can both calm and excite the mind. Match your music to the mood you're in—or want to be in. Music during meditation lets you go with the flow of melody and rhythm to mellow your mind. While music is a personal choice, Dr. Bill's five favorite meditation musical pieces are:

- "The Prayer" by Celine Dion and Andrea Bocelli
- An Emile Pandolfi piano album, *Once upon a Romance*
- Beethoven's "Moonlight Sonata" (the first movement naturally fits "Thank you God, thank you God.")
- "What a Wonderful World" by Louis Armstrong
- "Hawaiian Wedding Song"

Coach Erin's favorites:

- "My Beloved" by Kari Jobe
- "Somewhere over the Rainbow" by Katherine McPhee
- "After the Storm" by Mumford and Sons

I believe in music therapy, because I have felt the effects music has had in myself and seen its effects on others. Over four years ago, I sought treatment for alcoholism and was educated on the underlying issues that led to my drinking. While in treatment, I heard about music therapy. I believe that music has helped save my life, giving me an outlet for expression when I could not otherwise find one. It has helped me learn to cope with daily struggles, improved my self-esteem, helped me develop a sense of empowerment, and much more.

—ERIN CARDIN, CERTIFIED MUSIC THERAPIST

T5 MEDITATION STEPS: A SUMMARY

The meditation for you is the one you will daily do. Here are five starter tips.

1. **Pick a pose, select a setting.** As you start, get into your favorite position. Sit looking out a window at a garden, or whatever happy places you happen to be near. Eventually, you can learn to meditate anytime, anywhere.
2. **Take a deep, cleansing breath.** (page 132)
3. **Mind-mute.** This may start as only 5–10 seconds to clear your mind. (page 131)
4. **Mind your mantra.** Select a few of your favorites; add gratitude phrases. (page 146)
5. **Enjoy moving meditations:**

   - Flotation therapy (page 134)
   - Walk in the woods (page 136)

Just do it! Then later personalize and perfect it.

Meditation Makeover

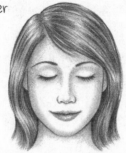

Calms mind clutter

Calms heart and
high blood pressure

Raises happy
hormones

Reduces stress

Improves attention

Helps problem solving

Increases
compassion

START YOUR DAY THE T5 WAY

How you begin your day often sets the tone for the rest of it. When we began eating the T5 way, we noticed that eating a healthy breakfast set the nutritional tone for how we ate the rest of the day. On days we started with our T5 smoothie, we had good gut feelings and less tendency to overeat. As a show-me-the-science doctor and a health coach, we wondered if there was science behind this observation. Sure enough, there was, and there was even a word for it—*frontloading*. People who start the day with a healthier breakfast tend to eat healthier the rest of the day. Could mental frontloading—starting the day with a joyful thought—promote healthier thinking?

THE FIVE-MINUTE WAY TO START YOUR DAY

As you ease out of bed, immediately click into an attitude-of-gratitude mindset: "I am thankful for . . . Today I look forward to . . ."

Pick five things you are thankful for and start the day focused on them. When you do that, you're telling your brain's gratitude center to light up. (Remember, the more you think about a subject, the more blood flows to that part of the brain.) At least for the first five minutes, trash any toxic thoughts or worries about things you dread having to do that day.

What can you say to brighten another's day? After your "five-minute way to start the day," think: "What can I say to the first person I meet to brighten his or her day?" It may be a server in a coffee shop, a stranger on the subway, or someone on the street who might look troubled. A smile or kind word might be all that person needs to stop dwelling on troubles and think about what's good in his or her life.

HOW T5 STRESSBUSTERS CAN LENGTHEN YOUR LIFE

Doctors who specialize in preventive medicine have long known that people with positive outlooks on life tend to live longer and healthier. Here's why:

Harmful stress effect	T5 effect	Health and longevity effects
• Higher heart rate	• Lower resting heart rate	• Heart lasts longer
• Higher blood pressure	• Relaxes stiff arteries	• Lowers high blood pressure
• Sleep disturbances	• Sleep better	• Repair system works better
• Dials up SNS too high*	• PNS predominates*	• More happy hormones, less stress effects
• Weakens immune system	• Immune system healthier	• Less often sick, faster healing
• Promotes inflammation	• Dials down inflammation	• Fewer -*itis* illnesses
• Depression/ anxiety (stress hormones too high)	• Happy hormones higher	• Happier moods
• Shortens telomeres**	• Lengthens telomeres**	• Live longer

*The sympathetic nervous system (SNS) has to do with fight-or-flight responses. It's involved with get-up-and-go and getting things done, and also with fear and anger. The parasympathetic nervous system (PNS) is your calm-down center, involved with "rest and digest" and "feed and breed" responses. SNS and PNS complement and balance each other.

** See "Telomeres and T5," p. 284 to learn why lengthening your telomeres, part of your chromosomes, helps lengthen your life.

To further motivate you to use the T5 stressbusters you just learned, let's consider what can happen to your brain and body if you let stress take over your life. You will now learn the meaning of "worried sick."

DON'T WORRY, BE HEALTHY: HOW STRESS HARMS YOUR HEALTH

In one important way, stress hormones are like blood sugar. When blood sugar is too low, the brain gets tired; too high and the brain gets inflamed and damaged by too much sticky stuff. The same is true of stress hormones, especially cortisol. It's interesting that the stress response that's meant to keep us alive in dangerous situations also can make us sick.

Cortisol isn't the only stress-related hormone, but we'll focus on it because its function is well known and a good example. The biochemical key to this discussion is *stress balance*. The stress dial in your brain is on alert 24/7. Stress balance means your brain dials up stress hormones to a high level when needed and quickly dials back down to a resting level.

The stress hormone dial turns down to its lowest level during sleep. (During the day, cortisol tends to be at the highest level around 6 AM and lowest around 6 PM.)

Stress can be lifesaving. The fire alarm goes off and jolts you awake. Your stress hormones instantly dial up to high alert. Your life depends on making quick decisions. You grab the kids and run out of the house, escaping the fire. You take a deep breath, thinking, "Thank God we're all safe." Gradually, the stress hormones dial back down. The next day you call your insurance agent and arrange for repairs, constantly thinking how fortunate you all are to have survived unharmed. This is a normal, healthy stress response.

But suppose your stress dial stays on high. After escaping the fire, you continue in panic mode: "If only I had . . ." "Will it happen again?" "Why me?" These "what ifs" drag on for weeks. When stress hormones stay too high for too long, they damage the brain in a process that has the scary name of *glucocorticoid neurotoxicity*. Feeling "frazzled" may be the result of early glucocorticoid neurotoxicity. There really is a neurochemical basis for words like *worrywart*, *negative person*, *pessimist*, as well as for *positive person* and *optimist*.

Our suggestion: To become un-depressed and un-obsessed, become de-stressed.

How stress strains the brain. Prolonged high levels of cortisol can literally shrink the memory and emotional centers of your brain. This is why you really don't want to go into an exam or business meeting stressed out—stress can neurochemically shut off the memory bank that you need to answer exam questions or solve problems.

High stress can cause you to go "blank," which can be good thing. It's your brain's signal that you need to take a deep breath and relax, settle down, and then return to your work. Prolonged stress and dwelling on negative thoughts causes glucocorticoid neurotoxicity, which is like spraying toxic chemicals on your brain.

THE OLDER YOU ARE, THE LESS STRESS YOU CAN HANDLE

As we age, our automatic dial-down stress-balancing mechanism becomes less reliable. Stress expert Dr. Robert Sapolsky defines aging as "the progressive loss of the ability to deal with stress." There is a growing science called *psychoneuroimmunology*; the word suggests that what you think affects your immune system. Environmental and personal stressors can suppress the immune system of the aging person more than a younger person's.

Not only do older people have trouble turning down the stress response, but their resting levels of stress hormones such as epinephrine, norepinephrine, and cortisol are higher. Chronically elevated epinephrine and norepinephrine levels contribute to high blood pressure and many of the common diseases of aging.

Putting on your brain's brakes. Most of this stress-control mechanism is located in the hippocampus, one of the areas of the brain that lose the most neurons with age. In the wake of a stressful event, the aged hippocampus is less able to put on the brakes to slow down those stress hormones. Since

the ability to handle stress lessens as we get older, it's important to learn more stressbuster skills as we age.

If you can't change it, don't worry about it. That sentence is the key to stress management. Happy, healthy centenarians report: "If I can't change it, I don't worry about it."

Be mindful. No matter what your age, equip yourself with a set of stress-busters that work for you starting now. Why wait until you're a senior? The sooner you begin, the better they stick, and the less you get sick from stress, throughout your life.

EXCESS STRESS CAUSES A NEUROTIC HEART

Cardiologists call the correlation between unresolved stress and cardio-vascular disease a *neurotic heart*. Chronic high levels of stress hormones can cause several physical problems:

- The arteries get *stiff.* Normally elastic arteries stretch and relax to open wider when the heart pumps harder. If the arteries get tense because the person is tense, the heart has to pump harder and beat faster than it should have to. Chronic high stress wears out the heart sooner, leading to *heart failure.*

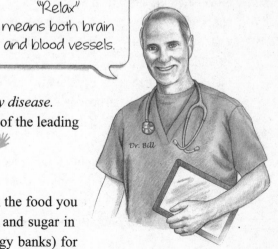

"Relax" means both brain and blood vessels.

Dr. Bill

- The blood flow and vessel lining get *sticky*, leading to clots—*coronary artery disease.* Unresolved stress is one of the leading causes of heart attacks.

STRESS CAN MAKE YOU FAT

The fatty acids and glucose from the food you eat are meant to be stored as fat and sugar in the liver and muscles (your energy banks) for later use. When you are overstressed, stress hormones release stored fat and sugar from the muscles and liver into the bloodstream and deposit them into belly fat. Another possible cause for stress-induced obesity is that stress blunts the *leptin effect* (the hormone leptin triggers satiety, increases metabolism, and burns fat). By hindering the appetite-control center of the brain, stress causes you to overeat. Being both overweight and overstressed is doubly bad for health.

STRESS BELLY

Bob, an investment banker, suffered from job-induced stress. All of Bob's vital signs were normal except for his waist, which was five inches too big. I began my T5 talk with: "Bob, your brain is getting foggy because of your big belly." Before I could launch into my T5 health sermon, Bob volunteered, "But I eat fine and I exercise a lot." To Bob's defense, I replied, "Yes, Bob, it's good you do that, but you suffer from glucocorticoid neurotoxicity." I went on to explain how stress that bothers the brain also bothers the belly, and gave him my stress-reduction plan. At the end of the consultation I said, "Bob, next time we meet I want to see less of you."

"The leaner, the lower" is becoming the motto for stabilizing insulin, because the insulin level of your blood is related to the obesity level of your waist. One of the main contributors to abdominal fat is high insulin levels.

Bigger belly, smaller brain. Suppose you go to your doctor for a brain-health checkup. The doctor is rushed, allowing time for only one measurement that would reveal your risk of getting a brain disease. That measurement should be your *waist size*. A 2010 study in *Neurobiology of Aging* showed that as waist size goes up, the size of the brain goes down. Simply put, excess abdominal fat becomes a harmful chemical factory spewing out sticky stuff: chemicals that stick to the walls of your brain's blood vessels and damage brain tissue.

Being overfat, especially around the middle, creates a downward spiral. Excess abdominal fat prompts you to overeat, because this type of fat secretes neurochemicals that travel to the appetite-control center in the hypothalamus to prompt the brain to eat more.

When I examine a reluctant transformer, I no longer say, "You're overweight." Instead, I shock my portly patient with the

> Shrink your belly to keep from shrinking your brain.

Dr. Bill

more scientifically correct terminology: "You're prediabetic." If the patient is still reluctant to transform, I upgrade to "You're pre-Alzheimer's." If brain-shrinking is not enough to motivate you to stay lean, consider that a person with excess body fat is by medical definition "prediabetic."

A waist size greater than forty inches in men and thirty-five in women is a red flag that diabetes may soon occur and is also associated with a five- to sevenfold increase in risk of Alzheimer's disease. 🖐

STRESS CAN MAKE YOU SICK, TIRED, AND DIABETIC

Wonder why stressed and anxious people often suffer chronic fatigue? A healthy stress response withdraws fuel from your body's energy storage bank (stored sugar and fat) and delivers it to the brain and muscles for quick decisions and fast moves. That's what these hormones are there for, especially the fast-acting adrenaline. Normally, this quick-response stress dial turns up and then turns down and stops withdrawing the energy money from the fat bank. That's a healthy stress response.

Suppose, however, this stress dial stays turned up too high for too long, and even worse, calls on its buddy stress hormones to add to the continued energy withdrawal. Eventually, your energy bank will be broke: you're sick and tired—chronic fatigue, *fibromyalgia*. Stress can make you weak. Chronic high levels of stress hormones can break down muscle protein as stress hormones are looking for any tissues to extract energy from, leading to muscle fatigue and pain—more fibromyalgia.

Because I was sick and tired of being sick and tired, I was motivated to change. Now I feel well and energetic!
—A TRANSFORMER

Ever wonder why stressed and depressed people get sick more often, or why you always seem to get a cold when you are stressed? Stress weakens the immune system. The fascinating new field of *psychoneuroimmunology* studies the effects mind has on immune system performance. The latest upgrade is even longer, by four letters: *psychoneuroendoimmunology*, how the mind, immune system, and endocrine system are all interconnected, each influencing the others. Stress hinders healing, because it uses up energy needed to help the body heal. Do you want better living through drugs, *pharmacology*, or better living through T5, *psychoneuroimmunology*?

Insulin resistance. Chronic stress causes more glucose and fatty acids to be mobilized into the bloodstream, more than the cells can handle. So the cells put a "closed" sign on their doors (receptors). That means you have excess sugar and fatty acids floating around your bloodstream—sticky stuff that gums up the blood vessels, leading to strokes, kidney disease, high blood pressure, and cardiovascular and cerebrovascular disease. Blood vessel damage is one of the main problems diabetics face. If you're fat and stressed, you have two strikes against you for becoming insulin resistant or getting type 2 diabetes. While type 2 diabetes seems to be the fastest-rising illness worldwide, the good news is that it's the disease most helped by T5. (See more about how T5 helps prevent and treat type 2 diabetes in chapter eight.)

STRESS CAUSES PAINS IN THE GUT

Stress first decreases secretion of saliva and the oral digestive enzymes it contains. Next, stress slows the stomach contractions that mash together food and digestive acids. Farther along, the intestines slow down, resulting in two problems: fewer food nutrients are absorbed, and food movement slows—constipation. The stress-induced decrease in blood flow to the gut further decreases digestion and mobility—more constipation.

Constipation and diarrhea can both occur during chronic stress. Constipation occurs when the whole bowel slows down, allowing the partially digested food to accumulate. Diarrhea occurs when the stress response causes the colon muscles to go on a contraction spree, evacuating the gut of its contents before the water is absorbed. This may be why people experience "the runs" during or even in anticipation of stressful events.

You stress, you leak! Chronic stress can also damage the lining of the small and large intestines, resulting in leaky gut, irritable bowel syndrome, Crohn's, and colitis. (See related section, "Leaky Gut," page 294.)

COACH ERIN: KEEP HITTING THAT RESET BUTTON!

Every T5 transformer has setbacks and disappointments. Don't let that get you down. Your inner critic can sabotage your transformation. What if Olympic athletes gave up the first time (or the hundredth time) they fell short? The difference between now and your old life is that you have the stressbuster tools to deal with it. Accept that these changes won't happen overnight. How long did it take you to form your unhealthy patterns? Your whole life, up to now. I give my clients and myself the permission to hit that reset button anytime, anywhere!

Never give up!

Don't give up no matter what! Keep hitting that reset button. Let go of past failures and take that next right step.

The biggest key for my sticking to this lifestyle is to lose the all-or-nothing attitude. In the past I would slip up on my diet, beat myself up, and give up. Erin has taught me to hit the "reset" button, which has saved me. Now when

I slip, I evaluate why and notice how I'm feeling, which motivates me to make a healthier choice next time.
—TRANSFORMER SUSAN PHINNEY

Coach Erin's Silicon Valley stressbuster. Even after we had practiced most of the T5 principles as a family for some time, my husband, John, still seemed to constantly get stuck in a mental fog caused primarily by his fast-paced, high-stress Silicon Valley work environment. He was caught in a stress-induced cycle that made it hard for him to use his healthy-living tools. However, over the last couple years I have lovingly observed him hitting that reset button in order to keep fighting for change. Now he is thirty pounds lighter, has better balance between work and his personal life, has space in his brain for healthy hobbies, and has a more positive outlook on life. How did he do it? He didn't give up. He kept taking little steps that eventually led to big changes.

Coach Erin's message for modern times. Too often today, people who are having trouble coping choose to lose themselves in the digital world instead of reaching out to a human being. One of the dangers of this is that almost everyone seems to put up a façade of happiness on Facebook and Instagram. It's easy to look at others' posts and think, "She has it so easy!" Comparing yourself to others is one of the quickest ways to fall into self-pity and even depression.

COACH ERIN HELPS YOU OVERPOWER YOUR INNER CRITIC

Your inner dialogue is very powerful. We need to manage it so that it's telling us the right things. If your inner voice is a constant, nasty critic—"You're not worth it . . . You can't do that . . . Why even try, you're just going to fail"—you need to change it, to retrain that voice to speak words of encouragement and self-love. This begins with acceptance.

Accept where you are at this very moment, do the best you can with today, and tomorrow you will be a little closer to your goal.

Your body responds to your thoughts, so what do you think is more empowering?

" Ugh, I hate the way I look—I have to get my butt to the gym . . ."

Or . . .

"I want to look and feel healthy, and I'm going to start with the workout I can do today."

This may be easier said than done, but once you decide to stop saying negative things to yourself, you will discover the power it had over you. Being honestly aware of your negative thought patterns is the first step to overcoming them. It takes practice! Now, go retrain that negative inner critic to become a positive one.

Unhealthy thoughts	Healthy thoughts
You can't get your body back.	I deserve a strong, healthy body.
You keep failing—how is this time different?	Today is a new day! I honor where I am today, and tomorrow I will be stronger.
You're selfish for taking time to work out.	I love my family so much that I want to be the best version of myself—for them.
You . . .	I . . .
You . . .	I . . .
You . . .	I . . .
You . . .	I . . .
(Fill in your own thoughts.)	

Don't sabotage with technology. Although I'm not technically a millennial (two years too old), I can relate to the glued-to-our-electronics way of life. A couple of months ago I realized my attachment to my iPhone was a bit out of balance. The biggest thing it was affecting was my ability to be completely present and connected with my husband. While technology is a great tool, it can also sabotage us. As with anything, there needs to be balance. Here are some tricks I have put in place to help me be more techno-balanced:

Life is not measu... in "likes."

1. I turn off my phone one hour before bed and only turn it back on in the morning after special time with my husband and morning meditation.

2. When I'm with a friend or fellow transformer, I put my phone away and out of sight. This helps me to really listen and be present.

3. I try to have three scheduled times during the day that I check emails and social media. This prevents me from mindlessly wasting large amounts of time.

4. Take a tech sabbath. Set aside one day, or even half a day, per week when you don't look at your phone. Imagine the space it creates in your brain when you turn that off.

5. Balance communication between texts, phone calls, and in-person connection times.

One of our top stressbusters is a high dose of what we call the Helper's High, which you will learn all about in the next chapter.

CHAPTER 5

SHARE WITH FIVE FRIENDS

ENJOY THE HELPER'S HIGH

When you believe it, do it, and feel it, you've got to share it. At this writing, I am in my fiftieth year as a doctor. What I call the *helper's high* is the main reason I'm still happy to see patients in my medical office. It's that priceless feeling you get deep inside when your advice helps people live happier and healthier. Remember our motto: "I thrive on T5." The helper's high happens when you transform your passion and caring into a purpose. In writing books, we think about what should we write and why are we writing it. The *why* never changes: to help many readers—and doers—feel better.

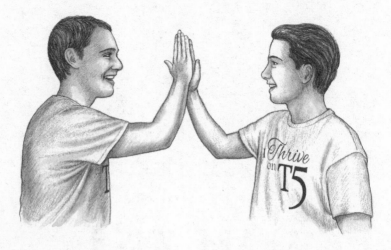

Coach Erin's helper's high. "The more you give it away, the more you keep it" is one of my mottos. Even before my transformation in 2011, I have always loved helping others find their joy. My background is in music, and I will never forget the joy I felt the first time I conducted a choir and saw the students' faces light up with the beautiful music they were making. Hearing my transformers' success stories fills me with that same joy and keeps me motivated every day!

After I had a particularly stressful day, I was talking to a friend who told me how T5 had given her much more energy to be there for her family, and how she finally felt hopeful again. I thought, "Now that's what it's all about!" One of my goals as a Certified Health Coach is to inspire a passion in each of my clients to share T5 with others.

Dr. Bill adds: My two tips for sharing T5 with someone new are:

1. Identify *their* personal needs first, before launching into *your* program. Most transformers have medical, social, psychological, and/or financial needs. T5 can help with all. (See "Mind Your Mirror Neurons," page 236, about how minds project.)
2. Speak from your heart. While this book will be your guide, tell people about it in your own language.

GETTING STARTED: T5's TOP WAYS TO SHARE

First, identify what your buddy-transformer needs. Most people needing a transformation have one or more of these needs:

Medical: *Help others transform their minds and bodies to heal their hurts.*

Social: *Feel good by doing good. Help others strengthen their social network.*

Financial: *Financial stress can worsen health. T5 can help you be more creative and productive and miss fewer work days. Share T5 to help others become financially secure.*

T5 helps meet these needs, and more.

TWO WAYS TO CHOOSE YOUR TEAM

Remember when we said you can choose between the T5 "fast track" or transforming one change at a time? You can approach sharing the same way, depending on what sets you up for success the best. How will you thrive? It's up to you:

- Get your T5 team together right at the beginning, or
- Share with friends only after you have caught the fire and feel transformed.

THE POWER OF YOUR T5 TEAM

Benefits of a buddy. Fellow transformers keep you accountable. They act as mentors, supporters, friendly nags, fun competitors, or whatever you need to keep you on the transformation track.

When you're ready to start the program, get a buddy—or two or three or four! There is power in numbers. Remember this recurring theme of T5: do what works for you! Are you a person who needs that safety net of accountability? In my experience, most people do. It is human nature to work in partnership. The transformers who have the most lasting success have embraced this, even when it hasn't felt comfortable. Most popular health-enhancement programs offer a coach and/or ways to connect with others for support. While many programs get this part right in theory, the connections you make with a coach or a group fade over time. But with T5, your team stays together and will be there for you.

Visualize your dream team. Who are the people in your life with whom you can be honest, no matter what? Who is strong but needs support, just like you? Who will motivate you when your self-motivating inner dialogue is in a funk? Think back on your life and visualize times when you had a goal for your health, or anything else important. Were you more successful when you had support? Birds of a feather flock together. The best partnership is where other people make you want to be better. Here are some examples of transformers' experiences with the T5 team model:

Who can you ac to your T5 tear

> *Several of my friends and I started our own support group focusing on meditation, smoothies, healthy meals, and mental clarity. I feel comfortable sharing what I've learned about my own health with others who also need support, and it feels amazing knowing they are going to experience all that T5 has to offer. I don't have to be an expert, I just share what I learned and help them find what works for them. Through my first five weeks on T5 my group was a huge key to my success. I loved hearing how others were handling challenging days, and loved celebrating our growth together.*
> **—KAREN LITTLEFIELD**

> *I felt way better about a tough, stressful situation at work after sharing it with my T5 team. It really took the burden off. I am very*

empowered by the group and used the support to get me though the week without giving in to my unhealthy food habits. The accountability and motivation have been so wonderful, as well as knowing that I'm not alone in this!

—ESTHER ALVA

I really didn't want to work out, but I had asked Coach Erin to help keep me accountable to my goal of four days of exercise this week. I knew she was going to ask me when we talked next, and I wanted to be able to say yes. I did work out four times!

—CLARA WALKER

Healthy in harmony. Four amazing ladies decided to start T5 as a team. They already had a strong bond, because they had been a singing group for years. They came to me and said, "Erin, we just want to stop feeling so unhealthy all the time." They had been through a lot of ups and downs through the years, and they saw the impact of grief on their health from losing loved ones. T5 challenged them to get control of their health from the inside out. The quartet included healthier food options during weekend retreats and worked out as a team. This experience made their bond stronger and deeper, because they were all in it together and lifted each other up when hard times hit. They enjoyed being one another's cheerleaders and found that being open about their shortcomings was powerful.

The danger zone of human nature. Group dynamics can be powerful in ways both healthy and unhealthy. What happens when you're hanging out with friends and there is junk food around? Everyone is eating it, so it doesn't seem like a harmful thing. Humans can be chameleons, adapting to their surroundings and taking on the traits of others. What if every party only had healthy food options?

"There is always food at my pity parties, and not the healthy kind." Let's un-invite ourselves from the pity party and *let go of self-pity.*

But that's easier said than done. Many of us have to find our way out of self-pity by trial and error. In addition to the attitude-of-gratitude tips you learned on page 135, here are some starting points:

1. Begin or end your day by listing the things you're grateful for (see "Start Your Day the T5 Way," page 149.)
2. Be of service to a fellow transformer or a friend in need.
3. Share your feelings with someone you trust; don't isolate yourself.
4. Focus on what you can control.
5. Enjoy your healthy hobbies.

Strength in numbers. Our culture has long valued individualism and applauded "self-made" people. Some people still see support groups as a sign of weakness. I believe the opposite is true. There is strength in knowing your shortcomings. As Clara pointed out, being honestly committed to her group pushed her to get that fourth workout in when she was looking for every excuse to skip it. I have experienced this in my own transformation and through the eyes of others in my support groups and T5 team. Hearing other transformers talk about their successes and challenges motivates me to keep my program going. Esther had a stressful situation that in the past would have led to stress-eating. Our secrets keep us sick, but she opened up to her T5 team, and that helped her balance stress the T5 way.

Have you ever wondered why most participants in those TV weight-loss shows don't keep the weight off, and many of them ending up even heavier? One reason is because the strong support system they had on TV wasn't there when they stepped back into daily life. Having friends and family on this path with you ensures your safety net of support and motivation is there for the good days and bad.

Why twelve-step programs are so powerful. In the gentle rooms of Alcoholics Anonymous you will hear phrases such as *rigorous honesty . . . carry the message . . . be of service . . . share our experience, strength, and hope.* We see three main reasons why these programs work:

1. They require honesty and willingness.
2. There is an admission that you cannot do it alone.
3. Lasting success depends on a connection with others and sharing the message of hope.

They link arms with a common purpose and support each other through thick and thin—like-minded people living a life that is happy, joyous, and free. In fact, some of our most successful transformers have turned their "addictive personalities" into a *positive addiction* by doing and sharing T5.

Also, we would be remiss if we didn't say that programs like Overeaters Anonymous, Alcoholics Anonymous, and Al-Anon might be the best path for many. An unhealthy lifestyle can be a symptom of deeper issues where the problem isn't merely bad habits but compulsive self-medicating, use, and abuse. If you think you need this level of support, contact the organization in your area or talk to your doctor. It can be very scary, yet we know firsthand how transforming it is to combine the twelve steps and T5.

Dr. Bill notes: I find some of the most ardent and successful transformers are those who are recovering from addiction. Instead of considering "addictive personality" a negative trait, I help move them toward positive addictions: "We're going to help you recover into positive habits."

Most people in recovery need a healthy purpose to recover into.

Dr. Bill

Erin's "saving race." Grab a buddy and sign up for a race! I remember a very stressful time in my transformation when I was derailed, overwhelmed, and grasping for help. I got married, moved, and changed careers, all in the same week. Even good change is stressful, and I was not prepared for how lost I would feel. Fortunately, because of the tools I have, this funk did not last long. Too many times before I had stood at a crossroads and decided it might just be easier to throw in the towel or take the unhealthy path. And boy, did I learn the hard way. Not this time! Here was my lifeline:

1. Take a really deep breath.
2. Admit to myself that I needed help.

3. Admit to a friend or family member that I needed help.
4. Grab an accountability partner.
5. Make a fun plan.

Okay, so the plan was in motion, which is always the hardest part. I instantly felt more empowered and less fearful, because I was honest and took action. My workout buddy and I decided to sign up for a half marathon. (If you're new to running or power walking, go for a 5K. Or choose whatever goal feels right for you.)

I was in a city new to me, so this was a chance to find some beautiful local parks and running trails as well as build a friendship with my workout buddy. We met a couple times a week, and every week I got stronger physically, which helped me relieve my emotional stress. There were times when I did not want to go, but knowing she was there waiting for me helped me get out of my own way. The marathon was challenging, but the amazingly beautiful trail run through the Santa Cruz Mountains just took my breath away. Running amid those tall redwoods made me feel strong yet humble, knowing that there is this big world and a loving Creator out there who has a plan for me. Suddenly, the trials of the past few months melted away, and I could see clearly the promise for my health and my life's path. Running and walking teach me to keep my head where my feet are.

It all starts with willingness. Are you ready to tr...

BE A "WALKING BILLBOARD"

Your face, your skin, your total-body transformation reflects your "business." When an admirer inquires, "What do you do for a living?" proudly answer, "I'm in the body transformation business." A likely reply: "That sounds interesting, tell me more." Your response: "What transformation do you need? T5 can deliver that!"

People will start noticing your transformation and become inspired to do it for themselves. You get to step into the role of mentor! Pass on what you learned and experience what Dr. Bill calls the "helper's high." There is something magical that happens when you share your experience, strength, and hope with someone who is struggling. Carrying the message brings new depth and power to taking control of your health. I've always said, if I can help just *one* person by sharing how I recovered, then the whole hard journey is worth it. Watching a loved one go through similar trials also brings a sense of ownership to how hard you have fought to find health. You know you can keep it as long as you keep working your program and sharing with others.

Another transformer (let's call her Jill) shares her story of sharing with friends:

I have been on the path for about three months now, and I am amazed at how much clearer and focused I am. I see those around me in a whole new light, and I feel like I have this secret that I just can't keep to myself anymore! After a particularly challenging day, I came home to find my sister in tears over the fact that she just couldn't find the energy to deal with her demanding schedule. She was feeling terrible about how she let her self-care go out the window.

Jill felt compassion for her sister, because she had been in the same predicament prior to T5. She listened to her sister and hugged her, saying, "I'm here for you a hundred percent, and I know you are going to get through this." Jill told her sister her own story of desperation, and this turned into hope for both of them. Jill shared how she committed to the simple changes of drinking more water and eating more fruits and vegetables. Her sister found comfort in how grasping a small thing can yield huge results. She said, "I can do that!"

The following week, Jill became her sister's accountability partner, checking in at the end of every day, and this helped them both stay on track. Those small changes added up, and now they are both experiencing life more fully and are thriving. Of course, a challenging day arose now and then, but they were able to share their struggles honestly and move on, instead of allowing those challenges to weigh them down.

MORE INSIGHT FROM ERIN

Birds of a feather flock together. Humans can be like magnets, drawing other people into their lives who are attracted by what they see. Think about your close friends. Do they share most of your core values, your outlook on life? Most likely, they do. When I was depressed, my negative energy drew depressed people to me. Now, after my transformation, I am more positive, and I have the most amazing circle of people around me, people who are continually striving to be their healthiest selves, and that rubs off on me in the process.

> I have removed toxic people from my life just as I am working on removing toxic food. I become those with whom I surround myself.
> —KIM BUCKNER

The power of a phone call. Get in the habit of calling a friend, relative, or fellow transformer every day, so on the days when you really need accountability the phone won't be as heavy. Our current culture of texting and social media "connections" is great, but there is nothing like a good old-fashioned phone call. Emojis are fun, but the nuances of the human voice allow for a more authentic interaction. I remember one conversation I had with a mentor who asked me, "Is there anything you *don't* want to tell me?" Yikes! My heart pounded as I answered her question and came clean about what was really going on. It is just too easy to put on those fake social-media smiles and never really get honest.

How to get and stay motivated. As a coach, I am my clients' biggest cheerleader. I wish there were motivation software that could be installed in you and me, but it *has* to come from within. I ask my clients two questions:

What motivates you toward healthy living, and how do you stay motivated? Here are their transformation tips:

1. "I want to feel good in my own skin."
2. "I look at my mom, who is overweight, overmedicated, and can't play with her grandkids. I am breaking that cycle today."
3. "I'm reaching inside and choosing to flip that switch. I've been selfish with my health choices, but now I will be there for my family the way they need me."
4. "It starts with having a clear vision of what I want and why."
5. "To enjoy retirement. I didn't work and save so long not to enjoy that investment."
6. "Focusing on small, attainable goals that stick. Success empowers me to keep going."
7. "Not beating myself up."
8. "Surrounding myself with like-minded people who are successful at healthy living."
9. "I learned the hard way and had to have a health scare, a wakeup call. Now I can choose to fight for my life through the choices I make."

COACH ERIN ON FINDING YOUR MOTIVATION

We all need well-defined goals. Olympic athletes are successful because they always have a definite goal or personal record they are working toward. Ask yourself what's missing for you: Energy, a clear head, flexibility, wellness? I wish you two kinds of motivation: personal and relational.

Personal motivation is something that burns inside you and drives you toward your goals, like wanting to have more energy or run a mile. Take a moment and write down five personal motivators:

1.
2.
3.
4.
5.

Relational motivation is driven by the people in your life. For instance, wanting to be able to run with your kids or grandkids, wanting to experience life to fullest with your spouse who is very active, or simply wanting to be a strong and complete person who can best serve those around you. Now list your top five relational motivators.

1.
2.
3.
4.
5.

My parents are incredible examples of this for me and my husband. They are in their seventies and truly living their retired years to the fullest. My dad, a.k.a. the Energizer Bunny, plays golf four times a week, swims, lifts weights, takes long walks holding his one-year-old grandson, and is present physically and mentally for all his children and grandchildren. As you read on page 105, the grandkids call his home gym "Grandpa's playroom." My parents achieve all of this because of the choices they have made to make health a priority and practice personal and relational motivation.

SOCIAL MEDIA HELPS YOU SHARE

As you just read, there's no substitute for a phone call or face-to-face communication, yet social media is still a great resource for you and your T5 team. You may feel the self-doubt and fear creeping in and say to yourself, "I don't want to post about my success, because if it doesn't stick, I'll be embarrassed." (See "what ifs," page 151.)

But what if it *does* stick?! Dr. Bill doesn't use social media much, but it's a big part of my life. I love seeing pictures and posts that show the progress of a young woman from sick, tired, overwhelmed, and unhealthy to a woman who is strong and living the T5 way. These posts are a constant reminder that I never have to go back to my old ways, and they help me celebrate my life now. It is like reading about two entirely different people.

> ▶ See DrSearsWellness.org/T5/Testimonies to view transformation testimonies.

Now I'll see a post from a friend saying, "I'm heading out for my run this morning even though I don't want to," or, "Help! I need some ideas for healthy eating, because I've been a little naughty over the holiday." I'm so glad they opened up, because I might be feeling unmotivated that day too, and it reminds me that if they can do it, I can do it, too. I have a friend, Jackie Ross, who has had an unbelievable transformation and who used the power of social media to open up her support group and gain thousands of cheerleaders. Initially, she shared with me her fears about bothering people or failing, but she got over that. Here is what she posted when she hit her weight-loss goal:

I hit my 100-pound weight-loss goal! I posted a lot on social media and in my T5 accountability group. I felt awkward many times and didn't want to share my journey. Now, looking back, I see how it was key for me in staying motivated. Hearing others' experiences and their cheers was awesome! Today was the day I met a HUGE goal. I'm officially down 100.2 pounds. ONE HUNDRED POUNDS. I don't think it has really hit me. I've read so many of these kinds of posts on social media and never thought I would be the author of one of them. Almost two months ago, I was feeling really down. I was stuck. But I didn't give in and pushed harder than I ever have, and I've lost almost fifteen pounds since then. The whole journey before that was no joke, though—thirteen months and not without its challenges. Surround yourself with those who support you. Be kind to yourself and love yourself. I am proof that it is 100 percent worth it.

Jackie has helped transform many people's lives by getting out of her own way and sharing her story, all of it, not just the roses and rainbows.

Be honest. Like Jackie, I had to decide whether I would share the struggles of my journey. I mean, who wants to read about that? The truth is, that's what connects with people. It is what everyone can relate to at some level. Support each other in the challenging times and cheer on each other as you grow. One client contacted me because she saw the same unfriendly number on the scale that prompted my own transformation mission (I call it my YOU-turn moment). People want to connect to success, but that really means finding a coach and healthy partners that they relate to—who have made this journey themselves. Otherwise, it would be like talking to a relationship counselor who has never been in a relationship. This is why I am grateful for the struggles I've had. They make me a more powerful and relatable coach.

A family transformation. Your family can be your best support system or your worst enablers. Women struggle more with this, it seems. It can be extremely tough to stick with your goals if others in the home want unhealthy food all the time. I get that. Fortunately, my husband is completely on board most of the time. Can you imagine a home where everyone supports one another all the time? We know this is easier said than done. However, there are steps you can take toward working together.

1. Set some house rules. For example, desserts like pie, cake, and ice cream are only for special occasions. Otherwise, have a piece of fruit for dessert.
2. Have everyone write down their favorite foods, including fruits and vegetables they are most willing to eat. This will make grocery shopping easier.
3. Make a rule that you all have to earn "screen time" by spending time outdoors—playing, walking, riding bikes. Make specific plans for outdoor playtime.
4. Have meals that include "build your own" elements like tacos and salad bar. Plan themed meals like meatless Monday and salmon Saturday.

5. Start a family healthy-living calendar where everyone can plan and input their activities. Hang a big paper calendar in the kitchen or use Google Calendar.

My whole family has jumped on board. I make an effort now to take the kids on bike rides, and we often hit the trails behind our house. We are enjoying making small changes in our eating habits, and it is so much easier when the whole family is on board. If you don't buy it, they won't eat it. My kids now enjoy air-popped popcorn instead of greasy potato chips.

—TINA EATON

Lead by example. Can't quite get your loved ones on the healthy living train? Stay patient and lead by example. Let their reluctance motivate you to be the family member who feels so good that your enthusiasm becomes infectious. Even if they don't jump on board right away, at least you have peace of mind knowing that when they are ready, they have a leader in you. Let family members' unhealthy choices be reminders of why you're transforming yourself. When my husband wakes up the morning after indulging in a bit too much celebration, I can't help but giggle to myself in gratitude that I can stay strong. Here is a great story from transformer Karen Littlefield:

> *I was sick and tired of seeing my family sick and tired. I started making small changes to my eating plan and started shaping my kids' tastes to like more plant-based foods by giving them a fruit and vegetable supplement like Juice Plus+ Orchard and Garden Blend Chewables. I went through the fridge and pantry, giving them a makeover, and slowly but surely my kids and I started reaching for more whole foods. They became more open to trying healthier options like lettuce tacos instead of tortillas. After my husband saw beautiful changes in us that were sticking, he began*

saying things like, "What's in that smoothie? Can I try it?" He still loves his unhealthy carbs, but we find middle ground. If he wants pizza, we make it thin crust with lots of veggies.

SHARE WITH TECH-SAVVY TRANSFORMERS

In this age when there's an app for everything, technology can play an important part in your T5 team and support system. You can share all the data with your group, for example by posting it on a group Facebook page. Support, accountability—even a little healthy competition—it all helps! My husband and I love to compete to see who recorded more steps, stairs, miles, and so on.

Fitness trackers. I had never used a fitness tracker before writing this book. Doing research for this chapter, I jumped into it and found that it's really fun. When you are embarking on the T5 lifestyle, you want to give yourself the best chance for success. Some people thrive on specific measures, like calorie counting and step-tracking, while others find that kind of discipline to be a burden. What kind of transformer are you? Will the extra accountability keep you motivated and on track, or will it trigger your obsessive thinking and end up sabotaging your success?

With a typical fitness tracker, you input certain information, and the device will suggest goals based on your lifestyle. Here is what to look for in trackers:

1. Step and stair counter
2. Sleep tracker
3. Intensity minutes (movements at a higher heart rate)
4. Calories burned
5. GPS
6. Ability to sync with your music
7. Ability to sync with other supporting apps. For instance, Garmin Fitbit syncs with MyFitnessPal, so you can monitor your activity level and your food intake.
8. Guided breathing sessions

9. Reminders to move (if you have been stationary too long, it sends a movement reminder)

Use your smartphone to track activity. There are free apps that track your movement and are wonderful motivators. Most transformers like MapMyRun. It stores your progress, tracks your distance, and posts to your social media outlets so your friends can cheer you on. I love that my music library can be linked to it as well, providing me with my workout tunes. Also, apps like this provide training plans to help you work toward a distance race, from 5K to a full marathon.

Food trackers—a slight disagreement between Erin and Dr. Bill. Do we count calories on T5? That is a loaded question. In short, no. When you follow the 5-S and mini-meal principle, you will likely stay within a healthy caloric intake in addition to balancing your carbs, proteins, and fats. And yet, while Dr. Bill doesn't count calories, I do. Again, the method for you is the one you will consistently do, and the one that keeps you motivated. If you want to count calories, there's an app for that.

How does not counting calories work? After six years on this program, there are still days when I have too many calories or too few. But the power of T5 is the education and awareness you will gain as you walk through the program. You learn what the healthiest calories are; calorie *quality* is more transforming than calorie numbers. In the beginning, you may need to be more diligent in tracking, reading labels, and looking up nutritional information as you build the list of foods that you thrive on. People have different nutritional needs, including caloric intake. If you are doing a lot of intense physical training, you will likely need more calories than normally recommended. (See "Counting Calories? No Need To!," page 282.)

Here's my calorie story. My five mini-meals each usually fall in the 200 to 400 calorie range, which add up to a healthy range for my moderately active lifestyle. (Remember, everyone has different needs.) I listed my favorite breakfast, lunch, dinner, snack, and dessert items and looked up the calories. After the first few weeks, I had a general sense of the amount of food that stayed within my range. But I have a tendency toward obsession, which has sometimes led me to be too restrictive in my food choices. So I had to ask myself if I was depriving myself of necessary nutrients. Was I choosing nutrient-dense foods—say, high-fiber whole wheat cereal over a Pop Tart?

It took a couple of weeks to dial in what worked. If I had an extremely active day I would listen to my body—if it told me I was hungry and needed more fuel, I would nourish my body with a healthy snack, even if I was over the "allotted calorie intake." I had an overall awareness of the nutritional value of the food I was putting in my body, but I did not become obsessive about it. That is what we always come back to—is this right for you? Also, because T5 foods, especially seafood, vegetables, nuts, and eggs are very nutrient-dense, you get more bang for your buck. A four-ounce piece of salmon will be much more filling and satisfying than a hamburger that has more calories. We go for quality over quantity. And remember, when you put the right fuel in your body, it becomes more efficient at burning that fuel instead of storing it as fat.

Don't trust the numbers 100 percent. I googled calorie trackers and tested three random sites. After inputting my weight, height, age, gender, and activity level, all three gave me a different calorie goal. So I use these as general reference points, not an ultimate authority.

Calorie piggy bank. You have a daily budget of calories to spend. You spend them by eating, but you earn more calories to eat by exercising. We do not recommend women consume fewer than 1,200 calories per day or men fewer than 1,500—those numbers are for people who don't exercise. And don't get too excited about the calories you "earned back" through exercise. The purposes of exercise are to relieve stress, improve cardio function, make our own medicines, and lose excess fat. Exercise is *not* an excuse to overeat. "Oh, sweet! I worked out. Now where's the burger and fries?" That kind of rationalization can lead to a never-ending roller coaster of guilt. It's very easy to overestimate calories burned, or not accurately log them. For example, an average one-hour walk will only burn 200–300 calories, depending on the intensity and your personal metabolism—not enough to justify that burger and fries. Unless you're exercising at moderate to high intensity for an hour or more several times a week, or are actively trying to gain weight, you most likely don't need to be worried about eating all of those calories burned in exercise.

Knowledge is power. One of the biggest advantages of using apps is that they keep food choices in perspective. You input your favorite meals and snacks, and the app tracks calories, fat, protein, and carbs. Then you go to your favorite restaurant, look up your go-to items, and find that they contain a stunning number of calories. That calorie app can be the tether that keeps you from falling off the wagon.

Here are some of the top tech items that transformers like:

Wearables: Garmin and Fitbit
Food tracking apps/sites: MyFitnessPal, CalorieKing
Activity apps: MapMyRun, 7-Minute Workout
Recipe organizing app: OrganizEat—this is my new favorite app! Who else is guilty of scrolling through Facebook and Pinterest for fun, healthy recipes, only to take a screen shot and then totally forget about it? This free app allows you to upload a picture and organize all your meals by category.
Recipe app: Forks over Knives (plant based)
On YouTube: FitPlus5—Erin Basile for workout ideas
On Pinterest: You'll find just about every type of recipe there. Just make sure the ingredients are T5-approved.

TAKE T5 INTO YOUR WORKPLACE

Eat healthier, move more, look better, and work better! An interesting study showed how this could happen in the workplace. Researchers divided employees into two groups: one began following a real-food, primarily plant-based diet, and the other got no dietary counseling. Result: the plant-eaters improved their work productivity.

SHARE T5 AT WORK

Are you too busy between work and home to find time for T5? No problem. Where there's a will, there's a way. Let's integrate T5 into every part of your day. Round up your like-minded office mates and work together.

1. Powerwalk to lunch.
2. Plan a walking conference call.
3. Hire a yoga teacher to offer lunchtime yoga.
4. Always have healthy snacks available in your desk and fridge.
5. Have an office salad-in-a-jar party.
6. Enjoy a healthy-living challenge: for example, everyone pays a small ante, and whoever walks the most steps in a week wins.
7. Instead of emailing a coworker who works across the hall, walk to his or her desk.
8. Invest in a standing desk.

SHARE WITH YOUR FOUR-LEGGED FRIENDS

Our family pets need T5, too! Enjoying a morning power walk or run with your canine buddy is a great way to fit in your cardio, and I have found it is a very peaceful way to start my day.

SHARE IT BY TEACHING IT

Want to get a really big dose of the helper's high? Become a Dr. Sears Certified Health Coach. Our goal: *to inspire health education around the world.* See how at DrSearsWellnessInstitute.org.

I WISH I WOULD HAVE

How many opportunities to feel the helper's high did you enjoy, or pass up, today? On a recent coast-to-coast flight I was working on putting the final touches on this book. Sitting next to me was a person whose body and habits clearly showed he needed T5. He guzzled several diet colas and

Grow Your Helper's High

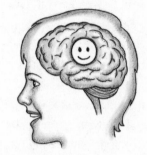

Share with 5 friends

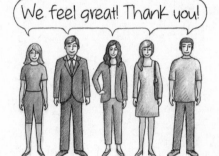

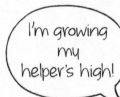 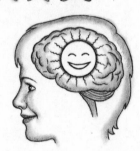

didn't move much while seated (he could have been doing isometrics), but I was too much in I-focus to tune into his needs. As I walked off the plane, I was rightly bothered by, "I wish I would have shared T5 with this seat-mate." Because I didn't like that "should have" negative thought, I made a point not to repeat it.

I recently attended a seminar and the person seated next to me—her name tag said "Angela"—obviously needed T5. After the meeting, I introduced myself and gave her an opener: "Angela, I was impressed how intently you were focused on this presentation. We have a program called Transform 5, and I would love to share it with you. Here is my phone number. Please call me soon." She then gave me her phone number and email address, and I followed up.

After being eighty pounds overweight, a sitter, and a compulsive overeater, Angela has now been on T5 for two months, periodically checks in with us, and Erin helps her keep on the right T5 track.

What a good feeling I enjoyed by just going out of my way for a few minutes to share T5 with a person in need.

You can feel that, too!

PART II

TRANSFORM 5 FOR THE "BIG SIX":

GUT HEALTH, BRAIN HEALTH, INFLAMMATION, HEART HEALTH, DIABETES, AND CANCER

T5 is a health plan for all ailments at all ages. If you or a loved one has health issues in the brain, heart, gut, joints, or hormones, you'll want to read Part II, our extra T-tips specific to these medical problems. The human body is the most beautiful symphony orchestra ever made. All the organs play in synchrony with each other. When the heart-health section plays harmonious music, so do the brain, gut, and all the other systems. What you do for one organ helps all your other organs stay healthier.

The T5 approach to disease prevention and healing is perfectly timed for the era in which technology has taken over modern living. Not so long ago, medicine functioned like an auto mechanic: "This part is broken, we'll fix it," with surgery and/or medications. In fact, we've become very good at replacing parts—knees, hips, and even hearts. But despite Americans spending more, and enjoying amazing advances in medical technology, they were getting sicker.

Enter the modern age of *personalized medicine*. As phones have become smarter, so have humans. We now see that we can make our own medicines and take charge of our health—with consultation from a trusted healthcare provider.

Most transformers feel their first health effects in the gut. The brain recognizes that something good is going on in the gut and says, "Whatever you are doing down there, I feel better up here. Keep it up!" The gut brain and the head brain are partners in your T5 transformation, as you will now learn.

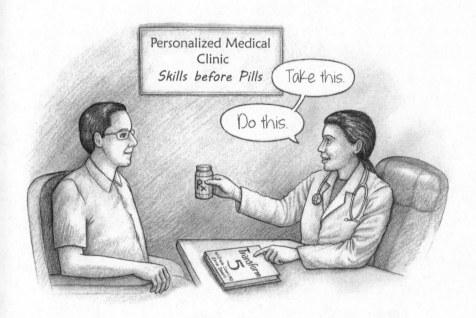

CHAPTER 6

T5 FOR GUT HEALTH

A ll disease begins in the gut," said Hippocrates. And that's where many transformers notice the earliest "feel-better" changes.

HOW T5 HELPS GUT HEALTH	
Gut Problem	T5 Solution
Heartburn, reflux	T5 grazing lessens reflux
Inflammation, colitis	Helps body make anti-inflammatory "medicines"
Constipation	Natural laxative way of eating
Infections	Supports a healthy immune system
Irritable bowel	Nourishes the gut lining
Leaky gut	Seals and heals the gut lining
Colon cancer	Lowers risk, helps recovery

Simply summarized, T5 helps ease the five "shuns": indigestion, constipation, inflammation, infection, and neurodegeneration.

Come along on a tour through your inside tract to see how T5 helps your gut feel good.

MEET YOUR MICROBIOME: WHAT IT IS, WHAT IT DOES, HOW TO MAKE IT WORK BETTER FOR YOU

Suppose you decide to make health your hobby. You consult a top preventive-medicine doctor.

"Doctor, I already do the dynamic duo, diet and exercise. Is there something more I can do to stay healthy?"

The doctor says, "I congratulate you on taking charge of your life by making health your hobby. How's your microbiome?"

"My what?"

"It's the organ in your body that is one of the most important, but the one you probably know the least about. Most of the patients I see have messed up microbiomes. By maintaining a healthy microbiome, you maintain your health."

Dr. Self-Care scribbles on a prescription pad:

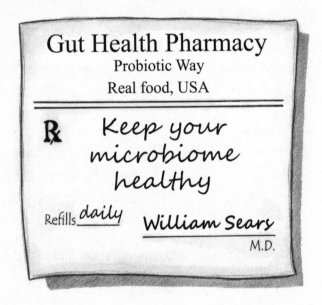

Gut Health Pharmacy
Probiotic Way
Real food, USA

℞ *Keep your microbiome healthy*

Refills *daily*   *William Sears*
M.D.

Microbiome (also called microbiota, or "little life") is now the number-one rising star of medical research topics and is the basis for one of the most doctor-recommended home medicines—*probiotics*. Get to know your microbiome!

"Microbiome" is the *community* of microorganisms, mostly bacteria, that reside mostly in your gut. In return for free food and a warm place to live, they do good things for their host. You will be surprised to learn what a powerful influence your microbiome has on your total body health. There is strength in numbers. These microscopic bugs outnumber our own human cells ten to one. (Obviously, they are very tiny compared to most of the body's own cells.)

Your microbiome is the biggest zoo in the world. An estimated 100 trillion bacteria reside in your gut, most of them in your colon, where more than a billion bacteria live in just one drop of intestinal fluid. These bugs weigh a total of around three pounds, making your microbiome one of the largest "organs" in your body.

T5 GROWS YOUR GUT GARDEN

If you want to grow a healthy gut garden, you need to do three things: plant the best seeds, feed and fertilize the soil, and keep the weeds and pests out. That's what the 5-S better-microbiome diet does.

- You *plant* the seeds (good bacteria) by feeding the gut lining (the soil) the foods it needs—high-fiber foods.
- You *fertilize* it with the 5-S diet.
- You keep the weeds and pests out by eliminating junk foods.

Having lots of good gut bugs helps with pest control. The lining of your gut has trillions of microscopic parking places. If the good bugs fill up the parking places, there's no place for the bad bugs to park and they simply get eliminated, pooped out. The best way to keep the bad bugs out is by encouraging more good bugs to grow, and that's what the 5-S diet does.

THE MIND–MICROBE CONNECTION

The "second brain." Your microbiome's influence extends from your bowels to your brain. The better we treat our microbiomes, the happier our minds. Call it your *mind–microbe connection*. Scientists call the gut "the second brain," because it has the most nerve cells of any organ other than your brain. 🖐

The gut brain is connected to the head brain. Throughout human history, the head brain and the gut brain have had a great working agreement for keeping each other, and the rest of the body, healthy.

The gut brain says to the head brain, "You've got to control those toxic thoughts—stress—that give me the queasies. The more relaxed I am, the better I can process the nutrients you need." So the head brain honors that request as best it can, and also prompts the human to eat real foods. That wasn't hard, since real food was all there was back then.

Then, very recently in human history, four radical unhealthy-living changes occurred:

1. The way we birth and feed our babies.
2. Children moved indoors where they sit rather than go outdoors, play, and get dirty.
3. The excessive antibiotics we give our children.
4. The artificial foods we invented.

Your second "personal pharmacy." The underlying theme of T5 is tapping into your own personal internal-medicine pharmacy to make your own medicines. On page 87 you learned about your internal pharmacy in the lining of your blood vessels. Meet internal pharmacy number two, the one in your gut.

YOUR MICROBIOME IS YOUR PERSONAL GUT-HEALTH PHARMACY

Think of your microbiome as your own internal biocomputer in the lining of your gut. These gut bugs manage your intestinal health. As the buggy figure below illustrates, you have trillions of tiny pharmacists working 24/7 in the lining of your gut to dispense "medicines" that you need, in the right dose, at the right time, custom-made just for you. And they're free! Also, these tiny pharmacists produce nutrients you need but don't usually get in your diet. Each person's microbiome is as unique as his or her fingerprints, *your personal bacterial thumbprint.* Just like people, the "pharmacy" staff needs to be housed, fed, and cared for. And the better you care for them, the better medicines they make for you.

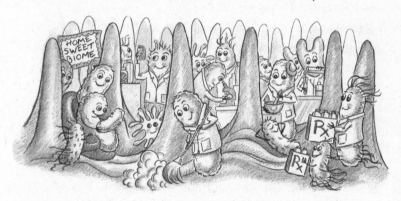

Gut Health Pharmacy

Intestinal lining

FIVE WAYS YOUR MICROBIOME HELPS YOUR HEALTH

Your gut is sensitive. Just as your head brain feels good when it thinks good thoughts, the gut brain is programmed to feel good when you eat well. One of the earliest gut feelings you may have after a few weeks eating the T5 way is, "That big burger bothered me." Good! It's supposed to! Your gut is now resensitized, transformed. Here's what your microbiome can do for you:

1. **Keeps bad bugs out.** Your microbiome fights the bad bacteria that enter your gut, keeping them from getting settled.

2. **Prevents leaky gut.** Your microbiome makes intestinal paints, sort of sealants (immunoglobulin A and butyrate), to keep invaders and foreign particles from leaking through the intestinal lining into the bloodstream. (See more about how T5 helps leaky gut, page 294.)

3. **Digests leftovers.** Your body does not like to waste food. So your microbiome lives off the leftover food that your stomach and small intestine can't digest, such as that chewy, fibrous asparagus stalk. (See more, page 205.)

4. **Sends biochemical messages to other organs.** Your microbiome communicates with other systems, especially your brain and immune system, to tell these systems how to behave. When this was discovered, the microbiome's status was upgraded to "the newest organ of the body."

5. **Dispenses nutritional "medicines."** Your microbiome turns food leftovers into nutrients your body needs, such as vitamins B and K, and others. It's especially important in making medicines your intestinal lining needs to heal and grow, nutrients you don't get enough of in your diet.

Microbial balance. Balance is critical to our health in many ways. For example, the maturing immune system has to learn how to fight germs to keep from getting infectious diseases, but not to "overfight" and attack your own tissues; that causes autoimmune diseases like allergies and asthma. Food allergies have increased 50 percent in the past decade, and one of the triggers for this is thought to be a microbial imbalance. You will always have healthy and unhealthy bugs in your gut. The goal of intestinal self-care is to make sure the good microbes far outnumber and outfight the bad microbes. Microbiologists estimate an 85:15 percent ratio of good bugs to bad bugs is fine, but they aren't sure. As one doctor explained microbial balance to me, "The good guys take up all the barstools so the bad guys can't get a drink."

AMERICANS, WE HAVE A PROBLEM	
Gut Problem	T5 Solution
Standard American diet (SAD)	Eat only real foods
Excess drugs unfriendly to microbiome	Self-care: more T5 skills, fewer pills
Gorge eating	Graze eating
Stress, anxiety	Meditate more, agitate less
Sitting too much	Move more
Germaphobia	Go outside and play—and get dirty!

SYNERGY: YOUR SYMBIOTIC SYMPHONY INSIDE

Synergy is another one of the top T5 concepts in healthy eating, and the reason why a multifruit smoothie or a multivegetable salad is so good for you. Synergy means, "We play better as a team." Eat a variety of nutrients together—or, as Dr. Mom said, "Put more color on your plate"—so each nutrient prompts the others to do a better job for the body.

Could synergy be important for a healthy microbiome? Likely so. When you put many different kinds of good bacteria together (the term is "microbial diversity"), each one having a unique biological function in the gut, they team up better to keep the bad microbes in check.

The hormonal harmony of health is the theme of many of my health lectures. Your body is a symphony orchestra, and all the hormones, when they are in balance, play beautiful music. When they are out of sync, you get sick. The same is true with your microbiome, which is why most of the bacteria in your bowels are called *symbiotes*, little bugs that play together for the health of their host.

"MEDICINES" YOUR MICROBIOME MAKES FOR YOU

A medicine, we believe, is any substance you take—or make—that improves your health. (In that sense the nutrients in food are medicine.) Researchers estimate that around *10 percent* of the nutrients you need come from your microbiome. Your healthy microbiome makes five groups of internal medicines:

1. WEIGHT-MANAGEMENT MEDICINES

Could your microbiome be keeping you lean or making you fat? Research reveals that your microbiome contains "lean bugs" and "fat bugs."

Lean mice and fat mice. Researchers transplanted microbiome samples, actually fecal samples, from the intestines of fat mice to lean mice, which consequently became fat mice. Why this happens is still under investigation, but one hypothesis is that the fat bugs are more efficient at transferring the calories from the food we eat to excess belly fat. It seems the same connection exists in humans. One of the main reasons why most diets don't work or last is they don't satisfy the microbiome. Both the head brain and the gut brain say, "We're still hungry."

Your internal weight- and waist-control managers. A personal weight-control trainer resides inside your gut, and it's your microbiome. These intestinal trainers help regulate how much food you need to eat to match the energy you burn. Body fat is affected not only by what you eat, but also by what your microbiome eats. Could it be that the more fuel your bugs burn, the more fat *you* burn? There are enzymes you need for food digestion that your body doesn't produce—you only get them from your gut flora. An imbalance of the gut bugs could lead to an imbalance of weight-control enzymes. The SAD diet feeds the fat bugs and malnourishes the lean bugs. Do you want that going on in your gut?

RED AND GREEN LIGHTS IN YOUR GUT

The gut brain, your microbiome, tells the head brain that it needs more food, or less. The head brain then triggers hormonal messengers, which prompt, "Eat less, you're satisfied, stop eating!" or "Eat more, go for it!" When the stop-and-go lights are balanced, your gut traffic, good gut feelings, and waist-control management run smoothly.

Our microbial prompts. The bottom line is that our microbiome prompts us to choose foods that meet our nutritional needs as well as theirs. For example, when we consume prebiotics, food that the bacteria like (see best foods for bowel bugs, page 209), the good bacteria thank us and increase the production of biochemical messengers that make us feel satisfied. When we were hunter-gatherers, these internal mechanisms helped us adapt to cycles of plenty and scarcity. Today, we hunt in the aisles of supermarkets and gather too much of what we like but don't need.

Activates "medicines" in food. An underappreciated role of our microbiome is that it upgrades compounds naturally found in plant foods to actually become internal medicines. Two examples are *sulforaphane,* an antioxidant, anti-cancer compound found in broccoli; and *lignin,* an estrogen-balancing nutrient found in flaxseeds. These two nutrients occur in plants as *precursors*, meaning they don't do anything for the body unless they're biochemically tweaked after we eat them. That's what the good gut bugs do. It's as if they press activation buttons in the nutrients.

2. HEALTHY FATS

If your microbiome could speak, it would shout, "I need a right-fat diet, not a low-fat diet!" Nutritional experts have finally realized that we don't get fat by eating fat; we get fat by eating junk carbs. The worst dietary advice ever given in America was the low-fat diet. We just got sicker and fatter. The microbiome realized the problem and came up with the solution: "We're going to have to make more fats for our own survival and make fats that our host needs to keep healthy."

Fabulous fats from fiber. One of the main fats the microbiome makes is short-chain fatty acids (SCFAs). These are some of the most healthful fats you can make. They provide nutrients to feed the lining of your large intestine to keep the cells healthy, including preventing them from turning cancerous. One of the most important gut-made fats is butyric acid, also called butyrate—more on this shortly. Also, SCFAs are among the body's quickest sources of energy, but the one deficient in most diets. Fiber from the spinach salad you chewed is digested by your microbiome into these fats, which then prompt you to feel fuller and not overeat. This is thought to be one of the reasons why people with a healthy microbiome diet tend to be leaner.

If you need it but don't eat it, we'll make it.

Fertilizing fats. Think of SCFAs as irrigators and fertilizers for your gut garden. They help the intestinal lining absorb water, repair and regrow cells, and protect the cells in the lining from becoming inflamed or cancerous. This is, providing that you feed them the foods they need to do their job, as you will learn on page 209. Another benefit of these good fats is that they help grow the villi bigger and stronger in your gut. Villi are tiny finger-like projections on the wall of the intestine, and each one is covered with microvilli. This greatly increases the gut's surface area for better absorption of nutrients. Healthy villi don't leak. Remember, "leaky gut" is a bad effect of the SAD.

Fermenting fats, making multivitamins. Your gut bugs don't like to waste food. Through *fermentation,* the gut bugs in your lower intestine digest the fiber, carbs, and protein that were not digested and absorbed in the upper intestine, and use these leftovers to produce SCFAs. 🖐 Your gut bugs also make vitamins A, D, K, and many of the B vitamins.

3. IMMUNE SYSTEM BALANCE

Immune system imbalance is the root of many "sick and tired" illnesses and a major challenge for modern medicine. Doctors call America the "inflammation nation." Nourishing a healthy microbiome helps train your immune system to act as it should, in balance. This is good design, since 70 percent of your immune system resides in your gut, right where your microbiome lives.

Your microbiome teaches the germ-fighting immune cells, such as T-cells, which germs are friendly and which are harmful. Once a T-cell has finished its training, it is ferried into the circulation and travels throughout the body. Say the soldier cells of your immune system are standing guard in the tissues of the airway passages when some germs come in. These cells are already programmed to identify whether these germs are friend or foe, and to deny entry to any bad guys. (Read about how your immune system soldiers shoot cancer cells dead, page 257.)

4. HELPS PREVENT COLORECTAL CANCER AND LESSENS LEAKY GUT

I believe I healed from colon cancer mainly because my 5-S diet nourished my microbiome. Colorectal cancer (CRC) is the second most commonly diagnosed cancer in the world. In Europe, it's also the second most common cause of cancer-related deaths in both men and women. The good news is that even though there is a genetic predisposition (my father died of CRC), new insights have shown that 85 percent of CRC is due to diet and lifestyle factors and less than 15 percent is due to genetic predisposition. What diet and lifestyle factors are preventive? The ones in Transform 5. Intestinal cancers are caused by the cells of the lining growing out of control. Your microbiome is the protector of these cells. The healthier your gut lining, the stronger your gut police are in number and the ability to *fight and protect.*

Having had CRC, I was motivated to learn why I got it, how to keep it from coming back, and how to help others heal from it and avoid getting it. At that time, twenty years ago, microbiome research was just beginning.

Now it has blossomed and produced fruitful findings: the healthier your microbiome, the lower your risk of CRC. Fear of cancer is a great motivator for people, even doctors, to make long-overdue changes in diet and lifestyle. It certainly was for me. Twenty years later I am free of cancer and colon polyps (which are seen as cancer precursors) and am a much healthier person with good gut feelings. I owe much of this good outcome to self-care—specifically to growing a healthy gut garden. I continue to enjoy a healthful cycle: learn it (study what's best for the bowel bugs), eat it, feel it, crave it, share it. My T5 story began in my gut.

Lessens leaky gut. When too much bad bacteria and other bad stuff enter the gut, the good bacteria find their neighborhood hard to survive in. The human host gets sick, mainly because those invaders cause the gut to leak. It's only in the past decade that the disease informally called "leaky gut" showed up in the doctor's dictionary. The gut lining, the main checkpoint for screening out harmful bacteria and chemicals, weakens. That's what gets strengthened by the Transform 5 program. One of the gut-friendly jobs your microbiome performs is *mucosal tightening,* an anti-leaking process involving butyric acid, a natural protective sealant made by your microbiome and found in certain foods, such as ghee, butter, and parmesan cheese.

When your microbiome is weakened or under heavy attack, it fails in its mission to stand guard over your intestinal lining. When the lining is exposed to attack and becomes inflamed, the spaces between its tightly packed cells open, allowing undigested food particles and chemical toxins to leak through. This is responsible for the modern epidemic of irritable bowel syndrome, colitis, and the host of other -*itis* illnesses and intestinal upsets now called "leaky gut syndrome." (If you suffer from leaky gut, see page 294.)

We lessen leaks.

5. YOUR MICROBIOME CAN MELLOW YOUR MOODS

Yes, your gut has a mind of its own. While "my microbiome made me do it" won't get you off the hook in court, your gut bacteria can produce neurohormones that alter behavior and emotion and release them into the bloodstream so that they go to the brain. ✋ If the microbiome is in a bad mood, it can put the head brain in a bad mood. So your anxiety isn't always "all in your head." There could be something "bugging" you in your gut. Let's take a trip along the lining of your large intestine to see how this works.

Your microbiome makes happy medicines. In fact, nearly 90 percent of your happy hormone, serotonin, is made in the gut and then shipped to the brain. While diseases of the heart have not increased, and some have even decreased, diseases of the brain are increasing at an alarming rate, and at younger ages. Hence the advent of the exciting, yet mysterious new science called *psychoneurogastroenterology*. Translation: Fix the gut to fix the brain.

The mind–microbe–leak connection. Let's start here: Psychoneurologists discovered that a leaky gut leads to a leaky brain. Neurotoxins (such as chemical food additives) get past the gut's security checkpoints into the bloodstream and travel to the brain. There they pass through a second checkpoint, the blood–brain barrier (BBB), and damage the brain.

Now let's talk about the effects of stress. It causes both security systems—the microbiome-protected gut lining and the BBB—to leak. The mechanism seems to be that stress prompts the microbiome workers in the intestinal lining to make chemicals that cause the lining to leak or self-destruct. You've heard about neurotransmitters, those magical medicines that your brain makes to govern your moods. As we mentioned, many are made in your gut.

Here's how this seems to work. Serotonin, the happy hormone, is made mostly in the gut. Gut bugs make the amino acid tryptophan, the main building biochemical of serotonin. One of the top gut bug "pharmacists," *Bifidus* (we call it "Bif") raises levels of tryptophan. This seems to be one of the ways in which our microbiome makes us happy. Preliminary studies suggest microbiomes may also make GABA, a top anti-anxiety nutrient. There is even a neurologic name for this psychotherapist inside: the enteric nervous system.

Gut skills over brain pills. So the pieces of the mood-managing microbiome puzzle are starting to come together. Most mood disorders are accompanied by gut disorders. We used to blame only the head brain for letting us "down" and anxiety for making us sick to our stomachs. Now we know we need to focus also on caring for our gut brain to help us stay happy. The mood-managing chemicals move in both directions between the head brain and the gut brain. Think of irritable behavior and irritable bowel as partners in unhappy health.

New insights in how the microbiome in the gut brain can affect behavior of the head brain are all the more reason for doctors to prescribe a healthful diet before rushing to prescribe pills. Your gut brain and head brain both prefer this approach, since mood-altering medications have the highest incidence of undesirable head and gut side effects (especially constipation and poor weight control) than any other group of prescription medications. Why trade troubles in the brain for pains in the gut if you don't have to?

Slow down, gut. For all we've learned about the way your gut brain affects your head brain's moods, the reverse is still true. How your head brain behaves affects the function of your gut brain microbiome. For example, suppose you are prone to anxiety attacks or just have prolonged, unresolved stress. The anxiety center of the brain gets dialed up, which naturally connects to the dials that signal the intestines to slow down and rest, because there is stuff going on in the head brain that requires more blood flow. The problem is, when intestinal mobility is slowed down, partially digested food remains too long in the intestines, causing constipation and increased growth of harmful bacteria. Or, sometimes the opposite happens; anxiety speeds up the intestines, causing diarrhea. Eventually, this contributes to inflammation and leaky gut. Some neuroscientists even use the phrase *melancholic microbes.*

Yet in a relaxed state, when the parasympathetic nervous system (PNS) predominates—it's your relaxation or cool-down mood center—intestinal movement and blood supply are normal, which promotes the growth of helpful bacteria and better digestion. Your moods affect how your bowels move.

PROBIOTICS: WHAT THEY DO FOR YOU

You've heard about probiotics, a bunch of good-for-you bugs in a pill. Probiotics (the word means "for life" or "for health") have been extremely popular nutritional supplements in Europe for decades, and have finally caught on in America. Supplying extra bacteria to your microbiome, these nutraceuticals now proudly reside next to a fruit and vegetable supplement and an omega-3 supplement in health-conscious people's medicine cabinets. Probiotics help build a better microbiome that does these good things for your body:

- Helps digest food
- Balances your immune system
- Makes nutrients your body needs
- Grows a nonleaky gut lining
- Trains your genes to behave (epigenetics)
- Helps prevent allergies
- Helps prevent intestinal *-itis* illnesses
- Mellows moods
- Eases pains in the gut
- Lowers risk of colorectal cancer
- Lessens diabetes
- Promotes weight and waist management
- More to come—the microbiome is one of the top research topics being studied.

From this list you can see that your microbiome does more than make gas. (See AskDrSears.com/Probiotics for how to choose a probiotic.)

DIET AND THE HEALTHY MICROBIOME

Suppose a research team of microbiologists wanted to do a population study to see which diets are best and worst for the microbiome. To study the worst, they wouldn't have to devise an experimental diet or study impoverished cultures in the developing world. The worst diet for the gut is right here: the standard American diet. To prove her point that SAD is bad for the good bugs in the gut, the lead scientist whips out her iPad and shows this slide:

FIVE OF THE WORST DIETARY HABITS FOR YOUR MICROBIOME	
Bad-for-your-microbiome diet	SAD (standard American diet)
• Low fiber	√
• High added sugar	√
• Processed, artificial foods	√
• High ratio of omega-6 to omega-3	√
• Gorging rather than grazing	√

A microbiologist from Asia might add more reasons why microbes don't live well in America:

- Higher use of antibiotics and antacids.
- Lower diet of prebiotic foods, such as garlic, ginger, turmeric, onions, tomatoes, cruciferous vegetables, chilies, green tea, and so on.

To make the point and close the meeting with a bit of culinary humor, the Asian scientist adds, "And Americans gobble fast with forks instead of eating slowly with chopsticks."

It's so SAD! Suppose our team of scientists wants to extend their experiment to study the effects of diet on the microbiome—and subsequently on the overall health of the body and brain. To devise the worst diet, they study the literature on the effect of diet on the brain, the gut, the heart, and all the major chronic diseases. What diet do they come up with now? You guessed it! Once again it's the SAD diet. For the past thirty or forty years we have been participating in one giant experiment in how to eat for bad health.

The SAD diet promotes sad intestines. How our diet and lifestyle affect our insides is shown by people who move to the United States from countries with diets that are much more plant-based, who then suddenly overwhelm their intestinal residents with feedlot-fed meat and highly processed foods. When they start eating like Americans, they get sick like Americans. The SAD diet starves the microbiome. It is high in animal fats and low in plant fiber, a combination that sets up the gut for *putrefaction*—literally, rotting. Microbe scientists estimate that 75 percent of the food in the Western diet is of little or no benefit to the internal pharmacy in your gut.

SAD from top to bottom. Most of the processed, "refined" carbs we eat are absorbed in the upper GI tract. What little gets to the lower end, where most of the microbiome resides, does not qualify as microbe food. This is a double-fault: unhealthy for human consumption in the upper intestine and unfit for microbiome consumption in the lower part.

GET YOUR GUT BACK: HOW THE 5-S DIET IS BETTER FOR YOUR MICROBIOME

Your microbiome should continually prompt you: "Feed me right, and I'll help you feel right." When you're tempted to take a bite of fake food, think: "Would my microbiome like this?" What is our T5 microbiome diet? Simply, it's a *real-food diet*.

There are two phases in growing your gut garden:

Phase 1: Remove foods—processed, unreal foods—that damage your gut garden.

Phase 2: Replant: reseed and fertilize your gut garden with foods that help it grow best.

You'll get your gut back into balance.

Five features of the Better Microbiome Diet:

1. *High* in foods most easily digested by your microbiome: fermentable foods,* friendly fiber, and prebiotic foods (see list page 293).
2. *Low* in processed fake foods, artificial flavor enhancers, and "carb-spike" foods, and *high* in "carb-steady" foods.
3. Higher in plant-based foods, lower in animal-based foods.
4. Rich in science-based probiotic supplements.
5. Right balance of omega-3 and omega-6 fats.

THE 5-S BETTER-MICROBIOME DIET: FIVE EATING CHANGES IN FIVE WEEKS

You read about the 5-S diet in chapter one, but let's briefly go back through those five Ss to see how they affect microbiome health.

---

* Fermentation essentially means your gut bacteria predigest the sugars so that your gut enzymes don't need to. Through fermentation, the bacteria use up the lactose in yogurt so that there is less of that spikey sugar than there is in milk. This is often why people who are confirmed lactose-intolerant can comfortably eat yogurt—usually in small amounts. This spike-less feature is also a reason why yogurt is healthier than milk, especially for people who are diabetic or prediabetic. If fermenting microbes could talk, they would boast: "We're helping you eat a lower-sugar diet." Fermentation, also called Mother Nature's refrigerator, helps keep food from spoiling by producing protective lactic acid, which gives yogurt the tart taste.

1. SALADS AND SPICES

If your microbiome could talk, it would say, "A salad a day keeps the doctor away." Fiber is the microbiome's favorite food, and that's where salads shine. When all that crunchy, chewy stuff that comfortably fills you up sooner and prevents overeating gets into your lower gut, your microbiome really enjoys the feast. The greens and beans in salads are top sources of your microbiome's favorite foods:

- Go green with organic arugula, kale, spinach, chard, and beet greens.
- Go red with tomatoes and peppers.
- Add a tablespoon of organic extra virgin olive oil to increase the synergy and intestinal absorption of the nutrients from the vegetables.
- Gut microbes love spices, especially turmeric, black pepper, ginger, rosemary, chilies, and cinnamon.

Check out the recipe for Dr. Bill's Delicious, Nutritious Microbiome Salad in Appendix C, page 332.

FIBER: FAVORITE FOOD FOR YOUR GUT GARDEN

Here's yet another reason to eat more fiber. You can't digest fiber, but the bugs in your microbiome can. It's their favorite food. You may not enjoy the stringy, chewy stuff in an asparagus stalk, but your gut bacteria thrive on it. It's as if your microbiome is saying, "Feed me your leftovers, and I'll turn them into really good food for your gut garden." The fiber-filled smoothie and salad of the 5-S diet is just what the gut doctor ordered. Fiber feeds gut flora.

There are two kinds of dietary fiber: soluble and insoluble. Soluble fiber is prebiotic. They feed our friendly flora, which is what the microbiome used to be called. Soluble fiber is readily fermented

(continued on next page)

in the colon to produce those "gut guardians," short-chain fatty acids. Insoluble fiber does not ferment, but it absorbs water and makes bowel movements easier. Good sources of soluble fiber are legumes, vegetables, apples, pears, oats, barley, flaxseeds, and beans. Good sources of insoluble fiber are whole grains, nuts, seeds, and skins of fruits.

Your microbiome affects food cravings. Your healthy bowel bugs crave what is best for you, and they send biochemical messages to the brain to crave good food. When your brain is trained to listen to those messages, you get hungry for real food. And when you eat it, your microbiome rein-forces your choice by giving you good gut feelings. Your microbes are just like your mother, urging you to eat more vegetables. They want you to eat the foods that are best for them and you.

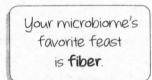

Your microbiome's favorite feast is **fiber**.

Dr. Bill

2. SMOOTHIES

The quickest way to get your microbiome in shape is to shake it up via the "sipping solution" (see page 8).

A smoothie a day helps your microbiome stay healthy.
Blending is better than juicing, because it preserves the fiber, your microbiome's favorite food. In our experience, our simple sipping solution will transform your gut microbiome and your gut feelings the quickest. It gets your gut used to a new way of eating by pleasing your gut brain in five ways:

1. The sipping solution resets the microbiome into balance, so eventually you will crave your smoothies at least five days a week.

2. It also resets your gut feelings so that you're satisfied with less.
3. It is a powerhouse of awesome antioxidants—natural, health-promoting nutrients that benefit your microbiome.
4. Your microbiome loves fiber-rich blended foods, because the fiber is already broken down into smaller, more easily digestible particles.
5. You get good gut feelings, because your microbiome is behaving as it should.

(See page 9 for Dr. Bill's gut-transforming smoothie suggestions.)

3. SEAFOOD

Go fish! Eat two servings (two fistfuls) of seafood weekly. If you're not fond of fish, eat it anyway. As described in chapter one, you'll gradually learn to love it. (See page 192 for how omega balance promotes microbial balance.)

MEAT-OUT YOUR MICROBIOME

Most commercially raised meat messes up your microbiome, because industrial feeding has messed up the meat. But regardless of how cattle, swine, and chickens are fed, people who don't eat them tend to have healthier microbiomes than those who do. Possible explanations could be as simple as the antibiotics fed to animals or plant foods being higher in fiber—your microbiome's favorite food—than meat. Plant-food eaters usually have more daily bowel movements, too, and constipation is not good for your gut. Also, it could be that some nasty chemical byproduct of meat metabolism sickens the microbiome. If you do eat meat, best to go with the organic, grass-fed kind whenever possible.

---

4. SNACK SMART

If your microbiome could talk, it would ask you to feed it smaller but more frequent meals. That's one reason why in chapter two we suggested using chopsticks and grazing according to Dr. Bill's rule of twos:

- Eat *twice* as often
- Eat *half* as much
- Chew *twice* as long

When you chew food more, it's easier to digest it in your stomach and beyond. Your microbiome will thank you!

5. SUPPLEMENTS

The natural supplements we recommend in the 5-S diet on page 32 also benefit your microbiome, especially probiotics, Juice Plus+, and omega-3s. As you are transforming your gut garden, add a daily probiotic.

MORE MEALTIME TIPS FOR YOUR MICROBIOME

Beyond 5-S microbiome-friendly food choices, change the way you start your meals:

- Take a moment to pray, meditate, or just quiet down before you eat, to get your gut brain and head brain in a relaxed frame of mind.
- Take a deep breath and relax.
- Think happy thoughts, smile, and make happy conversation between bites.

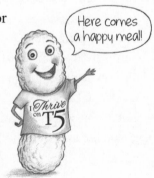

BEST FOODS FOR YOUR BOWEL BUGS

If your microbiome could write out your grocery list, here are items that would and would not be on it:

Green-light foods (eat more), organic when possible

- Apples
- Artichokes
- Asparagus
- Avocado
- Bananas
- Barley
- Beans
- Bee pollen
- Beets
- Bone broth
- Broccoli
- Coconut, unsweetened
- Cottage cheese
- Endive
- Garlic
- Ginger
- Green beans
- Honey, raw
- Jicama
- Kale
- Kefir
- Leeks
- Lentils
- Miso (non-GMO)
- Nuts and seeds
- Oats
- Oils: olive, coconut, avocado
- Onions
- Pomegranates
- Pears
- Quinoa
- Sauerkraut
- Squash
- Spirulina, Hawaiian
- Sweet potato
- Tempeh
- Tofu (non-GMO)
- Vinegar, apple cider
- Wild rice
- Yogurt

Yellow-light foods (eat less)

- White rice
- White potato (include the fiber-rich skin)
- White bread
- Pasta made with refined grains

Red-light foods (eat none)

- Artificial sweeteners
- High-fructose corn syrup
- Sugar-sweetened carbonated beverages 🖐
- Fast foods: fries, nuggets, burgers, hot dogs
- Deli meats, nitrite-preserved

T5 AND CONSTIPATION

Here's the scoop on poop. A third of the solid components in stools are gut microbes that have served their purpose and are ready, shall we say, to retire from their workplace.

One of the earliest gut-feeling changes I noticed was my bowel movements became softer, more numerous, and easier to pass. This had to be great for my gut, right? But why? I surveyed what stoolologists, poop experts, had to say. A person's poop reflects his or her intestinal health. People who poop more often generally enjoy a healthier gut and a healthier body. Since my first six months on T5, I have continued to enjoy at least *five bowel movements a day*. The better you care for your microbiome, the better you poop. Here's the science:

- People who eat the most plant foods poop more often, and people who eat the most meat poop the least.
- People eating the SAD diet (low in fiber, high in processed food) averaged *only five ounces* of stools daily. Those on a traditional high-fiber diet pass three times this amount.
- "Intestinal transit time" (the time it takes for food to move from mouth to out) is an indication of how friendly your diet is to your gut health. People on the SAD diet have a much longer transit time. The longer partially digested food stays in the gut and presses on and stresses the lining of your intestines, the more likely it is to cause diverticulitis, a disease in which partly digested food gets sealed off in a fold of the colon, causing severe inflammation and infection.

All this adds up to what I call microbial *intestinal turnover*—the rate at which old, worn-out microbes are eliminated and replaced by new healthy ones. The 5-S diet improves that, too.

Enjoy fun and informative tips for better bowels—download a free copy of the book *Dr. Poo* at AskDrSears.com/DrPoo.

Now that you know how T5 smartens your gut brain, let's see how it helps your head brain.

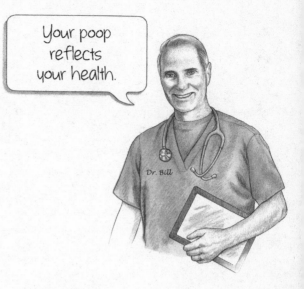

Your poop reflects your health.

Dr. Bill

CHAPTER 7

TRANSFORM YOUR BRAIN HEALTH

W hich organ needs transforming the most and which is likely to feel the most lasting effect? The gut, being the loudspeaker of the body, wins the *quickest effect* award. The heart is happy because T5 lowers its workload. But the brain wins the award for the biggest and most lasting transformation effect.

FIVE WAYS T5 IS TERRIFIC FOR BRAIN HEALTH

1. The brain is 60 percent fat. T5 says to eat a smart-fat diet.
2. The brain is richly vascular. T5 protects blood vessels.
3. The brain needs more healthy blood vessels. T5 *grows* blood vessels in the brain.
4. Brain tissue is most vulnerable to oxidation damage. T5 says to eat foods high in antioxidants.

(continued on next page)

---

5. The brain is bothered by stress and sticky-stuff spikes. T5 blunts spikes and stress.

STAYING SMART: FIVE SIMPLE BRAIN FACTS YOU MUST KNOW

What's your *brainspan*? Americans are living longer, but we are not living *smarter*. Our *brainspan*, the years we live before losing some of our mind, is getting shorter. The good news is the brain is the most "transformable" organ in the body.

1. WHY OUR BRAINS ARE SO VULNERABLE

The smartest organ in your body is also the one most vulnerable to getting sick, because we're all "fatheads"—the brain is 60 percent fat. Fat is the tissue most vulnerable to attack from oxidation, the top source of tissue damage. Oxidation of fat is also referred to as "turning rancid." Remember how that fatty fish fillet smelled after you mistakenly left it out all night?

I'm a fathead!

We rust. Which organ uses the most energy? Most people would guess the heart, but in fact, it's the brain. The heart is a relatively simple organ that does the same thing 24/7, but the brain is amazingly complicated and changes continuously. Even though the adult brain weighs only three pounds, 1 to 2 percent of your entire body weight, it uses

- 25 percent of all food energy,
- 20 percent of the oxygen you breathe,
- 15 percent or more of the blood your heart pumps, and
- 20 percent of all the antioxidants that you eat.

All this hypermetabolism causes a lot of wear and tear, *oxidative stress*, so the brain needs a high dose of anti-oxidants to blunt oxidation's harmful effects. T5 is terrific, because it is full of antioxidants—anti-wear-and-tear, anti-inflammatory, anti-rust foods. Again, antioxidants are awesome.

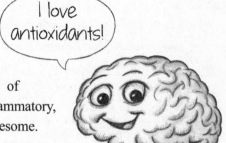

2. HOW THE BRAIN NATURALLY PROTECTS ITSELF— AND DOESN'T

As you might expect, the organ that runs the show is the best-protected one. Besides being enclosed in a thick skull, most of its tissues are defended by the *blood–brain barrier* (BBB), a protective wrap one cell thick that acts like a smart filter, letting in the nutrients the brain needs, yet screening out neurotoxins and other harmful stuff. The problem with the BBB is that sometimes it leaks. In fact, many neurodegenerative diseases can be attributed to a leaky BBB—similar to what we discussed in the last chapter, leaky gut. The T5 brain health plan helps keep your BBB from leaking.

Eye feel safe. Since the eyes are really an extension of the brain, there is also a protective wrap in the vessels of the retina, the blood–retinal barrier (BRB). We know much more about the BRB than the BBB, because eye vessels are easier to study. Scientists can look directly at the tiny capillaries in the retina by shining a light through the pupil the same way your eye doctor does during an exam. Neuroscientists know that fruits, vegetables, and seafood help keep the BRB from leaking, because these smart foods contain neuroprotectant bioflavonoids and DHA. While we can't shine a light on the BBB of the brain, it seems safe to assume that these same foods are good for the brain. (See "Eye Feel Good!," page 117.)

3. THE BRAIN CAN CHANGE

Another function that protects the brain is *neuroplasticity,* its ability to repair damaged and worn-out cells, and grow new and smarter cells. Yes, you can teach an old brain new tricks. People who are disabled in one part of the brain often become super-abled in another part, a testimony to how the brain adapts to increase our chance of survival. A vivid example is that in blind people the area of the brain normally devoted to vision increases its sensitivity to touch, hearing, and smell. I remember a blind mother bringing me her baby for treatment of a rash. I couldn't see any rash, but I trusted the mother's instinct enough to have her bring her baby back a day later. Sure enough, now there was a rash. She could feel it a day before I could see it.

You can think yourself into brain health. In chapter four you learned how worry robs the brain of the very neurochemicals that make it smart and happy. One of the most fascinating revelations in recent years is how our thoughts can dial up neurochemicals that nourish the brain and make it smarter and healthier. Conversely, our thoughts can dial up neurochemicals that damage brain tissue.

You are what you eat, and you are what you think. A major aspect of our brain health plan is how you can think yourself happy, well, and smart.

4. THE BRAIN CAN SHRINK AS YOU AGE—IF YOU LET IT

The good news is the brain doesn't have to shrink as we get older. The bad news is that in 40 percent of persons over age sixty, it does. The brain doesn't have to get weaker with age the way muscles do. We can grow new brain cells, repair worn-out ones, and even make lots of new connections between brain cells *at any age.*

Scientists used to think that brain cells couldn't be replaced. This is because nerve growth factor (NGF), the natural neurochemical that repairs worn-out brain cells and grows new ones, can, without a preventive maintenance program, decline with age. As you will soon learn, you can increase your levels of NGF, which can both repair and regrow worn-out cells.

Live lean and clean. The older we get, the smarter we need to be about how our food, thoughts, and lifestyle affect our brain, mainly because the natural neuroprotective mechanisms may weaken with age. As noted, even the BBB tends to get leaky. But new insights reveal that as we get older, healthy diet and lifestyle help us maintain bone, muscle, and brain tissue. The older we get, the more we have to work at eating smart, staying active, and keeping our minds active and positive.

5. THE BRAIN IS THE MOST VASCULAR ORGAN

An organ is only as healthy as the blood vessels nourishing it, and because it works the hardest, the brain has the richest blood supply. Our T5 brain health plan helps you grow more blood vessels to the brain *and* keep the vessels healthy. Remember, stroke is one of the leading causes of disability and death. Some persons demonstrate memory loss due to multiple small strokes, "mini-strokes." Dementia is aptly described as hardening of the brain arteries.

The brain accumulates sticky stuff. A simple yet scientifically correct explanation of the cause of brain disease is: *The more sticky stuff you put in your mouth, the more sticky stuff gets into your brain.*

Alzheimer's, which we call *cognitivitis,* is caused by inflammation that results from accumulation of sticky stuff. There is an accumulation of amyloid plaque—brain sticky stuff—in two vital structures: the brain tissue itself, where it interferes with nerve transmission; and in the linings of small blood vessels. (The latter is one of the most common causes of nearly all brain diseases, especially neurodegenerative diseases and strokes—and it's preventable.) Also, when sticky stuff accumulates on brain cell membranes, the "doors" get stuck so that insulin can't open them. This, as you've learned, is called insulin resistance, and it causes high blood sugar, which affects the brain, among other tissues. This is why Alzheimer's is also called type 3 diabetes. In a nutshell, our T5 brain health prescription is as simple as this: keep sticky stuff out of your brain. (See more about sticky stuff, page 39.)

So it follows that you shouldn't wait until you're old to think about protecting yourself from Alzheimer's. One day I was playing golf with famed neurologist Dr. Vincent Fortanasce, author of *The Anti-Alzheimer's Prescription.* I asked Vince, "When does Alzheimer's begin?" His not-so-surprising answer: "Alzheimer's begins in childhood."

For that reason, and because other neurodegenerative diseases, especially multiple sclerosis, are occurring at younger and younger ages, the earlier you begin the T5 brain health plan, the better.

HOW FOOD AFFECTS BRAIN FUNCTION

The quickest way to change your brain is to change your diet. These special features of the brain make it the organ in your body that is most affected, for better or for worse, by what you eat:

Brain Function	Brain Food
Brain tissue is 60 percent fat.	Eat a *smart-fat* diet.
Brain uses around 25 percent of all food energy.	Eat a nutrient-dense diet for energy.
Brain produces lots of harmful *oxidation*, "exhaust," from a high metabolic rate.	Eat lots of *antioxidants*, plant-based foods.
Brain tissue is sensitive to artificial foods and chemical additives.	Eat a pure, "real-food" diet.
Brain is sensitive to sticky-stuff spikes.	Graze: Eat smaller meals, more often.

THE TRANSFORM 5 BRAIN-HEALTH PROGRAM AT A GLANCE

Our three most important goals in growing good brain health are:

1. Feed your brain *smart foods*.
2. Nourish your brain with more healthy *blood vessels*.
3. Increase your happy thoughts to make the *right connections* among brain cells.

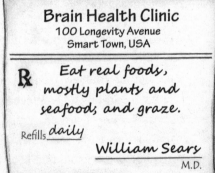

Brain Health Clinic
100 Longevity Avenue
Smart Town, USA

℞ *Eat real foods, mostly plants and seafoods, and graze.*

Refills *daily*

William Sears
M.D.

The T5 brain health plan is about how you *eat*, *move*, and *think*.

That is smart!

Growing a Healthy Brain: How You Eat, Move, and Think

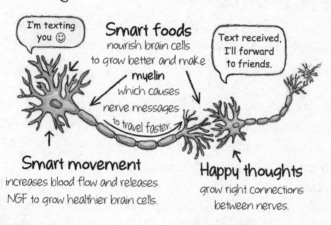

I'm texting you 😊

Smart foods nourish brain cells to grow better and make **myelin** which causes nerve messages to travel faster.

Text received, I'll forward to friends.

Smart movement increases blood flow and releases NGF to grow healthier brain cells.

Happy thoughts grow right connections between nerves.

Brain Health Problems	T5 Brain Health Solutions
Brain volume shrinks.	Exercise your body, grow your brain.
Fatty tissue wears out.	Eat a right-fat diet.
Brain tissue rusts.	Eat plenty of antioxidants.
Blood flow slows.	Move more to increase brain-growth fertilizer.
Stress wears out brain tissue.	Stress less.

T5 HELPS YOU GROW YOUR BRAIN GARDEN

The brain is smarter than any computer, because brain circuits can change themselves, form new pathways, and prune away disabled nerves. That mostly happens without your knowing, even while you're sleeping. You can never entirely unplug your brain as you can a computer.

Think of your brain not as a computer but as a garden—the greatest garden ever grown. *T5 is a brain-garden growth and maintenance plan.* You plant healthy seeds, feed, fertilize, and water them, prune the plants, pick the weeds, and keep out pests. You can do all that!

To truly appreciate how great your brain garden is, let's see how T5 helps your garden grow, step-by-step. The brain structures that are most affected by food are the four M's: membranes, mitochondria, myelin, and messengers.

T5 FOR SMART "PLANTS"

The plants in your brain garden are brain cells, or neurons. A neuron's outer protective membrane is composed mostly of fat. The 5-S diet is full of smart fats.

Feed the brain-cell membranes. *Every organ is only as healthy as each cell in it.* And each cell is only as healthy as the outer membrane protecting it. Think of the brain cell as a water-filled bag. The bag is the membrane that protects the inner structures of the cell, which are suspended in the fluid inside. Besides being protective, the membrane is *selective.* Throughout the membrane are many microscopic doors called receptors that act like delivery drop-off areas. Nutrients delivered by the blood come in through the doors and are stored and used inside the cell. Those tiny doors are smart and selective, like bouncers at an exclusive nightclub, magnificently designed to let in nutrients and other things the cell needs while screening out the bad stuff. Your diet affects how well these doors function. One example of this is the insulin resistance—type 2 diabetes—we discussed earlier (see page 156).

Feed the mighty mitochondria. Mitochondria are the cells' energy generators. Ever experience "brain fog" from low blood sugar? Your generators have simply run out of gas. Note that the mitochondria in your brain cells are some of the hardest working in your body. In fact, energy-deprived mitochondria are now described as a disease: *mitochondrial dysfunction.* (See related section, "Mighty Mitochondria," page 110.)

BECOME A SMART "FATHEAD"

Nerve cell fibers are like electrical cords. They do in fact carry electrical impulses, and like electric wires, they are insulated to keep current from escaping. The insulation is called *myelin.*

Make more myelin. Myelin protects and nourishes your neurons and keeps nerve impulses flowing along their intended pathways rather than leaking out—100 times faster than circuits that are not myelinated. Guess what the main component of myelin is. Fat. The epidemic of some neurodegenerative diseases such as multiple sclerosis are considered to be diseases of weakened myelin.

The high concentration of fat in the myelin and the rest of the brain cell is why brain tissue is 60 percent fat. This has two practical implications for brain health: (1) we need a smart-fat diet, not a low-fat diet; (2) because fat is the tissue most prone to oxidation, the brain needs a diet high in antioxidants, which is the 5-S way of eating.

NERVE CONNECTIONS: AN AMAZING TANGLING OF TENDRILS

Neurons, the brain plants, become "bushy" by growing branch-like nerve fibers. Each bush gets a genetic prompt to connect with others nearby. To picture it another way, lay your arm flat and spread your fingers. This is sort of what a nerve fiber looks like. At the fingers' ends are many smaller projections called axons (at the outgoing end of the neuron) and dendrites (at the incoming end). The axons of one nerve connect with the dendrites of the next, forming lines of communication throughout the brain and the rest of the body. These pathways let us make quick, sometimes lifesaving decisions; store memories; and tell the body to walk, talk, turn around, watch its step, and so on.

Smart means having the right connections. Each brain cell may send out as many as 10,000 to 15,000 branches connecting with branches on other nerve cells. Our T5 plan helps your brain grow smarter and more imaginative and creative by *making the right connections.*

Just by reading this book and studying these diagrams, you are making new brain connections.

Care about your connections. Another component of brain cell function is the *synapse,* which is the gap between the axon of one cell and the dendrite of the next. Put your two hands together so that your fingertips just about touch one another. The gap between your fingers is like the gap between brain cells. For nerves to communicate, something has to bridge this gap. Enter *neurotransmitters*, biochemicals that act like sparks flying across the gaps between nerve cells. The end of one branch is a sender that emits sparks looking for the receptors on the other cell.

Of course, the senders and receptors have to fit together right, like a key in a lock. If there's a misfit, the connection misfires, and your thinking goes haywire. Neuroscientists believe that the majority of mood disorders, such as depression, bipolar disorder, and anxiety, are caused by misfiring synapses. Guess what neurotransmitters need to keep them firing on target: real food. Nutritional neurologists explain it this way: fake food clogs the locks so the keys can't fit. Real food helps the locks and keys fit.

Be nice to your neurotransmitters. Over sixty neurotransmitters have been discovered thus far. Neurotransmitters, how many you have and how and when they fire, may actually be the neurochemical basis of "you."

FEED AND FERTILIZE YOUR BRAIN GARDEN

Nutrition affects the brain, for better or worse, more than any other organ. Nourish your brain with smart foods, and you'll grow a smart brain. Eat dumb foods, you'll go the other way.

Smart Foods	Dumb Foods
Wild salmon, sardines, anchovies, and other cold-water seafood	Sweetened beverages
Berries, especially blueberries	Chemical flavor enhancers, e.g., MSG
Greens	Factory-made sweeteners
Nuts	Foods high in "added sugar"
	Fiberless processed foods

Easy way to remember smart foods—go fish, go blue, go green, and go nuts!

Dr. Bill notes: At a recent conference on brain health, neurologists recommended eating *four fistfuls of greens* daily for optimal brain health.

HAPPY FOOD—WHAT SCIENCE SAYS

The lead article in the April 2016 issue of *Scientific American Mind,* titled "In Search of the Optimal Brain Diet," revealed a long-overdue scientific connection: the smarter you eat, the smarter and happier your brain. Neuroscientists are just now finding a scientific basis to the notion of "happy food." Population studies of diet's effect on happiness showed that three traditional diets are associated with the healthiest and happiest people: the Mediterranean diet, the Japanese diet, and the Nordic diet. What do these three have in common? First, more seafood. *Go fish!* Next, more antioxidant-rich vegetables. *Go green!* Finally, more nuts. *Go nuts!* And all these happy diets are *low in added sugar and processed foods.* In other words, they are *real-food diets*—just like the 5-S diet!

THE SAD DIET SHRINKS THE BRAIN

More and more neuroscientists are finding a direct link between the SAD diet and sad feelings. In the last five years, neuroimaging techniques have silenced the skeptics. Persons who consumed a Western diet not only suffered more mood disorders, but, according to MRI scans, *they showed a smaller hippocampus,* the brain's happy center. One proposed explanation is that a diet high in processed food causes neuroinflammation, which literally shrinks the brain. This would go along with the finding that depressed persons generally have higher blood levels of what are called inflammatory markers, sticky stuff. In other words, some "comfort foods" will eventually make you, shall we say, uncomfortable.

My fish story. I had the privilege of being a co-presenter at an omega-3 conference in Japan. Dr. Michael Crawford, the renowned neuroscientist who has studied the association between our evolving brains and eating more seafood, explained to me that our brains prefer what he calls "ready-made DHA" from seafood and use it much more efficiently than the omega-3 fatty acids from plants.

To make sure I understood this, I said, "So, Michael, the brain likes the tall guys, long-chain fatty acids with twenty to twenty-two carbon atoms, and those are only found in seafood. Land plants only have the short guys with eighteen carbon atoms, so the body has to run the short guys through the liver to add on two or four carbon atoms so the brain will let them in."

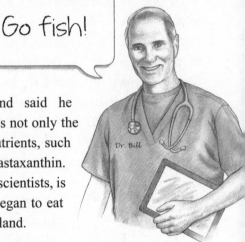

Crawford confirmed my science-made-simple explanation and said he liked it. He went on to explain that it's not only the omega-3s; fish give us other smart nutrients, such as iodine, selenium, vitamin D, and astaxanthin. His conclusion, shared by other neuroscientists, is that humans got smarter when they began to eat food from the sea as well as from the land.

MOVE MORE TO GROW YOUR BRAIN GARDEN

While movement makes medicines for all organs, the two that movement most helps are the heart and brain. Good science and good sense usually grow together. Movers tend to be leaner. Movement increases nerve growth factor (NGF), or as I call it, brain growth fertilizer (BGF). Conversely, obesity is often associated with lower BGF. Also, less movement leads to slower blood flow, which leads to a smaller brain.

If you asked me, Dr. Bill, what was the one change you could make that is scientifically proven to have a profound and lasting effect on your brain health, here is the prescription I would write for you:

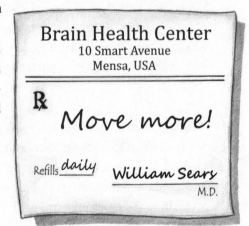

Brain Health Center
10 Smart Avenue
Mensa, USA

℞ Move more!

Refills daily   William Sears
M.D.

I'm not the only one who thinks so! In June 2017 I attended a fantastic medical conference on brain health hosted by the Institute of Functional Medicine, where two top brain scientists remarked specifically on exercise's beneficial effect on the brain.

Exercise is the number one brain growth factor.
—DR. DAVID PERLMUTTER, NOTED NEUROLOGIST AND AUTHOR OF *BRAIN MAKER*

Exercise is the mother of all brain growth factors.
—DR. JOHN RATEY, PROFESSOR OF NEUROPSYCHIATRY, HARVARD MEDICAL SCHOOL

YES, EXERCISE GOES TO YOUR HEAD

If you planted a garden, you would need two things to keep it growing and healthy: *irrigation* and *fertilizer*. Movement grows more irrigation channels, blood vessels. And it pumps into your garden natural neurochemical fertilizers, like BGF.

Activities like dancing and ping-pong require both movement and quick adjustments, which help strengthen the cerebellum and the prefrontal cortex. They also increase the volume of the basal ganglia, which helps the way you process visual-spatial information and is good for balance and preventing falls. These types of movement build strong memory, reduce stress, and reduce depression. One of the ways this seems to work is by increasing blood flow and delivery of blood sugar and oxygen to fuel the hungry brain. (See "Gotta Dance!," page 107.)

Movement makes more blood vessels. Once again, an organ is only as healthy as the blood vessels supplying it. This is especially true of the brain. The more blood vessels you grow, the better your brain works. Exercise decreases the *hypoperfusion syndrome,* a recently defined disease, that simply means the brain garden isn't getting watered and fed. Many people diagnosed with a neurodegenerative disease such as Alzheimer's have been found to have had multiple mini-strokes. In other words, their brains aren't functioning because they aren't getting enough blood supply.

Movement makes healthier blood vessels. It's not only the number of blood vessels, it's how wide open these vessels are. Sitters tend to have constricted blood vessels, and the lining of their blood vessels tends to be sticky. This is why diet and exercise are buddies in brain health. Diet keeps the sticky stuff off the tops of the medicine bottles in your body's pharmacy, and movement opens the medicine bottles to release natural medicines. (See page 91; see also the endnotes.)

Movement makes brain food. Increased blood flow to the brain increases the release of NGF, which is like Miracle-Gro for the brain.

A visit to Veggieland. One evening I had a memory mix-up. When I arrived at a venue to give a brain-health talk to what I had assumed would be mostly adults, I was surprised to be greeted by lots of kids. Solution: Brain switch. Take the kids on a smart trip to "Veggieland" where their brain grows like a garden. One of my favorite brain fertilizers is vascular endothelial growth factor (VEGF), a natural biochemical that helps keep the lining of the vessels smooth. It sounds like "Veg," so Veg became the hero of my story. After the talk, ten-year-old AnnaBelle showed me her drawing (see next page) of Veg popping up out of the endothelial medicine bottles to help her brain garden grow smarter.

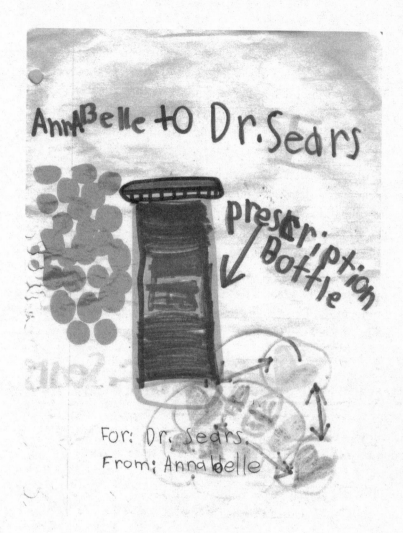

ALZHEIMER'S BEGINS IN YOUNG ADULTS

Like spacecraft, our bodies are designed with a lot of "redundancy" in case of damage. We have extra lung, kidney, and intestinal tissues, so that we can live well if parts of those organs fail. Critical exceptions are the *heart and brain*. We only have one

(continued next page)

each of those vital organs, and damage to even a small part of the heart or brain can be disabling or fatal. Heart and brain diseases both begin in childhood. Yes, autopsy studies have revealed the beginnings of Alzheimer's in the brain tissue of twenty-year-olds. I believe the obvious explanations are sitting too much and eating too much sticky stuff.

Researchers are now gradually coming to the conclusion that Alzheimer's disease is due to accumulation of sticky stuff and inflammation not only in brain tissue, but in the vessels that feed that tissue as well. In other words it's at least partly due to the same mechanisms that cause heart disease: stiffness and clogging of the vessels. And the slow but gradual loss of brain tissue may be mostly due to a gradual decline of blood flow. What is one of the top features of T5? An increase in blood flow to your tissues—all of them.

MOVEMENT MAKES MORE BRAIN MEDICINES

Next time you're walking for exercise with a group of friends, proudly exclaim, "It feels so good to be making my own brain medicines!" When they ask what in the world you're talking about, say, "I'm making my own personal neurochemicals to fertilize my brain garden. That makes my brain smarter and healthier and happier." You'll really sound smart if you add, "This discovery won the Nobel Prize."

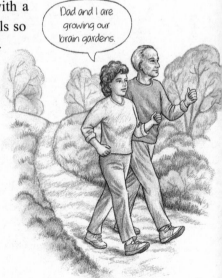

Dad and I are growing our brain gardens.

SCIENCE SAYS: MOVEMENT MAKES BRAIN MEDICINE

The new science called *psychoneuroendocrinology* reveals that exercise makes:

- Antidepressants
- Mood mellowers
- Happy hormones
- Anti-inflammatories
- Growth hormones for brain and body

(See the endnotes for more brain medicines movement makes.)

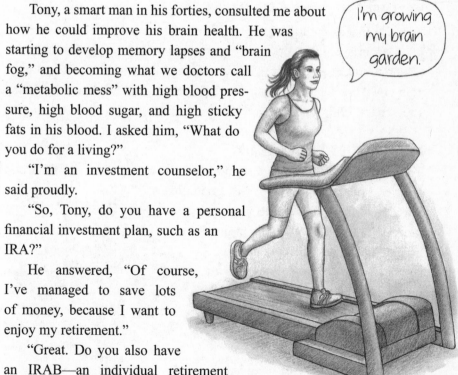

Tony, a smart man in his forties, consulted me about how he could improve his brain health. He was starting to develop memory lapses and "brain fog," and becoming what we doctors call a "metabolic mess" with high blood pressure, high blood sugar, and high sticky fats in his blood. I asked him, "What do you do for a living?"

"I'm an investment counselor," he said proudly.

"So, Tony, do you have a personal financial investment plan, such as an IRA?"

He answered, "Of course, I've managed to save lots of money, because I want to enjoy my retirement."

"Great. Do you also have an IRAB—an individual retirement account for your brain?"

I'm growing my brain garden.

He was astounded, "No, I hadn't thought of that. That makes sense."

I won my case, and he went home with my "retirement plan for brain health." I ended our conversation by telling him, "Keep that silver lining healthy, so you can better enjoy your silver years." Really, movement is the fountain of youth medicine for all ages.

MOVEMENT IS YOUR SMART FOUNTAIN OF YOUTH

One of the top youthful hormones in your brain's symphony orchestra is *growth hormone*. Sadly, the older we get, the less growth hormone we usually produce. Exercise helps you make more youthful hormones.

MOVEMENT MELLOWS YOUR MOODS

Exercise makes natural mood mellowers. This could be why exercisers often suffer less depression, since movement makes newer brain cells and newer connections that are "less depressed," sort of like getting out of your down brain and into your up brain. (See related section on mellowing stress, page 128.)

MOVERS ENJOY BIGGER BRAINS

You'll be happy to know that movers have bigger and smarter brains than sitters. The brain, like muscles, shrinks if you don't get physical exercise. As noted, brains tend to shrink as we get older. But movers' brains shrink less and grow smarter. As with muscle, the more you use it, the less you lose it. Movement increases blood volume and brain growth factor especially benefit the hippocampus, the area most involved in maintaining memory and thought

I'm getting smarter!

processes. (See related sections on best exercises for the brain, pages 107 and 228.)

GROW YOUR GOD CENTER: THE NEUROSCIENCE OF SPIRITUALITY

Can you *believe* your way to better brain health? Yes! Over my fifty years as a doctor I have noticed a strong relationship between a person's spiritual health and their mental health. This is why we include *spiritual fitness* in our T5 brain health plan for mental fitness.

SCIENCE SAYS: SPIRITUAL PERSONS ARE MORE LIKELY TO . . .

- Have happier brains
- Have healthier bodies
- Live longer
- Heal faster

(See DrSearsWellness.org/T5/References.)

When you focus your mind on God, you get out of yourself, your rut, your negative thoughts. You feel in control. You can choose the path of spirituality that best fits your mind, your family, your relationships, your life. This is why there are 18,000 different religious denominations in the United States. There are many common spiritual paths and themes, and we often choose different paths at different stages in our lives.

When you grow the "spiritual center" of your brain, you lower anxiety and depression, enhance social awareness and empathy, and think more clearly.

When I read neuroimaging studies of prayerful people, a light bulb went on: I realized why some of the best memories of my life were those spent with the most deeply religious people, especially my memorable mentors. What these studies show, and the results were not surprising, is that we can change our brain to more easily let God in.

My spiritual soul mate of 50 years, Martha, advised our teens to choose a spiritual person for a life mate. This takes on new meaning when you realize that a person actually has "spiritual" pathways in the brain that influence moods, sense of self, and how we treat others and see the world and beyond.

Growing your God center fits naturally into growing your happy center. It gives you hope: "God listens and heals." In fact, the scriptures of most faiths focus on taking charge of your inner self—that "you turn" again—and following scripture as a roadmap. The sacred texts of the great religions could appropriately be called "the greatest brain-health books ever written."

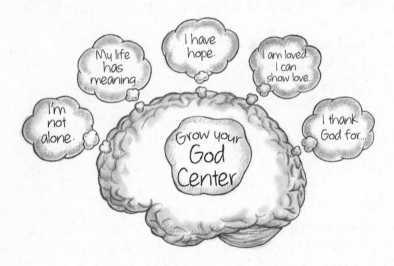

We should be helping infants, children, and teens grow their God centers at the times in their lives when their brains are most fertile.

"I'll just wait until my child is older . . ." Not smart! I was with a group of parents who prided themselves on being "modern" and "free thinkers." A mom said, "I'm not going to teach my child all this stuff. I want her to be a free thinker and make decisions on morals and habits when she's older." That thinking goes against both common sense and neuroscience. By that time, I really understood how children's brains developed. I had survived raising eight children and was in recovery from parenting eight teenagers. I listened respectfully to these parents' views, just waiting for an opportunity to explain why they were missing important windows of opportunity to help build growing brains. You plant seeds at the age when the ground is most fertile. You then fertilize those seeds at the age when they are genetically programmed to grow the smartest. *After* you've planted the seeds and nourished the roots, they're ready to try out free thought.

In the first five years of your child's life, you plant seeds and fertilize the roots. This is the age at which children usually just do what you ask and follow your example, despite the occasional, normal outburst of preschool rebellion. They learn the *we* principle: "In our home this is how *we* talk . . . how *we* act . . . what *we* eat . . . and what *we* believe." Children this age naturally accept "how we do things" as normal, whatever that might be in your family. That's why seeds and roots tend to grow best in the first five years, and why those children need the most parental guidance.

From five to ten years, children may begin to question these roots, but they still, for the most part, continue to accept the *we* principle. So you need to nourish these roots even more so they grow stronger and deeper. It's in the teen years that children become "free thinkers," naturally questioning parental guidance and wanting to do "their own thing." This is normal in the development of the brain—they may deviate from the family *we* principle into the *me* principle.

Here's where things can go happy or unhappy. Teens and young adults may go astray and get into trouble, but those with the deepest roots are the ones most likely to get back up when they fall, correct their mistakes and learn from them, bounce back, rediscover their roots, and follow the path their parents set them on when they were younger.

Still not convinced? Mental illnesses, especially depression, anxiety, addictions, and general feelings of "What is my life worth?" are at an all-time high among young adults. Growing a personal God center is good medicine for young, troubled minds.

FIVE EFFECTS OF BELIEF
ON MIND AND BODY

A healthy trend is that transformers are becoming more spiritual. A study of a group of churchgoers from nineteen Baltimore churches showed that more exercise and a healthier diet actually improved their spirituality.

Here are my observations and conclusions why the T5 effect and the belief effect are partners in mental health.

1. BELIEVERS HEAL BETTER

Science reveals that believers, regardless of specific religion, heal better physically and mentally. One reason seems to be that we are "wired" for God. Many neuroscientists believe that there are God centers in the brain where resides a natural impulse to believe in and call upon a supreme spiritual being. When you sincerely believe that God will help you heal, you're more likely to heal. It may even help to hear someone say, "I believe God will heal you." This is why statements like "I'm praying for your healing" are so helpful. Yes, prayer is good medicine.

A person who has a well-developed personal God center, or who is "open minded," has a head start in personal healing. Many doctors, your authors included, have noticed the more deeply spiritual a person is, the more likely they are to heal from physical and especially mental illness.

He makes the whole body fit together perfectly.
As each part does its own special work, it helps
the other parts grow, so that the whole body
is healthy and growing and full of love.
—EPHESIANS 4:16

In June 2015, I was invited to be a speaker on an important part of a brain-health prescription, relieving family financial stress. This course was held at the 610-acre Padgett's Farm in Waynesboro, Georgia. I was pleased to speak at a farm, not in a hotel conference room or big auditorium. My favorite themes, the neuroscience of nature and "go outside and play," naturally fit. The host asked me to talk about brain health, which was another natural fit: the better your brain health, the better equipped you are to manage your finances.

Upon driving into the farm it became immediately obvious that this was a spiritual place. The biblical verse on the side of the big barn said it all: "Seek ye first the Kingdom of God." Translation: The big thing is to seek God; do that first, and all your worries will be small. I realized that this family had learned the relationship between growing your God center and growing your business sense. On some speaking occasions, I don't bring in spirituality, because my audience isn't likely to accept it or even see it as "politically correct." However, this was the South, the Bible Belt. At this farm, I had home-field advantage.

2. BELIEVERS GROW THEIR EMPATHY CENTERS

Growing your God center grows your empathy center. Neuroimaging techniques, those windows into the brain, showed that meditation stimulates the empathy or social awareness center. Where in your brain is the compassion center? It seems to be in the anterior cingulate, a tiny structure that sits near the junction between the frontal lobe, which processes thoughts and behavior, and the limbic system, which governs feelings and emotions.

The anterior cingulate tends to be larger in women than in men, which may explain why women are generally more sensitive, empathetic, and socially skilled, but also more likely to react to fearful situations. Please note that differences between the sexes are only that. They don't mean that one gender is better than another. But this particular difference probably explains why women are more likely to be labeled as "sensitive." And that's a good thing! It means women typically have a greater capacity for caring and for empathy—sensing others' feelings. Yet higher sensitivity can have a downside. It may produce higher levels of anxiety, which could be the reason why more women than men are prescribed anti-anxiety medications.

While empathy and compassion are similar, compassion goes a step further by dialing up our ability to respond to another person's emotions and pain. Compassion allows us to be more tolerant and accepting of others' quirks and our own. Perhaps the larger and more active this compassion center is, the greater empathy you'll be capable of, which may be the neurological basis of "social skills." This compassion center is the one that is most stimulated by spiritual practices and meditation. (See the related section on growing your empathy center in chapter four, page 126.)

SET YOUR SENSITIVITY DIAL

Being called "sensitive" is a mixed blessing. Over my years in medical practice I have noticed that "sensitive" persons are more prone to anxiety. Here's my theory why: When your sensitivity dial is set just right you are compassionate, empathetic, caring, and appropriately bothered by injustices. Yet you can become "too" bothered by relative smallies and become overly anxious. This is why sensitive persons need to carry a larger toolbox of stressbusters to keep their sensitivity center set just right

---

Mind your mirror neurons. Mirror neurons are part of the brain's empathy center that fire in response to others' emotions; for example, as we watch someone laugh or cry. Empathy often translates into social action. Members of religious organizations that practice meditative prayer are more likely to serve in community charities. It also explains why monks who devote a great deal of time to contemplative practices are often activists in social or peace movements. The Dalai Lama, a monk, won the Nobel Peace Prize. For an in-depth discussion of the neuroscience and neuroimaging of empathy, read the books *The Mindful Brain* and *Mindsight* by Daniel J. Siegel. (See references for chapter seven, DrSearsWellness.org /T5/References.)

3. BELIEF BUILDS A YOUNGER BRAIN

Interesting studies from the Psychiatric Neuroimaging Research Program at Massachusetts General Hospital show that spiritual meditation can build a younger brain. The cerebral cortex usually gets thinner with age, but these studies showed that it actually thickened in older meditators. This means that by enjoying a rich spiritual life you can delay brain shrinkage and preserve your gray matter as you turn gray.

4. BELIEF BUILDS A HAPPIER SENSE OF SELF

Spiritual persons may have a better sense of self. Researchers who wired up meditators discovered that even when they were not meditating they generally had more activity, compared with nonmeditators, in the happiness center of the parietal lobe, the area of the brain that gives you your sense of self-worth.

Are God-centered brains neurochemically different? Yes! A study of people who routinely practiced a type of meditative yoga were found to have a marked increase in dopamine, the pleasure hormone, which is also very involved in stimulating positive thoughts. In short, dopamine is essential to our "sense of peace." This could also explain why people who have mastered the art of meditative prayer to the point that they feel like they are "in another world" actually have higher dopamine levels. (Remember, some of the increasingly common brain disorders, such as Parkinson's, are neurochemically dopamine deficiencies.)

Believers and nonbelievers. Suppose you were a neurologist, and the sort of pure scientist who has the "show me the God" mentality. You want to study the biology of belief. So you walk into a convent and ask Mother Superior if you can wire up some of the nuns to see how belief has wired their brains. Then you go across town to a monastery and ask the abbot if you can wire up a bunch of monks to see what's going on in their brains. You would discover that the worry centers in the prefrontal lobes of the monks' and nuns' brains are *less active* while they are praying. Your conclusion: *The prayerful believers are better able to quiet their minds to let God in.*

Then you gather together a bunch of self-proclaimed atheists, wire them up the same way you did the holy folks, and ask them to pray. Not surprisingly, you'll find that their brains don't change much during "prayer." Their brains are not primed to the God prompt: "Be quiet and let me in." Brain scan studies of atheists don't show an active center in the brain that lights up when they contemplate about "God," because God may have no value to them.

Actual studies of nuns and monks have concluded that meditators are more cerebrally able to "feel at one with God," or any thought or object on which they focus. Another conclusion of these studies is that people who master the art of meditation are able to dial down the "self center," the pre-occupation with and worry about what's happening to self, and are able to more easily and automatically dial up contemplation of God. In a nutshell, less about me, and more about everything else, God.

"Quiet the mind!" Isn't that what we all crave?

5. HELPS YOU TRASH TOXIC THOUGHTS

Psalm 46:10: *"Be still, and know that I am God."* How few of us master those two peaceful words, *be still*!

Early on in my transformation I worked hard at quickly trashing toxic thoughts before they festered and infected my mind. By practicing daily meditation, daily prayer, and more communal spiritual exercises, I learned to quiet my mind more quickly by repeating this sequence:

Toxic thought begins . . .one second later I think, "Mind-mute." A few seconds later I click into a prayerful meditation: "Thank you, God, for . . ." (See "Trash Toxic Thoughts," page 129.)

WHERE IN THE WORLD OF THE BRAIN IS THE GOD CENTER?

Brain scan studies suggest that in some people the God center is in the *thalamus,* a walnut-shaped structure in the center of the brain. The thalamus sits on top of your emotional center, the hypothalamus, and is like your brain's air-traffic controller. Each thought must pass through the thalamus, which tells it where to go or where to land. In many people who have dysfunctional thinking, their trouble is in the thalamus. A worrying thought gets into the brain and instead of quickly redirecting it to the trash bin, the thalamus redirects it all over the brain, causing anxiety.

In other people, the God center (or centers) might be more in the frontal lobe, which is the CEO of the brain, governing logic, decision making, and perceptions. Some people may use one predominant center or many to connect with God. This is why there is unlikely to be a specific God center in the same part of everyone's brain. There are times when your frontal lobe focuses on God, such as when you're trying to figure out in an intellectual way who or what God is. Other times it's in the emotional center, as when you simply want to listen to God, thank God, and feel God: "Dear God . . . whoever or wherever you are . . . please answer my prayer . . ." Meditation, "centering prayer," is a way of cleansing the cluttered mind to make room to listen to God.

The more you meditate, the spiritually stronger you get. Just as in muscle building, the longer and more deeply you practice meditation, the better your brain changes. Some studies show beneficial brain changes after only eight weeks of daily meditation. The greatest effect was found in those who practiced thirty minutes or longer a day for many years. Meditation and prayer are synergistic. Meditation is more about using techniques to clear your mind to make your prayer to God more meaningful and to make you more receptive to God's response. The famous studies of Catholic nuns and Buddhist monks showed that individuals in both groups grew a God center, neurologic changes in the brain that were observed in radiologic scans. And the longer their daily meditation practices, the more permanent these changes were likely to be. (See more about meditators, page 139.)

While many neuroscientists are understandably skeptical, Erin and I believe in a God center. Our belief is based on our personal experiences and on the neuroimaging studies that show how those parts of the brain involved in a sense of peacefulness and meaningfulness light up during prayer to the God of one's understanding.

Meditators have larger thalami, which enable them to have increased awareness of God as part of their lives. God is real, not just a fiction that your mother or teacher pounded into you to keep you on the straight track. The more you meditate on God, the more your God center—parts of your thalamus—grows, enabling you to gradually increase your belief and sensation that God is real and, even better, a personal God who is connected to you.

Whatever kind of spirituality you do or do not subscribe to, it's becoming increasingly difficult to turn your back on the science that says spiritual beliefs can have profound health benefits, mental and physical. (See scientific references: DrSearsWellness.org/T5/References.)

Make *spiritual fitness* your partner in health.

CHAPTER 8

T5 FIGHTS INFLAMMATION

The biggest topic in modern medicine is inflammation. Often heard at medical conferences: "The U.S. is an inflammation nation. Welcome to the inflammation age."

HOW T5 EASES INFLAMMATION	
Causes & Effects of Inflammation	**How T5 Helps**
Immune system out of balance.	Balances immune system.
We "rust."	T5 loaded with "anti-rust" antioxidants.
SAD* is full of sticky sugars.	Free of sticky sugars.
SAD produces sticky-stuff spikes.**	Blunts sticky-stuff spikes.
SAD diet is pro-inflammatory. ***	The 5-S diet is anti-inflammatory. ***

Excess sitting aggravates arthritis, makes you stiff.	T5 movers stay loose and mobile.
Anti-inflammatory pills have many side effects.	T5 helps make your own anti-inflammatory medicines.
SAD increases inflammation-producing belly fat.	Leans out your waist.
Pains in the gut.	Good gut feelings.
Thinking toxic thoughts, stress.	Think-changes your brain, manages stress.

* Standard American diet.

** See page 41 for explanation of "sticky-stuff spikes."

*** Some important semantic notes: The term "pro-inflammatory" means "causes excessive inflammation." "Anti-inflammatory" means dialing down excessive inflammation to help put the body in inflammatory balance. "Anti" can be misleading, since the body can't heal or even live without some inflammation—it's a component of a healthy immune system. We use the term "anti-inflammatory" to mean "promoting inflammation balance."

INFLAMMATION—IT'S ALL ABOUT BALANCE

Inflammation is the response of your body's immune system to help you heal from injury or infection. A healthy immune system means *inflammation balance*. A body in balance heals; a body out of balance hurts. You experience wellness when your body enjoys inflammation balance. Your body hurts when you suffer from inflammation imbalance—all the disorders that end with *-itis* are examples of inflammation. T5 keeps your body in balance.

Inflammation made simple. Chronic or excessive inflammation signals that your immune system is weak and/or confused. Most of your immune system is strategically positioned just beneath your gut lining, on constant alert to identify real foods: "Yes, we recognize veggies as good guys, we'll welcome them in." But, SAD (standard American diet, or "spikes all day") eating eventually makes the immune system sad through inflammation: "That boxed stuff is not real food and we're going to fight it." Soon the immune system gets sick and tired, and you get sick and tired. Next, the immune system gets confused and starts attacking your tissues—*autoimmune diseases.*

When the T5er gets sick and tired of being sick and tired and starts eating real foods in real gut-friendly amounts, the immune system sends "likes" to its friends all over the body: "We're back to normal. We'll fight just right for you, so we don't drain your energy. We feel good, you feel good, and we're back in inflammation balance."

Your immune dial. Look closely at the dial. When your immune system is hyperactive, dialed up too high, the excessive biochemicals it releases cause wear and tear on the tissues—colitis, arthritis, all the diseases whose names begin with a tissue and end in -*itis.* Dialing up too high leads to allergies, which have doubled over the past twenty years, and the current epidemic of autoimmune illnesses. When the immune system dials down too low, you get sick and tired. T5 helps keep your immune system dialed just right.

Inflammation Balance

Just Right

Too Low
Sick and tired

Too High
Autoimmune diseases
Allergies

T5

T5 BALANCES BODY AND BRAIN

Illness, mental and physical, is basically a body and brain out of balance. In this book's introduction, we invited you to think of your body as a symphony orchestra. Beautiful music—health—happens when all the players in the symphony orchestra are balanced, playing the right notes at the right time. There is a synergy in this. When the musicians all play well together, the music is greater than the sum of its parts—the body and brain feel better.

SAD is an unbalanced diet that puts our bodies out of balance, including our immune systems. Hence the epidemic of inflammatory diseases. The mushrooming epidemic of mental illnesses is the result of neurohormones out of balance. The T5 program is like bringing a new orchestra leader—you—into your body and getting it back into balance: hormonal harmony, beautiful music, good health. You can feel it!

Balances blood sugar. The root cause of most inflammation illnesses—from diabetes to Alzheimer's—is spikes of sticky stuff in the blood. (See our explanation of sticky stuff—the root cause of most illnesses—on page 39.) This is especially true of blood sugar, which, when it gets too high for too long, sticks to arterial walls and slows blood flow. The best transforming foods are naturally low in fast-release sugars and high in fiber, which slows the release of the natural sugars in foods. "Low and slow" is just what the inflammation doctor ordered. We'll add a third word, *steady*. Remember, the brain does not store sugar, so it needs a steady supply of smart carbs. It gets exactly that when you sip and graze steadily throughout the day, as you learned to do in chapter two.

Balances your immune system. While a hyperactive immune system contributes to chronic inflammation, a weak immune system leaves you sick and tired. If the immune system could talk, it would say, "The 5-S diet keeps me in balance."

Giovanna, the young trial lawyer you met in chapter one, initially consulted me for healing of her *-itis* illnesses. Gio has a hyperactive intestine, or what I call an ultrasensitive intestine (which is more common in very kind, empathetic and, yes, "sensitive" people). She said, "When I feel stressed, my whole body locks up. My joints ache, and my gut feels awful. When I relax, all that goes away. I've learned so much by practicing the T5 stressbusters, and I use those in my work. Unlike my colleagues, who during a trial stress about what they will say in the closing arguments, I go outside for a walk. The thoughts naturally flow better, and my closing arguments turn out better." And T5 helped heal her irritable bowels caused by inflammation of the gut lining.

Balances omega fats. Omega imbalance (omega-3s too low, omega-6s too high) is one of the top causes of inflammation imbalance.

GIVE YOURSELF AN OIL CHANGE

To protect yourself against most major illnesses, including cancer, eat more omega-3 fat and less omega-6 fat.

Diets high in omega-3 fats	Diets too high in omega-6 fats
Promote immune balance	Promote immune imbalance
Decrease inflammation	Increase inflammation
Suppress tumor growth	Increase tumor growth
Decrease blood stickiness	Increase blood stickiness
Improve brain function	Depress brain function
Decrease depression	Increase depression

(See explanation of omega balance in the endnotes.) 🖐

HOW T5 PROMOTES INFLAMMATORY BALANCE

The answer is those two healing words that are now permanently engraved in your healthy-living vocabulary:

Avoid spikes!

Sticky-stuff spikes trigger excessive inflammation, which triggers *-itis* illnesses. T5 keeps your blood sugar and insulin in balance. No spikes with T5!

We are lumping the major illnesses, heart disease, cancer, and diabetes, into inflammation, since new insights reveal that nearly every illness has its roots in inflammation.

- Arthr*itis* (joint pain)
- Bronch*itis* (asthma)
- Card*itis* (cardiovascular disease)
- "Cognitiv*itis*" (Alzheimer's)

- Colitis (intestinal illnesses)
- Dermatitis (skin inflammation)
- Endothelialitis (clots in blood vessels)
- Gingivitis (gum disease)
- Nephritis (kidney disease)
- Retinitis (vision loss)
- Thyroiditis (Hashimoto's disease)

Each one of those illnesses is triggered by the accumulation of sticky stuff in tissues.

T5 HELPS YOUR BODY MAKE ITS OWN ANTI-INFLAMMATORY MEDICINES

In chapter three, you learned that moving and eating the T5 way opens your internal pharmacy. That's because T5 keeps the endothelium smooth and supple, so you can effectively make your own medicines, some of which are natural anti-inflammatories. In fact, in recent years a new *-itis* illness has infected the doctors' dictionary—*endothelialitis*, wear and tear on a sticky endothelium.

Your third silver lining. You've learned about the internal pharmacies in the linings of your blood vessels and intestines. Here's a third one. It's in the linings of your joints. When you move, the lining of your joints makes natural anti-inflammatories.

Let's peek inside the joint that bothers people the most, the knee. There is a lining around the joint, a little like plastic wrap, called the *synovial membrane*. This magical membrane makes a medicine called *synovial fluid*. Moving the knees squirts synovial fluid into the joint as you flex it to keep it lubricated. Also, unlike most tissues, the cartilage in your joints doesn't receive a rich blood supply. Instead, synovial fluid nourishes the joints and removes metabolic waste products.

HOW T5 BALANCES INFLAMMATION—A SUMMARY		
	Inflammation Balance	**Inflammation Imbalance**
The 5-S Diet	Loaded with antioxidants. Low in sticky stuff. High in healing nutrients. Promotes omega balance.	Omega imbalance promotes inflammation. Diets low in plant-based antioxidants.
Graze to the rule of twos	Lowers sticky-stuff spikes.	SAD raises sticky stuff and causes spikes.
Movement	Mobilizes blood flow and balances inflammation. Helps you make your own medicines, including anti-inflammatories.	Sitting stiffens joints and builds up sticky stuff in tissues.
T5 stressbusters	Lower pro-inflammatory biochemicals, help balance inflammation.	Stress increases buildup of pro-inflammatory biochemicals, dials up inflammation.
Sharing	Helps you rely on your T5 social network to develop more skills to need fewer pills.	The more alone you are, the less likely you are to heal and the more likely you are to need more pills for your ills.

Now that you understand inflammation as the root cause of most chronic illnesses, let's see how T5 helps prevent and heal the "big three" illnesses that we haven't discussed much so far: cancer, cardiovascular disease, and diabetes—all of which are caused by inflammation imbalance.

HOW T5 PROMOTES HEART HEALTH

Whether the brain or the heart is the sickest organ of the body depends upon whether you consult a neurologist or cardiologist. Diseases of both these vital organs are widespread for the same reasons: If you sit too much and put too much sticky stuff in your mouth, you get sticky stuff in your arteries. That makes them stiff, causing high blood pressure, and wears out the pump—heart failure. It's as simple—and preventable and reversible—as that. T5 can help you have a change of heart.

STICKY ARTERIES—THE ROOT CAUSE OF MOST CARDIOVASCULAR DISEASE

We believe the top T5 anti-inflammatory benefit is keeping sticky stuff off the walls of the arteries. The more open and smooth your arteries are, the better they nourish all the tissues, and the less inflamed these tissues get.

Remember that each organ in your body is only as healthy as the blood vessels supplying it. Blood vessel health is a central theme of T5, and the organ that benefits most from T5 just happens to be the blood vessels.

Heart disease is the number-one killer disease the world over. High blood pressure is a primary cause of heart disease and is almost as common as type 2 diabetes—one-third of Americans now have it. We are a nation of stiff blood vessels. The good news is that, like diabetes, high blood pressure is one of the most preventable and reversible diseases. High blood pressure was once assumed to be just another unavoidable effect of aging. False! Age has little to do with it. It's a function of how we eat and live, and you can change that at any age. At seventy-seven, my average blood pressure is 112/78; Martha's is 110/76.

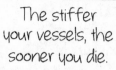

The stiffer your vessels, the sooner you die.

Our heartfelt message to young people. Cardiovascular disease, coronary artery disease, high blood pressure—whatever you want to call it—is happening in *teens*. Eat well, move more, stress less *now* for your best chance at a long, healthy life.

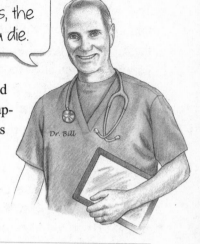

Dr. Bill

CAUSES OF CARDIOVASCULAR DISEASE	
SAD diet and lifestyle	**How T5 helps**
Too high in sodium	Lower in sodium
High in sticky-stuff spikes	Lower in sticky-stuff spikes
Sticky stuff deposits on arterial walls	Smoother arterial walls
Shrinks blood vessels	Grows blood vessels
Stresses and weakens the heart	Relaxes and strengthens the heart
Lowers vessel-relaxing nitric oxide	Promotes more nitric oxide
Raises blood pressure	Optimizes blood pressure

FIVE WAYS T5 HELPS THE HEART

Yes, it's the same scenario that helps every other organ: eat less sticky stuff, avoid spikes, relax the blood vessels, grow more blood vessels, strengthen the heart.

1. PASS ON THE SALT, PLEASE

T5 eating is a "right-salt" diet, because real, natural foods seldom contain excessive salt. Sodium is not bad. It's in nearly all plant foods. It's the *excess* that is bad for our blood vessels. Why? Ever notice how, after gorging on oversalted food at an all-you-can-eat buffet, you got up to pee four or five times during the night? To dilute excess salt, your body retains water. This is why you get thirsty after eating a big bag of salty popcorn at the movies. Getting rid of the excess water requires the heart to pump harder, pushing the fluid through the kidneys, which increases pressure on the artery walls.

Why do Americans eat so much salt? Because we have programmed our taste buds to like it. Restaurants and processed-food companies know this.

The good news is, since *taste-reshaping* is a prime feature of T5 eating, you will come to love the "right-salt" taste of real food, and unreal foods will soon taste too salty.

You know how a garden hose gets stiff and sometimes leaks around the fittings when you turn down the flow at the nozzle? If you could turn up the pressure enough at the spigot, the hose would rupture. That's what happens to your blood vessels when your blood pressure keeps rising. Except, instead of a broken hose, you're risking stroke, aneurysm, heart attack, and heart failure. This is why lowering salt is one of the earliest interventions promoted by the American Heart Association.

A double fault for added salt. Excess salt plus excess sugar equals double trouble. Fortunately, you can now find "low sodium" labels on soups and other foods, to help you choose wisely. Like sugar, salt triggers an "eat more" craving. It also triggers thirst, which is the likely reason you get free salted nuts at a bar or chips with your sandwich. Salty chips and sweetened soda (not to mention maltose-rich beer) are partners in crime against your health.

BEWARE OF THE SALTY C'S

- Chicken
- Chips
- Cheese
- Canned soups

* Sorry, chicken lovers, but you'll know what I mean if you ever visit one of those big industrial chicken factories and see how the birds are fattened with fake food and infused with salt. Buy your chicken from a farmer you trust to raise his birds naturally, and bake it, don't bread it.

We reshaped our tastes to enjoy less-salted foods, the same way we did for less-sweet chocolate with a higher percentage of cocoa. (See "Confessions of a Chocolate-Lover," page 61.)

Gradually change over from regular canned soup to the low-salt kind—or gradually back off the salt in your homemade soups. After a few weeks, you will notice that what once tasted bland now tastes fine. Tastes are easier to reshape than you might think, but it takes persistence. Try these de-salting tips:

- Put the salt shaker in the spice cabinet—not next to the stove and certainly not on the table. A shaker out of sight means less salt on the food.
- Try not adding any salt to your food for three weeks. You'll be amazed how your taste buds come to like the real taste of real foods.
- As you're using less salt, use more healthy spices and herbs, such as garlic, turmeric, pepper, and oregano.
- Insist on no added salt at restaurants. You might even tell the waiter, "My doctor put me on a low-salt diet. I'll have to send it back if it's too salty." They'll get the point.

- Buy foods labeled "low sodium" or "no added salt." The easiest way to do this is to buy fresh produce. If you eat only real foods, you'll get the right amount of salt.

2. EAT MORE PLANT-BASED FOOD AND SEAFOOD, LESS ANIMAL-BASED FOOD

This is Heart Health 101. The greater the percentage of plant-based foods in your diet, the happier your heart. That's what the 5-S diet is—mostly plants and just the right amount of safe seafood.

Thank you, Dr. Dean. When I was poring over medical journals to learn the science-based changes I needed to save my life, I read about fascinating research done by Dr. Dean Ornish, who proved that changing to a plant-based diet could unclog coronary arteries, often sparing a person with coronary artery disease from bypass surgery. Credit Dr. Dean with giving scientific credence to what mom always said: "Eat more vegetables." (See more on Dr. Ornish, pages 272 and 359 and at DrSearsWellness .org/T5/References.)

3. GRAZING MAKES THE HEART GROW STRONGER

Again, it's the "sipping solution" that helps you "avoid spikes." (See page 8.) And here's a great tip—one or two tablespoons a day of ground flax-seeds added to your smoothie can lower your blood pressure more (and more safely) than some of the drugs prescribed for hypertension by making the blood less sticky.

4. STRESS LESS, ENJOY A STRONGER HEART

Lowering stress reduces heart rate and blood pressure. Stress hormones can increase blood pressure by causing the heart to beat faster and blood vessels to narrow. (See "Excess Stress Causes a Neurotic Heart," page 153.)

5. MOVE YOUR HIGH BLOOD PRESSURE DOWN

Sitters are more likely to suffer from high blood pressure than movers. Movement relaxes arteries and lowers blood pressure.

Pulse more pleasing. When sitters become habitual movers, they often notice their resting heart rate drops. After six months of doing T5, my pulse went down ten beats per minute. That's 600 fewer beats less per hour, 14,000 fewer per day. In two months, your heart would beat nearly 1 million fewer times. That kind of change means your heart stays stronger longer.

T5 FOR PREVENTING AND HEALING TYPE 2 DIABETES

Type 2 diabetes, now the fastest-rising ailment in America, is also the one most preventable and curable by T5. Wow! In the past thirty years, the incidence of type 2 diabetes has tripled. Within the lifetime of most of you reading this book, *one-third of Americans are likely to get diabetes.* That sad statistic alone should be a big motivator for you to do T5—and stay with it.

DAVE THE DIABETIC

Dave went to the doctor and got a diagnosis he didn't want to hear: "You've got diabetes." That dreaded word drove fear into Dave's already aching body. He imagined himself slowly withering away: vision loss, amputations, weak heart, frail bones, dementia. Eventually, everything hurts and nothing works. That was not the dream life Dave wanted to live. So he asked his doctor, "What is diabetes, how did I get it, and what can I do about it?"

Diabetes made simple. Type 2 diabetes is not a death sentence, but it *is* a warning sign. Here's what Dave's doctor told him:

- Replace *spikey* and *sticky* foods with *steady* and *smooth* foods.
- Stop eating processed food and junk carbs.
- Stop eating too much too fast.
- Start eating more seafood and fruits and vegetables and foods with lots of fiber.
- And start grazing instead of gorging.

DANIELLE THE NONDIABETIC

Danielle eats a salad, sips on a smoothie, and nibbles on a palmful of nuts. Most of her meals are plant-based. The sugars in her diet steadily seep through the gut into her bloodstream. Her pancreas gets the signal to squirt out just the right amount of insulin to escort those sugar molecules to the cells in her body.

When this insulin–glucose couple arrives at the cell membrane, they meet a doorman called a *receptor*, whose job it is to let in only the amount of glucose the cell needs. The doorman says, "Glucose, come right through. The mitochondria [the energy generators inside the cell] are waiting for you." The cell then signals, "Insulin, thanks, you've done your job. Tell your master, the pancreas, to dial down and rest until needed." The blood is happy because it contains just the right amount of sugar. The organs are happy and healthy because they get the right amount of sugar. For Danielle, life is well!

Dave, on the other hand, eats far more sugar than his body needs. Even worse, he eats types of sugars that are especially bad for his body. Too many insulin-and-sugar couples arrive too fast at the cells, overwhelming the doormen. To protect the health of the cell, the receptors have to resist the entry of the excess sugars: "We're overloaded already. No vacancy." So the insulin–sugar couple is turned away, resisted, and a crowd of sugar couples accumulates in the bloodstream. Dave has high blood sugar.

Worse yet, the sticky fats and sugars Dave eats jam up his cells' receptors, making them even more resistant to letting in needed glucose. This is a very simple explanation of type 2 diabetes.

Drugs don't do it. *You* have to! In 2008 the medical community was shocked by a study published in the prestigious *New England Journal of Medicine*. It showed that drugs for lowering blood sugar didn't always help patients get better, and that aggressively drugged patients often got sicker. No wonder! These drugs treat the effects of high blood sugar, not the cause. That's the beauty of T5. It teaches patients how to make their own medicines to regulate blood sugar. Even in patients who still need medication, T5 plus prescription meds—skills plus pills—works better.

The real-food diet prevents and reverses type 2 diabetes. Of course you could cut the risk of getting diabetes—and even increase your chances of reversing it—by severely restricting how much you eat every day. Decades ago, researchers discovered this correlation in people living amid war, whose blood sugar levels were forced down by starvation. There is an easier way, and one that will last—eat the T5 way. Remember the T5 basics:

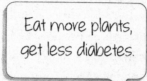

Eat more plants, get less diabetes.

Dr. Bill

- Plant-based foods fill you up, with fewer calories.
- T5 lowers sticky stuff.
- Move more, burn more.
- Graze according to the rule of twos to avoid spikes.

STAY LEAN FOR LOWER DIABETES RISK

In counseling patients with big bellies, I no longer talk about obesity. Instead, I say, "You're prediabetic"—a term that's more scientific and motivating. Lean waist, less risk of diabetes.

How big bellies and type 2 diabetes become partners in illness. Your body is normally programmed to store excess fuel as fat. Think of each fat cell as a balloon. If you eat too much sugar, the balloon fills up. If you keep putting sugar into them, they get bigger and bigger. When fat cells get way too full, they dump sticky biochemicals, pro-inflammatories, into your bloodstream, causing inflammation illnesses.

HOW T5 HELPS PREVENT AND BEAT CANCER

"Dr. Bill, you should write a book about cancer," readers often tell me. T5 is the book. Cancer is a disease your authors know a lot about, unfortunately, from personal experience. I am a colon cancer survivor. My father died of colon cancer, as did Martha's mother. One of our daughters-in-law is a twenty-year survivor of Ewing's sarcoma, a very malignant and usually fatal bone cancer. And, as we write this book, another daughter-in-law is recovering from brain cancer. You're about to read not only of our passion, but the keys to preventing and recovering from cancer.

At a recent T5 lecture, my daughter, Hayden, opened with this introduction, which left me with tears in my eyes:

Almost twenty years ago, when I was in college, I got a call from my mom. It was that dreaded call. She said, "Hayden, Dad has colon cancer. It's serious, and you need to come home." Thank the Lord, he made it through the surgery. The hardest part was after that, the chemotherapy, the radiation, literally watching the hero of my life become so broken. But during that very difficult time in my family's life, something very beautiful started to happen deep inside my dad. It was his passion, his fire, his obsession. He had to figure out how he could heal himself. But even more than that, he had to figure out how his eight children would never have to experience cancer. His dad died from colon cancer, and my mom's mom died of colon cancer, so genetically it would appear that we Sears children were doomed. But the Lord gave us a secret weapon, my dad. He spent the next few years of his recovery just poring over research journals. Luckily, he was in a position of his career that gave him access to top minds in health and nutrition. He was able to glean from all of these resources. He had a new mission, a new passion in life. So he has spent the last twenty years of his career sharing with others what he learned way back then for himself. So what you get to hear tonight is not only from the mind of a brilliant scientist, but also from the heart of a father.

WHY WE GET CANCER

Cancer used to be blamed on "genes." But more and more studies are discovering a variety of causes. Yes, genes are an important factor, but in cancer, as in most other illnesses, new insights reveal that genes get less than 20 percent of the blame. The other 80 percent is due to deficiencies in LEAN, our acronym for lifestyle, exercise, attitude, and nutrition.

Significantly, all of these are under our control. Imagine that your genes have a "cancer dial." If the gene's dial is turned up—if the gene is "expressed"—your chances of getting cancer go up. But if its dial is down—if it's not expressed—you are less likely to get cancer. According to the growing science of *epigenetics*, while you can't get rid of those "dials" or "tendencies," you can influence them. LEAN affects how your genes are expressed, and therefore reduces your chances of getting cancer.

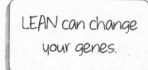

LEAN can change your genes.

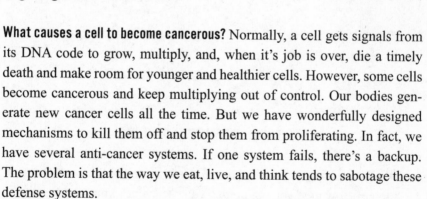

Dr. Bill

What causes a cell to become cancerous? Normally, a cell gets signals from its DNA code to grow, multiply, and, when it's job is over, die a timely death and make room for younger and healthier cells. However, some cells become cancerous and keep multiplying out of control. Our bodies generate new cancer cells all the time. But we have wonderfully designed mechanisms to kill them off and stop them from proliferating. In fact, we have several anti-cancer systems. If one system fails, there's a backup. The problem is that the way we eat, live, and think tends to sabotage these defense systems.

Natural killer cells. These are the main backup system. Natural killer (NK) cells are heavily armed, well-trained soldiers that are constantly on a search-and-destroy mission for cancer cells that get through some of the body's other checkpoints. In most people, NK cells overwhelm whatever cancer cells arise in the body and prevent disease. They fire biochemical bullets into cancer cells to blow them up. T5 feeds these NK soldiers so that they fight better for you.

Unlike other immune cells, NK cells don't need prior exposure to an antigen in order to mobilize. They patrol the body watching for cancer cells as well as harmful bacteria and viruses. As soon as they detect a cancer cell, NK cells attach to it, then poke holes in its cell membrane and fire their bullets (basically cancer-dissolving enzymes) into it. The dead, deflated cancer cell becomes garbage, which is removed by macrophages, the garbage collectors of the immune system. One of the top natural cancer-fighting medicines your body can make is stronger NK cells.

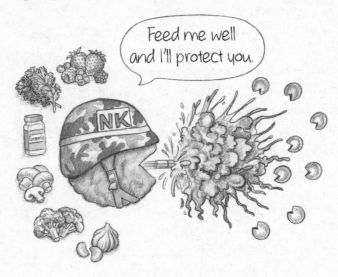

MAKE YOUR OWN "IMMUNOTHERAPY"

Immunotherapy is now the hottest word in cancer treatment. Doctors can now give you a drug that educates your immune system's cancer-fighting cells to selectively kill cancer cells while sparing healthy cells. The T5 anti-cancer program also enables your immune system to fight smarter, making healthy cells more cancer resistant and cancer cells more vulnerable to NK destruction.

YOUR CHOICE: FEED CANCER OR FIGHT IT

Here's how the standard American diet (SAD) feeds cancer, versus eating the T5 way:

The SAD Cancer-Feeding Diet	The 5-S Diet
High in added sugar	Low in added sugar
High in omega-6 fats, low in omega-3 fats	The reverse: healthy omega balance of these fats
Low in antioxidants (cancer-fighting nutrients)	High in antioxidants
High in chemicals that throw the immune system out of balance	Promotes immune system balance
Science says SAD causes cancer	Science says 5-S decreases cancer risk

CANCER CAUSES	
Causes of Cancer	How T5 Helps Beat It
High animal-based, low plant-based diet	Much more plant-based than animal-based diet
Low-fiber, high-sugar diet	High-fiber, low-sugar diet
Sedentary lifestyle	Moving more
More processed food with additives	More real foods
Stress feeds cancer	Less stress

Why smoothing out sugar spikes with a plant-based diet helps fight cancer. Sugar is a "grow food" for cancer cells. Also, a plant-based diet lowers excess IGF-1, another cancer-cell fertilizer. Every minute of the day, old cells in your body die and new cells are born. If cells kept reproducing unchecked, they would grow out of control—cancer. But your body has a beautiful set of checks and balances. Cancer cells only spread when they find a fertile garden in which to grow. The standard American diet is basically chemical fertilizers for tumor growth. To paraphrase Hippocrates, let food be your anti-cancer medicine.

Dr. Bill's big fat change. In the 1990s, nutrition scientists placed a lot of emphasis on the fact that carbs feed cancer. During my crash-course in lifesaving nutrition, I pictured a cancer cell saying, "Yum! Feed me those fast carbs and I'll grow and multiply." Just what I didn't want. That was my motivation to go on a right-carb diet. My dilemma was that I would be going against the conventional wisdom (and diet craze) of the time, which was low-fat, high-carb. Our whole culture was under the delusion that eating fat makes you fat. Now we know that's wrong! Carbs make you fat. After changing my diet from low fat to right fat, I felt better, had more energy, was satisfied with my meals without being stuffed, and was getting leaner. Why did one simple cancer change make such a difference in my health—one that has lasted for nearly twenty years? This was how the 5-S cancer-preventing diet was born.

SWEET FOOD-LABELING NEWS

Currently planned for sometime in 2018 are long-overdue changes in science-based and consumer-friendly food labeling. The Nutrition Facts label on foods is getting these upgrades:

1. **The meaningless "calories from fat" line is gone.** This change is based on a statement by two of my favorite nutritional scientists, Dr. Walter Willett, professor and chairman of the Department of Nutrition, Harvard Medical School, and Dr. David Ludwig, professor of pediatrics at Harvard Medical School: "We don't get fat by eating healthy fats. We get fat by eating unhealthy carbs."
2. **A sweet addition.** The Nutrition Facts label will state the *added sugars* in grams. The Sears family is excited about

---

this, because it will tell the consumer how much "real sugar" was contributed by Mother Nature and how much was added by food makers. Manufacturers will now compete for the lowest "added sugars" numbers. We will reshape our tastes to prefer the natural sweetness of real foods and no longer be prompted by added sugars to overeat, overbuy, and become overweight.

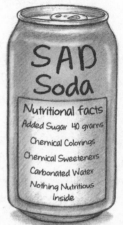

However, consumers beware. According to the August 2017 issue of *Nutrition Action* health letter, the FDA, bowing to pressure from Big Food lobbyists, may delay this label-truth upgrade. Please support the Center for Science in the Public Interest to help lobby for these changes.

Once again, avoid sugar spikes. Sugar feeds cancer growth. And oncologists have told me that high-fructose corn syrup feeds cancer cells more than table sugar (sucrose). So should you avoid *all* sugar? No. You need carbohydrates for energy. But absolutely avoid "added sugar," chemical sweeteners, sweetened beverages, high-fructose corn syrup, and so on. And remember, these sugars are worse yet if you gulp and gorge too much too fast. Don't worry about the "sugar" in blended fruits and vegetables in your slowly sipped smoothie, as they're partnered with the right fats, fiber, and protein to blunt the sugar spikes. These foods help *prevent* cancer. Consider these points:

1. Our bodies cannot live without sugar. It's the fuel that powers everything, including the brain. Have you ever experienced foggy thinking or even fainted when your blood sugar was low?

2. In a typical healthful diet, half the calories come from sugar—but they're from the natural carbohydrates that Mother Nature puts in her plant foods. And that healthy diet also includes fiber, fat, and protein.

3. The brain does not store sugar as well as muscles do, so it needs a constant supply of energy. 🖐

4. It's the sugar *spikes* we want to avoid.

Here's how I explain smart sugars and dumb sugars to kids: "A smart sugar plays with its friends, protein, fat, and fiber. It never plays alone. So, when the sugar holds hands with its friends and enters the intestines, the friends hold the sugar back from being absorbed too fast, so you don't get spikes. A dumb sugar, like a sugar-sweetened soda, has no friends to hold it back. Your blood sugar spikes, and cancer cells say, 'Here comes my food.'" Also, sugar spikes trigger insulin growth factor, which is one of the top cancer cell fertilizers.

Avoid sugar spikes is one simple tip that could cut your chances of getting cancer and greatly increase your chances of healing from cancer. Added sugar is cancer fertilizer. It's as scary as that. Let's follow two sugars in two eaters . . .

Suzy eats a salad. *The vegetables naturally contain various kinds of sugar, carbohydrates. They're absorbed into Suzy's bloodstream slowly, in moderate amounts. Any cancer cells that are waiting for sugar spikes go hungry. They either die or go dormant.*

Chuck guzzles a cola. *Sugar rushes into his blood and causes an insulin spike. The cancer cell says, "Yum! A feast! I'm going to grow and multiply."*

The incidence of cancer in America went up as our consumption of unreal foods went up—refined sugar, corn syrup, refined white flours, and so on. Any correlation? Yes! If you want to grow cancer cells, SAD is the ideal diet.

Sugar is a cancer cell's favorite food. A cancer cell can gobble up glucose at ten times the rate of healthy cells. X-ray studies have proven this. One of the ways of detecting where cancer is and how fast it's growing is to do a PET scan, in which you're injected with radioactive glucose. Tumor cells light up much faster than healthy ones, because they gobble up the glucose. Excess sugar not only feeds cancer cells; it suppresses the very immune cells that fight cancer cells. This is called the "Pac-Man" effect, after the old video game. Certain white blood cells patrol the body looking for cancer cells. They wrap themselves around the cancer cells and essentially gobble them up, like Pac-Man. Excess sugar reduces the ability of these cells to do that. Experiments have revealed that eating ten teaspoons of sugar (the amount in a 12-ounce soda) reduces the ability of white blood cells to gobble up cancer cells by over 50 percent.

T5 KEEPS YOUR GARDEN FROM GROWING CANCER: A SUMMARY

Cancer has been aptly compared to a garden growing out of control. Sometimes a genetic mix-up causes a "seed" (a cell) to become a cancer seed. How much and how fast the cancer seed multiplies depends on the soil around it. If the soil is fed cancer-fertilizing foods, then the seed grows into a cancer plant, a dangerous weed.

When those weeds grow out of control, they steal nutrients, fertilizer, from the normal plants and crowd them out. Eventually, they grow beyond the boundaries of the garden—the cancer metastasizes. The best ways to control the growth of cancer in your body's garden is to:

- Keep the seeds from becoming cancerous, and
- Shut off their food and fertilizer so they can't grow.

Cancer specialists call this improving our *biological terrain*, making it unfriendly to cancer growth.

Two simple changes to lower your risk of getting cancer, and support healing from cancer, are how you *eat* and how you *think*.

TOP ANTI-CANCER FOODS SUPPORTED BY SCIENCE

- Asparagus
- Berries: blueberries, tart cherries, strawberries, raspberries, cranberries
- Broccoli
- Brussels sprouts
- Cabbage
- Cauliflower
- Chili peppers
- Garlic
- Green tea
- Kale
- Leeks
- Mushrooms: shiitake, chaga
- Onions
- Scallions
- Spinach
- Turmeric

(See Dr. Bill's Anti-Cancer Salad recipe, page 331.)

HAVE AN ANTI-CANCER MIND

This is the most challenging part of our anti-cancer plan. There is a new specialty in psychiatry called *psycho-oncology*, the study of how the mind affects, for better or worse, the growth and spread of tumors. When I was healing from cancer, I was profoundly influenced by Norman Cousins's book *Anatomy of an Illness*. This must-read book is an introduction to the world of mind-body medicine. It helped trigger the fascinating new field called psychoneuroimmunology, the study of how the mind can tell the cancer-fighting immune system how to behave. Feelings of helplessness, hopelessness, worry, and stress dial up inflammation, which facilitates tumor growth.

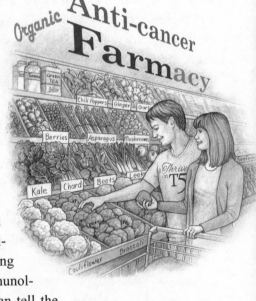

Studies have shown that in cancer patients who had the anti-cancer mentality—courage, hopefulness, and a belief that they will beat their cancers—NK cells were much more active than in patients who felt depressed and helpless.

It turns out that our circulating NK cells (see page 257) are sensitive to and controlled by our emotions. (See related section, how meditation helps make your own medicines, page 141.)

Moreover, stress increases circulating pro-inflammatory chemicals, which dial up the stress hormones adrenaline and cortisol. These act like cancer-cell fertilizers and also can awaken cancer cells that have been dormant. The body makes cancer cells all the time, but the immune system finds and destroys them. However, uncontrolled stress and a defeatist attitude can dial down the built-in anti-cancer mechanisms that are meant to protect us.

T5 is an anti-cancer mentality, an anti-cancer diet, and an anti-cancer lifestyle. Do T5!

CHAPTER 9

ANSWERS TO COMMON T5 QUESTIONS

I f you've read this far, you may have some questions about Transform 5. We have compiled and answered the most common and important questions transformers ask us. We hope the experience of others helps you adapt the T5 program to your life.

GETTING HUSBAND ON T5

I'm on T5, but my husband won't do it. His family tree is littered with early heart attacks. How do I get him to make changes?

The best way to a man's heart is not through his stomach. If you really want to motivate him, start here: the United States has the highest incidence of erectile dysfunction of any country where such statistics are available. The standard American diet hardens arteries but softens the penis. (There's a direct correlation: restricted blood flow keeps the penis from becoming fully engorged.) The "Viagra vegetable effect" is an actual medical term meaning that the men who eat a plant-based diet have better blood flow to two of the principal sex organs—the brain and the penis.

ALCOHOL

I love wine. Will it interfere with T5?

Does a glass a day keep the doctor away? Not necessarily. Headlines such as "Drink Wine, Live Longer" are not backed by good science. As a doctor who enjoys a glass of wine with dinner a couple evenings a week, I might be tempted to do a selective literature review, choosing alcohol-friendly articles that support my biased wine-lover's taste. Not being under the influence, I resisted this temptation and came to these conclusions:

If you don't already drink wine, don't start. The alleged health effects aren't proven and are not worth the risks.

Drink smart. Remember, alcoholic beverages, like soda, contain fast-spike sugar. The alcohol itself is quickly absorbed into the bloodstream and goes into the liver, the first organ damaged by excess alcohol. (The brain is a close second). Tips for smart drinking:

- Never drink alcohol on an empty stomach. Skip before-meal cocktails.
- Sip *slowly* and only after you have partially filled your stomach.
- Try to limit yourself to one five-ounce glass of wine per day.
- Take an occasional vacation from wine for a few weeks. You'll miss it less than you think. If you find that you miss it horribly, that might indicate a problem even more serious than your diet, and you may want to consider a trip to your friendly neighborhood Alcoholics Anonymous meeting.
- Out of sight, out of bloodstream. Keeping the wine bottles out of sight lessens the temptation to have "just one more glass."

Don't get your microbiome drunk. Excessive alcohol may harm the health of your microbiome. That's why it helps to stay within the American Heart Association's guidelines of no more than one drink per day for women and two for men. Greater amounts have been shown to harm the good bacteria in the gut while feeding the bad guys, a condition called dysbiosis.

Beware of beer belly. Beer is typically higher in carbohydrates and calories than hard liquor or wine. Because of its lower alcohol content, drinkers tend to consume more of it, accounting for the term "beer belly." Ever wonder why that term is directed mostly at men? It's not only that men tend to drink more beer; they're genetically programmed to store more fat in their paunches. Women, on the other hand, are programmed to store more of their fat in the hips and thighs.

VEGAN* DIET OKAY?

As a vegan, I am concerned about getting enough nutrients.

People used to think that they should eat more meat than plants, because meat has more iron. The concern was that vegans (and vegetarians) could suffer anemia (iron deficiency in the blood). In fact, some vegans do occasionally become borderline anemic, but in general, studies have debunked the notion that veganism leads to anemia. On the other hand, while too little iron makes you sick, too much can be toxic. Intestinal lining to the rescue! If the iron in your blood is too high, your intestinal lining, with help from your microbiome, limits the amount of iron you absorb from food. If iron is low, the lining dials up to absorb more. Here's what vindicated the vegans: the built-in iron-regulating dial in the intestines works better with plant sources of iron, or what is called nonheme iron. (See DrSearsWellness.org/T5/plant-sources-iron.)

---

*   "Vegan" means not eating any foods of animal origin. For many, veganism is based on ideology rather than nutrition. Vegetarianism precludes meat, but eggs and dairy are okay.

We believe for most people a pesco-vegetarian diet is more nutritious than a strict vegetarian or vegan one. Our 5-S diet is vegetarian plus seafood, much like the *traditional* Mediterranean diet (as opposed to the pasta-loaded *modern* Mediterranean diet). Vegans are particularly prone to deficiencies in omega-3s and vitamin B_{12}.

Nonetheless, a vegan diet can lower, even reverse, cardiovascular disease (my friend and mentor Dean Ornish proved that; see pages 272 and 360), and also decrease diabetes, cerebral vascular disease, metabolic syndrome, obesity and its consequences, and more. While I am not aware of any studies showing that a strictly vegan diet can prevent brain-health problems, neuroscientists do conclude that eating mostly a plant-based diet plus seafood can help prevent and treat neurodegenerative diseases.

Our top nutritional concern is that a vegan diet can be too low in smart fats needed for children's brain development and for maintaining brain health in seniors. In a nutshell, or in this case a seashell:

1. Consider becoming a pesco-vegetarian. See the endnotes for selecting the safest and most nutritious seafood.
2. If you wish to remain a healthy vegan:

   - Measure your omega-3 blood levels. (See page 350.)
   - If your omega-3s are below 8 percent, consider taking 1,000 mg daily of an algae-based omega-3 supplement.
   - If your B_{12} levels are low and you wish to remain vegan, consider taking a B_{12} (cobalamin) supplement or eating foods enriched with B_{12}.

ORGANIC FOODS

Are organic foods healthier and worth the extra expense?

Yes, most are. While vitamin and mineral content is about the same either way, organic produce has 20 to 40 percent higher antioxidant levels. Also, organic foods have lower levels of toxic heavy metals, such as mercury and lead, and of pesticides and phosphates. If expense is a concern, choose organic for the "dirty dozen" and conventional produce for the "clean fifteen." (See these lists on EWG.org.) For the best nutritional value—and best taste—grow your own garden. (See how, page 22.)

MEASURING STICKY STUFF

I love your sticky-stuff analogy, but I feel a little funny asking my doctor to measure my level of sticky stuff.

Doctors love to laugh. When your doctor asks the purpose of your office visit, don't be shy. Say, "I'd like you to measure the level of sticky stuff in my blood." After the eyebrows go up, add, "I mean my HbA1c or sticky red blood cells." (Read about frosted hemoglobin, page 40, and also see the next item.)

MEASURING YOUR HEALTH MARKERS

I'm going in for my annual blood tests where they measure my blood fats and cholesterol. What do I need to know?

Think of "markers" as your level of sticky stuff and as warning signs that you may need to make T5 changes before you feel what your blood tests show. If people ask you what you got measured at the doctor's office, surprise them by saying, "My blood level of sticky stuff." Here are the "sticky markers" your doctor is most likely to measure:

- High sensitivity C-reactive protein (HsCRP)
- Hemoglobin A1c (HbA1c)
- Homocysteine level
- Fasting insulin level
- Oxidized LDL (OxLDL), the sticky cholesterol. Better yet if your doctor orders the most meaningful cholesterol test, which measures the number of *small-particle* cholesterol-carrying molecules in your blood. These are ones that worm their way

into the walls of your arteries and contribute to cardiovascular disease. Cholesterol particle size has proven to be a more meaningful marker than total LDL value. It's really the small particles that count. (More on this later in this chapter.)

Your *triglyceride levels* may be a better marker for heart disease risk than cholesterol, since triglycerides are most affected by how much junk carbs you eat, not fat. The profile you don't want is high small-particle cholesterol and low HDL (the protective cholesterol that mutes the harmful effects of sticky stuff in your blood.) An even worse profile would be high triglycerides, low HDL, and high small-particle LDL—known among cardiologists as the "killer triad."

Another new finding is that just as you don't get fat by eating healthy fats, you don't get high cholesterol by eating cholesterol-containing foods (except for a small percentage of people who have a genetic quirk). The whole notion that cholesterol causes heart disease is being reconsidered by the most trusted scientists. The real culprits are sitting too much, eating too much too fast, and eating too much unreal processed food.

HEALING HEART DISEASE

There's a lot of disease throughout my family—heart disease, brain disease, and cancer. What health change can we make to see the results the fastest?

If you're sick and tired of being sick and tired, and you want to feel better soon and for a long time, science says make one simple change: *eat more plant foods and less meat*. Again, my friend and health mentor Dr. Dean Ornish proved this in his landmark study of people with coronary artery disease who were candidates for surgery. His research showed that within a few weeks on primarily a plant-based diet, these patients showed improved arterial health. Your body can be a rapid-response healer if you feed it the right "medicines." Do it and feel it! (For more about Dr. Ornish's heal-heart-disease diet, see our recommended reading list, DrSearsWellness.org/T5/recommended-reading, or google Dr. Dean Ornish.)

TRANSFORMING WHILE TRAVELING

I travel a lot for work and find it so hard to keep on my T5 track. Help!

Where there's a will, there's a way. I have logged more than 100,000 flying miles each of the last ten years, mostly for lifestyle lectures. Naturally, I wondered if I was harming my health by traveling on airplanes to lecture about health. I now replace some travel with webinars and video conferences, but I thought up ways I could still do T5 while traveling:

- I load up with antioxidants right before the trip. I make a big smoothie and sip it on the way to the airport. My preflight smoothie has double the kale, a top source of anti-radiation antioxidants.
- After arriving at the gate, I take a brisk walk in the concourse.
- I load my briefcase with antioxidant-rich trail mix.
- During the flight, I do as much isometrics as possible. (See isometrics, page 99.)
- I pack exercise bands. (See page 106.)
- If possible, I choose a hotel that has:
  - windows that open for fresh air,
  - a quiet setting, away from traffic noise and exhaust,
  - a gym and/or pool, and
  - a healthy breakfast buffet to start my day the T5 way. (Smoothie tip: ask the bartender to make you a smoothie from foods you choose from the buffet.)

Finally, I figured everything in America is studied, often overstudied, so there is bound to be a study about the effects of nutrition on pilots, who, because they do most of their work at 35,000 feet, are exposed to a lot more radiation than most of us. Sure enough, the pilots who ate the most fruits and vegetables seemed to be less harmed by such exposure. Other aspects of the 5-S diet helped, too, especially spices like garlic and turmeric. (See DrSearsWellness.org/T5/References.)

GOOD GRAINS

I notice you don't recommend wheat in the T5 eating plan. Why?

For the same reasons we badmouth beef, chuck chicken, and downgrade dairy: What we eat is not *real* wheat.

Remember, as you learned on page 203, our intestines are designed to digest real food—welcome it, metabolize it, and usher it healthfully into the body. Yet, when the genes of the wheat are changed, as is the case with today's commercially grown wheat crops, the nutrient profile plummets. Books such as *Wheat Belly* and *Grain Brain* explain what's wrong with our wheat. While messing with the genome of real, good wheat caused yields and profits to increase, there was a corresponding sharp rise in disorders of the intestinal linings: celiac disease, gluten intolerance, and leaky gut problems.

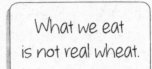

In addition, grinding wheat into fine particles and removing some of the fiber and protein downgrades it from a slow-release carb to a spikey carb—sticky stuff.

We, Dr. Bill and Coach Erin, are the last members of our family to go almost wheat-free, since many of the others are gluten-intolerant. We have replaced wheat with quinoa, amaranth, and wild rice. (For a complete ranking of grains, see DrSearsWellness.org/T5/Grains.)

DOWNGRADING DAIRY

Should I go dairy-free on T5?

Not necessarily, yet we do prefer organic yogurt, kefir, and goat's milk as more intestine-friendly than the regular cow's milk. As with meat and wheat, the problem is the way Big Agro has messed with milk that has made the guts of milk lovers unhappy.

While writing this section, I was invited to give a healthy-living lecture at a venue next to a family farm (read story, page 234). After the talk, a local farmer took me to his home for a glass of freshly pumped goat's milk. Wow! What a difference in taste, consistency, and likely also in nutrient profile and digestibility! The raw, real, whole, unhomogenized milk made my microbiome happy. When I shop for kefir and yogurt I look for these five healthy features:

1. 100 percent grass-fed
2. Organic
3. Whole milk
4. Non-GMO
5. No added sweeteners or artificial colors

(See more about dairy products: DrSearsWellness.org/T5/dairy.)

BADMOUTHING BEEF?

In recent years, I've read a lot about how bad meat is for you. Is this true, and why?

While I am not a vegan, I am also not a meat-eater, except for my monthly venison steak my hunter friends graciously give me. Without belaboring the point, one simple fact that nearly all nutritionists and scientists agree on is: *the more meat you eat, the more of just about every disease you get.* But don't blame the meat. It's what we've done to it that makes it bad. Like how the processed-food and agricultural industries have chemically changed wheat and diary, Big Agro has messed up our meat.

When Americans started feeding junk food to cattle and raising them in stalls, so they can't freely roam, the cattle started getting fat. And the additional fat is disease-promoting fat. Caging and fattening cattle increased economic returns, while increasing the weight and waist size of beef eaters—us. My wife, Martha, grew up on a farm, and I spent many childhood hours working on farms, so I love farmers and farming. If you know how a farming family cares for their cattle, consider eating their products. If you don't, hold the beef.

Here's a sad statistic, which Dr. Michael Greger had the wisdom and courage to point out in his book *How Not to Die*: rising belly-fat accumulation parallels rising meat consumption. One of the largest studies ever done on the effects of eating meat showed that it wasn't just the amount of calories that caused people to get fat, it was the type of calories. The more meat people ate, the more likely they were to get fat. It was as simple as that.

Eat different fats—store different fats. As I was transforming my diet to fewer animal-based foods and more plant-based foods, the research that sealed the deal was the discovery that the fat stored in the tissues of people who eat a lot of animal food was different—and less healthy—than the tissue fat of those who ate mostly plants. I had suspected this all along because I knew that the stored fat of breastfed babies was different, healthier, and more easily shed when in excess than the fat of formula-fed infants. When you eat good fats you're likely to store good fats, and vice versa. People who eat more plant-based foods and less animal-based foods tend to store fewer trans fats (the bad fats) in their tissues. The largest study ever on the effect of diet on health, the NIH/AARP Study, followed half a million men and women, ages fifty to seventy, for ten years. You could call it "the meat and mortality study," because the more meat people ate, the more likely they were to die prematurely, especially from cancer and heart disease. Sorry, carnivores: *Meat-eaters get sicker and die sooner.*

IS MEAT OKAY TO EAT?

To do T5, do I have to give up my meat?

Not necessarily. *Real* meat, in moderation, can be a healthy food. If you know where that steak comes from and how it was fed, it's probably okay. The problem is what they do to good meat to make it bad for you.

Cows' intestines are designed to digest grasses, not corn. But industrial cattle operations feed them corn, and the cows suffer "indigestion," get more intestinal infections, and thus need more antibiotics to treat the infections. The meat we eat therefore not only contains more fat from the corn, but the antibiotics are bad for our microbiomes. We eat the meat and we get fat and sick and need more antibiotics. So the USDA is fattening Americans *and* the profits of the food industry. There should be a USHA—United States Health Agency—that can't be bought.

Okay, in case you're wondering, I'm mainly an herbivore, but I do enjoy a monthly dinner of wild game (venison or elk) and a glass of Zinfandel. The difference between wild game that eats real food and feedlot-fed animals who eat foods not meant for animal consumption is partly in the taste, but mainly in the nutrients.

Try this fun learning demonstration with your children or grandchildren, as I have done. The supermarket is a giant nutritional classroom. One day I showed our grandson Jonathan a typical sirloin steak. "Jonathan, see how this steak is full of flab and fat—the white streaks. That animal sat around and ate junk food all day." We later compared the flabby steak with a lean venison steak. "This animal ate real food and ran a lot. Notice how much stronger the muscles are. Would you rather your muscles look weak and flabby or strong?" He got the point.

CHUCK THE CHICKEN?

I'm cutting down on beef. Is chicken okay?

We omitted chicken from our list of healthy foods for the same reason we bad-mouthed beef. Modern chicken is not the same nutritious, free-roaming meat we ate when we were free-roaming youngsters. It is now much more fatty, and most of the calories are from less-healthy fats. Also, industrially raised poultry is one of the most mistreated animals and one of the most likely foods to be contaminated with bacteria.

Further, mass-produced chicken has a lot of added salt. It's a cheap way to inflate the weight (by inflating the water content), and it prompts you to crave more and eat more. It's another sly little way the food industry shapes our tastes toward eating more and buying more. I have kicked chicken out of our kitchen—unless I know the farmer and how the chickens were fed and cared for.

GLYCEMIC INDEX

I've heard about choosing foods according to the glycemic index. Is this necessary with T5 eating?

No, for two reasons: First, because we don't eat the way the carbs are measured and, second, we want to eliminate as much "counting" as possible. The glycemic index ranks carb-rich foods by how fast they cause blood-sugar spikes. The higher the GI number, the higher the spike. Remember, this is based on laboratory measurements of an individual food item. The baseline is table sugar, sucrose, which has a GI of 100. Generally, the more processed the carb, the higher the GI. "White" foods—white bread, white rice, white potatoes—and low-fiber, low-protein breakfast cereals tend to have the highest GI. A more meaningful number is the *glycemic load* (GL), which indicates how the *meal* affects the sugar spikes. This is more meaningful, because you could pair a high-GI vegetable, such as a white potato, with olive oil or cheese, and the glycemic load, or the effect on the blood sugar, would be lower. So it's really the company a food keeps that is the most meaningful measure. T5 naturally has a low glycemic load. It's "spike-less" eating.

FAMILY FATNESS

My mother worries that the reason I'm always struggling with weight control is because she overate and got overfat while pregnant with me. Is this true?

How much excess fat a mother gains during pregnancy can determine whether or not her baby is born with a tendency to store excessive fat she'll have to deal with throughout life. Sorry, Mom, but you can influence, for better or worse, your child's tendency toward leanness or obesity.

Notice I said tendency, not destiny. We're not talking about a life sentence. What genes you have are beyond your control. How your genes behave is highly under your control. That's what T5 helps you do: control how your genes behave. So don't be too hard on your mom. It's now up to you.

Modern geneticists teach that less than 10 percent of obesity is due to genetic predisposition. That's good news! Ninety percent is under our control. Epigenetics is the science of how the environment in which your genes grow up and live affects how they are expressed—how they behave. *T5 promotes healthy epigenetics.* (See more about epigenetics and cancer, page 257.)

Geneticists compare epigenetics to a dimmer switch. Perhaps the light bulbs on your ceiling are too bright. You can dial down the dimmer switch. When it comes to body fat, T5 helps you dial the dimmer switch to just the right light—or fat storage—for your well-being.

Finally, too little body fat can be just as unhealthy as too much. This was revealed during World War II, when women who were undernourished during pregnancy were more likely to have babies who would become obese children and adults. Maternal epigenetics can affect baby and child epigenetics.

Again, the 5-S diet is right-calorie, not low-calorie; right-fat, not low-fat. You retain the right amount of body fat to help you feel good and look good.

FUNNY FAT PHRASES

Fat scientists have coined some amusing terms for weight-loss fiascoes. Here are a few of my favorites:

- TOFI: thin outside, fat inside—describing an apparently lean person with excess fat stored inside the abdomen.
- "Baloney mass index." This is our spoof for how meaningless body mass index (BMI) is for many individuals. Lean, muscular persons with large bones will flunk the BMI test, especially because muscle and bone weigh more than fat.

Our own definition of BMI: belly matters instead.

SUGAR-SENSITIVE PEOPLE

My doctor says I'm sugar sensitive. What does this mean?

It means you really need T5, to blunt your insulin spikes. Researchers are realizing that insulin spikes can be as individual as personality. Two people can eat the same carbohydrate-containing food, yet spike different sugar and insulin levels. Sugar-sensitive people spike more quickly and are the ones who tend to store more sugar as fat. Less sensitive persons spike more slowly and tend to gain less weight from carbs. In fact, in sugar-sensitive persons, even a month on a right-carb diet dials down the insulin, as the pancreas stops overreacting. (See related section, "How Unhealthy Carbs Make You Fat," page 45.)

INSULIN INSULTS

Consider the consequences of high insulin. As discussed on page 3, the main metabolic goal of T5 is stable blood sugar and insulin levels. When insulin is off, your organs get sick:

- Your *liver* produces too much fat and gets inflamed with sticky stuff. There is now an epidemic of a disease we doctors never even heard about until recent years—nonalcoholic fatty liver disease.
- Your *blood vessels* get stiff and high blood pressure results. (See page 156.)
- Cancer risk increases. Excess insulin causes the cells' genetic machinery to malfunction. Excess sugar and insulin is known as a cancer feeder, as you learned on page 257.
- The *ovaries* start producing more testosterone and less estrogen—not what women want. This accounts for the epidemic of polycystic ovarian syndrome (PCOS). Our daughter was diagnosed with PCOS in her early twenties. Her endocrinologist warned her, "Hayden, you will need to take metformin [medicine for blood sugar control] for the rest of your life." Hayden

insisted, "No I won't!" She did T5, and within two years her PCOS resolved. She no longer needed medicines and became a proud mother of three.

SCALE WATCHING

How often should I weigh myself?

Skip the scale. Okay, we know you're going to step on the scale anyway, no matter how much we discourage it. So, cut back to once a week or month. Instead, use a more meaningful measurement, such as a tape measure for waist size or the way your pants fit.

Weight is not the primary issue. It's *where the weight is* that counts. T5 will shrink your belly but *increase* muscle and bone mass. Because muscle and bone weigh more than belly fat, the scale won't tell you how well you're really doing. Waist-to-hip ratio is one of the most meaningful measurements doctors are now adding to the list of "vital signs." (See values, page 372.)

CHEATING ON EATING

Sometimes I give in to my favorite sweet treat. Is this okay?

The answer depends on how fast you want to thrive on T5. Our scientifically correct answer and a T5 mantra is *don't cheat for five weeks*. You want to rewire the food-craving pathways in your brain; that's the basis of T5. We came up with this advice based on a rough estimate of the time it takes to change brain pathways.

Say you crave pastries—you love to pick up a Danish on your way to work. Every time you think about or see a Danish, those neuro-pathways are going to light up, prompting you to "just cheat this once." Remember, the brain, like muscle, is "use it or lose it." If you don't let the eat-pastry pathway continue firing, it starts rewiring into "bad pastry." It usually takes five weeks for the pastry craving pathway to dial down and form a new pathway: "lettuce wrap instead."

Remember, the reason T5 works and lasts is that you are changing your body and brain from the inside. Eating by the 90/10 rule (10 percent treats) is okay after the first five weeks, and by that time your craving to cheat has been dialed down and should stay that way.

I discovered this when one of my biggest cheats was a couple teaspoons of honey in my morning coffee. I convinced myself that I would absolutely not give this up, that it was my treat, and that it was okay to enjoy it. Besides, it wasn't much of a nutritional problem anyway, especially since I used organic, raw honey.

After many years of daily honey coffees, my dentist shocked me by showing me my gum-bone decay: "Some bacteria must really love what you're eating, because they're growing and eroding your bone." Aha! They were after the honey!

I went off honey-sweetened coffee for four weeks. My cravings changed. Although it was a bittersweet change, I now enjoy the real taste of coffee itself. After a month, my gums thanked me.

Another way to keep from cheating is to change food-pairing associations. The sweet-craving center in my brain stubbornly recorded: "Coffee must be paired with honey." So, I replaced coffee with green tea for a couple weeks and, sure enough, both my coffee cravings and honey cravings diminished. Remember, changing your brain changes your cravings. *Crave-change your brain.* Above all, avoid all binge eating. (See the end-notes on *endothelium dysfunction* after binge eating.)

COUNTING CALORIES? NO NEED TO!

I notice that the 5-S diet doesn't promote counting calories. Why?

Good news: With the 5-S diet you don't need to count calories. Remember, T5 is a no-numbers plan. You are not required to eat less, but rather eat smarter. The T5 food choices balance calories naturally. These nutrient-dense foods fill you up with fewer calories, so you will become satisfied with less. For example, calorie restriction advocates (sometimes called CRs) claim you must eat 20 to 25 percent fewer calories to feel the full health effects. T5ers will naturally do this without counting calories.

In fact, the current language in trusted obesity-control teaching is *calorie deception.*

Try this test of eating a 75-calorie slice of white bread (mostly carbs) one day when you're hungry and the next day an egg or half an avocado. Same number of calories, but you'll stay satisfied longer with the egg or avocado, which also contain fat and protein. This is why I strongly believe in adding healthy, preferably plant-based fats and protein to the two S's, smoothies and salads. Besides, fats taste better. You'll enjoy your food on T5.

Calorie-counting diets are going the way of the low-fat diet. The primarily high-fiber, plant-based real-food diet is just what the weight-control doctor ordered for those waist watchers who can't stick to calorie counting and portion control, the double dogma of weight control.

Another problem with calorie counting is we don't all burn calories the same way. Some people are "burners," others are "storers." Both are normal—people just metabolize foods at different rates. The calorie-burning number in a chemistry lab doesn't necessarily reflect what happens in your individual body.

That doesn't mean you should ignore calories altogether. One of my 90/10 treats, especially while on vacation, is dipping bread in olive oil and balsamic vinegar. I rationalized that the fatty olive oil would blunt the sugar spikes from the bread. One day I decided to count the calories in my treat. Wow, 400 calories! I cut back to one slice of high-fiber bread and downsized to one tablespoon of olive oil, which cut calories in half. Numbers make sense when they prompt a healthy change. Count calories *if and when* it actually helps you cut calories. You can count calories if you want, but you don't need to. Mother Nature does it for you. 🖐

MEDITERRANEAN DIET

Is the 5-S diet like the Mediterranean diet?

Yes and no. The T5 way of eating is close to the traditional Mediterranean diet, not the modern misconception of it. In my trips to coastal Mediterranean towns in Italy and Greece, I observed that the real Mediterranean diet isn't laden with pasta. Moreover, it isn't just a matter of the foods themselves, but Mediterranean people's mental, social, and sometimes spiritual approach to their cuisine. They are proud to know which farms their food comes from. Nearly all of it is from local plant and seafood sources, along with a little meat. But even their meat is real. Healthy Mediterranean towns are where the real "happy meals" are served.

TELOMERES AND T5

I've heard about telomeres being important to health. What are they and how does T5 help?

Telomeres are protective protein structures at the tips of each chromosome, sort of like plastic shoelace tips. They shrink as you age and serve as a measure of physical aging. Telomere measurements will soon be as common as blood tests.

Who are likely to have the longest telomeres, and therefore live the longest?

- Meditators
- Plant eaters (compared to meat eaters)
- Transform 5ers

Who have the shortest telomeres?

- Worriers
- Junk-food and animal-food eaters
- Couch potatoes

EGG WHITES ONLY?

Is it necessary or healthy to eat egg whites only instead of the whole egg?

I cringe when I'm at an omelet bar and hear "egg-white omelet, please." More often than not, the cook plops that tasteless, cholesterol-less omelet on a plate next to a wheat pancake drowning in high-fructose corn syrup. The truth is, a couple of egg yolks, which are rich in several valuable nutrients, would have made no difference at all in their blood cholesterol. It's the carbs in the syrup and the pancake that are likely to raise their cholesterol. So, the guy sits down and eats a breakfast that triggers giant sugar and cholesterol spikes, while the next guy enjoys a delicious, healthful whole-egg omelet. Also, I'm always suspicious when that "egg white" comes in a carton. I like to see real eggs cracked open and beat into an omelet.

CHOLESTEROL CONFUSION

I'm due for my annual checkup, and I've heard that cholesterol may not be the culprit for heart disease after all.

Let's clear up your cholesterol confusion.

A big, fat, sweet lie. A recent flurry of books and articles published in reputable journals by some of the top "fat scientists" have revealed shocking evidence that consumers have been duped into believing that dietary fat is the cause of heart disease, obesity, diabetes, and almost everything else. For many years, false reporting by the food industry and false science funded by the food and weight-loss industries pushed the idea that eating fat makes us fat, when in fact refined carbs are the culprit. The food industry has taken out fat and pumped up the carb content, and the nation has become fatter and sicker as a result.

More about cholesterol and the carb–cholesterol relationship. Another big fat misconception is that your blood level of cholesterol reveals how sick your heart is. Now we know that the standard cholesterol tests that most doctors use, a simple measure of HDL and LDL levels, don't tell the whole story. HDL is called the "good" cholesterol, and higher levels of it do seem to have protective value. LDL is mislabeled "the bad cholesterol." Here's the new way "fat scientists" explain it.

When it comes to LDL particles, size matters. LDL particles come in two sizes—large and small. The large particles are sort of like balloons that are fully blown up, light and puffy. They float through the bloodstream, mind their business, perform the normal, healthy function of transporting fat for energy and nourishment, *and they don't stick to the walls of the blood vessels*. They are too big to worm their way into and through the lining of blood vessels to build up plaque. Small particles—think of them as balloons that are only partially inflated—present two problems: (1) they may stick to the lining of the blood vessels; and (2) are small enough to worm their way through the lining. This is why the meaningful measurement is of *cholesterol particle size*. This can be done by Quest Diagnostics via their Cardio IQ Test, or by LabCorp's NMR LipoProfile test. So if your doctor orders a blood cholesterol test (lipid panel), ask, "Does this include my cholesterol small particle size?" Doctors love savvy patients who take charge of their health.

Carbs are the cause. When you eat less fat and more processed carbs, you deflate those large, puffy particles into smaller ones, *and* you make more new small particles. The more sugar, the more small-particle LDL, the more blood vessel and heart disease. It has been proven that people who eat more sugar tend to have higher triglycerides, LDL, and total cholesterol, *regardless of their weight*.

Not all fat is good for you. Even though fat is now seen as a good guy, don't be too quick to welcome more fats into your diet. It's more scientifically correct to say that *good fats don't make you fat*. Good fats lower your risk of nearly all the top diseases. The good fats are those naturally found in plant foods and seafood. (See DrSearsWellness.org/T5/Traffic-Light-Eating for a list of good fats and bad fats, and see related chart, "Give Yourself an Oil Change," page 245.)

High-fructose corn syrup. "Added sugars" are finally being recognized as a top cause of most diseases, and the most sickening sugar of all is high-fructose corn syrup (HFCS). Excess of other kinds of junk sugar is very bad, because it builds up sticky cholesterol in your blood vessels. But

HFCS is the worst, because it goes directly to the liver and is stored there as fat and cholesterol, raising your risk of fatty liver disease.

My cholesterol story. I decided to capitalize on my transformation by seeing if I could upgrade my life insurance policy. Since I was now healthier, I reasoned, I should get a better rate. The insurance company decided to take a chance on that, but they required some blood tests. Naturally, a sixty-five-year-old man isn't the type of risk insurance companies welcome. So, they sent a doctor to my home to do a thorough physical examination. I passed the in-home part, and he drew blood for a whole list of tests, including cholesterol, which at the time was still "the bad guy."

A couple weeks later, the doctor called with good news and bad news. "The bad news is the computer rejected your application for a better rating on your insurance policy, because your total cholesterol was high. The good news is we decided to upgrade your policy, because your good cholesterol (HDL) is so high." That made sense since one of the most accurate predictors of heart disease is the ratio of total cholesterol to HDL. Cardiologists like it to be no greater than 3:1. Mine was 2:1, even though my total cholesterol was high.

You should also know that new research has proven that for most people, a right-fat diet does not raise the blood cholesterol level or your risk of heart disease. It's the cholesterol that's made in the liver that contributes to most of your blood level measurement, and as you just read, that excess cholesterol starts out as extra sugar in your diet, not fat. While dietary cholesterol can raise cholesterol levels in some people, it raises the LDL and the HDL proportionately, so there's usually no harm done.

T5 FOR DEPRESSION

Like many of my friends, I suffer from mood swings, depression, and anxiety, and I'm taking medication for it. How could T5 help?

T5 is just the skills to partner with your pills.

Depression symptom	How T5 helps
Can't get off the couch.	Motivates you to move.
Negative thinking.	Promotes positive thinking; you can think-change your brain.
I can't help myself.	Empowers you with self-help skills.
Poor appetite.	Promotes smart food craving.
Sleepless.	You learn sleep-better tools.
Mood swings.	Promotes stable moods.
Low self-worth.	You make a project out of your problem.
Feeling alone, hopeless, and helpless.	T5 team supports you.

I don't believe I'm hearing this. Coincidentally, while writing this book I was invited to attend an international seminar on brain health. Many of the speakers were the top scientists in neuropsychiatry. Before the conference, I wrongly assumed this would be like the same old theme—what's the new wonder drug? Man, was I wrong! Let me summarize the science-based take-home messages. The renowned neuroscientists thoroughly studied the top medical studies on what works best for depression in the most people. Get ready to be surprised. Here's their priority list:

1. Exercise
2. Eating healthy
3. Avoidance of dietary and environmental neurotoxins
4. Cognitive behavior therapy—think-changing your brain
5. Being part of an accountability group
6. Professionally supervised medication

As I listened to these treatment priorities, I kept thinking, "That's T5!"

(See "Think-Change Your Brain," page 124; also read chapters four and seven.)

> Never self-wean off mood-altering medications. Always consult your doctor *before* changing your prescribed dosages.

SLEEP DEPRIVED

I have trouble sleeping. Can T5 help me sleep better?

Many T5ers report they sleep better within a few weeks. Here are the benefits of quality sleep and how T5 can help.

Sleep helps hormones. Human growth hormone peaks at night. You may not think you still need growth hormone, but you do. You're constantly regrowing and repairing worn-out cells all over your body. Cortisol, the get-up-and-go hormone, is naturally lowest during sleep and peaks around 6 AM to turn your brain and body back on.

Sleep regulates your turn-up and turn-down dials. During sleep, your sympathetic nervous system naturally dials down, while the parasympathetic nervous system dials up (see page 201). Basically, this means that sleep dials down hormones and nerve firings you need while awake and alert, and dials up those you need to rest and restore.

Your heart rests. Heart rate naturally decreases during sleep.

The gut rests. Remember when we said the earlier you eat, the better you sleep? That's because gastric acid secretion often peaks just after you go to bed, usually between 10 PM and 2 AM, and is lowest in the early morning. Also, intestinal motility, the force by which the gut moves food along from top to bottom, decreases during sleep. That combination is a set-up for reflux, especially in seniors.

Your brain gets better. The brain is one part of your body that *doesn't* totally sleep while you sleep. During sleep, the brain re-sorts all the confusion and clutter during the day, trashes what you don't need, and selectively files memories for you to keep. During sleep, the brain sorts out decision making, which is why people often go to sleep with a problem and wake up with a solution. Also, while blood flow may decrease to other parts of the body during sleep, it increases in the brain. Further, toxins that have accumulated during the day get washed away at night. Your brain recycles waste during sleep, removing waste products from hardworking brain cells and dumping them in the waste waterways of your lymphatic system.

It's fascinating how many messages the brain sends to the rest of the body during sleep. The brain tells the bladder to hold more urine so you can sleep through the night. The liver gets messages to deliver whatever extra glucose the brain needs, while the brain tells the heart, "Rest—you worked hard all day."

FIVE TRANSFORMATION TIPS FOR BETTER SLEEP

1. Move more during the day, sleep better at night. For most people there is a real correlation between how much they move during the day and how well they sleep at night. However, it helps to dial yourself down. During the last couple hours before bed, avoid heavy exercises that increase heart rate, blood pressure, and body temperature. Heavy exercise late in the evening confuses the body and brain by dialing your metabolism up when it's supposed to dial down.

2. Eat earlier. As a general guide, *the earlier your evening meal, the better you'll feel*. Try to end your supper no later than *three hours* before you retire. This correlation varies with age and is more necessary for seniors prone to reflux (heartburn). Log in your T5 journal the correlation between what and when you eat and how well you sleep. This will help you adjust to your perfect personal eat-sleep rhythm.

3. Discover your personal snooze foods. Some scientists teach that the longer you fast—the more hours between the evening meal and breakfast—the lower your insulin spikes and the better for your insulin sensitivity. But longer nocturnal fasting is harder for some people than for others who might need a light, healthy snack before bed. Discover your personal snooze foods, those that help you sleep. Dr. Bill's is an egg.

SNOOZE FOODS

These foods are high in the sleep-inducing amino acid tryptophan:

- Dairy products: cottage cheese, cheese, milk
- Soy products: soy milk, tofu, soybean nuts
- Seafood
- Meat
- Poultry
- Beans
- Greens: spinach, kale
- Hummus
- Lentils
- Hazelnuts, peanuts
- Eggs
- Sesame seeds, sunflower seeds

---

4. Unplug. For most people the more time you spend staring at artificial screens—phones, tablets, computers, and TV—the less you sleep. The lights in most electronic devices mess with *melatonin*. This is especially true of the new energy-efficient LED—light-emitting diode—light bulbs, which have high-blue wavelengths. Your brain's master clock (in the hypothalamus) constantly monitors the intensity of light around you. When light goes up, so do your get-up-and-go hormones. When light dims down, the drowsiness and go-to-sleep hormone, melatonin, increases.

Dial down the dimmers. Savvy transformers put dimmers on all their light switches throughout the house, especially in the bedroom. They start dimming their whole house a couple hours before bedtime. The brain is naturally programmed to dial down when the natural light outside fades at sundown. But if we keep the artificial lights bright when we should be dialing down, the brain gets confused and doesn't rest as it should during sleep. Sleep researchers describe this scrambling of brain rhythms as the dark side of too much brightness in the evening. If you just *have* to use your screen devices at night, use software such as f.lux, available free at JustGetFlux.com, to automatically adjust your computer or phone screen.

Many smartphones have a settings option for a built-in blue light filter that's good to toggle on at night. And use *amber* night lights. Remember, "Lights down at least an hour before lights-out."

5. Enjoy a before-bed ritual. Don't ignore your natural "crash time." Most people will naturally get sleepy as the evening progresses, and that's when you should go to bed. If you wait an hour or so later for a specific "bedtime," your body will start to reawaken when you should be going off to sleep. Many people find it helpful to have an evening wind-down routine. Enjoy after-dinner yoga and meditation, a family board game, or take your pet for a walk. Write in your gratitude journal and enjoy a calming cup of herbal tea and some relaxing music. Take a warm-to-cool shower or bath twenty to thirty minutes before bed—your body's cooling off triggers melatonin. Keep your bedroom cool, less than 70 degrees. Practice deep-breathing while drifting off to sleep. And let your mind cool down with happy thoughts. Savor the moment. Don't rehash the day's events or think about the next day. Drift off to sleep only in the present, or even in your imaginary happy place.

FIVE TERRIBLE EFFECTS OF SLEEP DEPRIVATION

Sleep, like food, should be valued by quality over quantity. Poor-quality sleep increases the risk of just about every ailment you don't want to get. T5 living, eating, and thinking puts your body into balance. Sleep deprivation puts it out of balance in several ways:

1. Disrupts appetite-balancing hormones, leptin and ghrelin. Under-sleepers tend to be overeaters and prediabetics.
2. Causes carb cravings, making you prone to prediabetes and insulin resistance.
3. Increases the stress hormone cortisol to a higher level than you really need.

4. Leads to immune system dysfunction, increasing the risk of inflammation and even cancer.
5. Brain fog.

PREBIOTICS

What is a prebiotic?

Prebiotics are high-fiber foods that promote the growth of beneficial gut bacteria: oats, bananas, onions, garlic, leeks, asparagus, artichokes, and the list of best foods on page 209. *Synbiotic* foods have a combination of probiotics and prebiotics. These are primarily fermented foods, such as kefir. When fermented to sauerkraut, cabbage (a good source of indigestible plant fiber to begin with) also provides lactobacillus and so becomes a synbiotic. Some probiotic preparations come packaged with prebiotics with names like *fructooligosaccharides*.

Where do you find the most prebiotics in your grocery store? Dr. Mom could have told you this long ago. In the produce section. Onions don't come from the farm with nutrition facts labels on the skin, but they are rich in prebiotics nonetheless. (See illustration, page 264.)

GUT HEALTH AND AGING

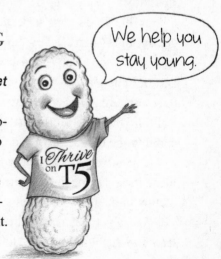

We help you stay young.

Do probiotics become more important as I get older?

Yes! The older you get, the more probiotics you may need, because your ratio of good to bad microbiome bugs tends to decrease. This means your microbiome won't be as effective at preventing disease unless you start taking better care of it. Further, as we get older, many of us take more medicines like antibiotics, antacids, and anti-inflammatories, all of which are unfriendly to the microbiome. All the more reason to step up the probiotics.

LEAKY GUT

I have a leaky gut. Help!

As you read in chapter six, a top job of your microbiome is to *heal and seal*. Let's take a really close look at the intestinal lining for a better idea of how that works. The lining of the intestines looks like a shag carpet. The individual shags are called villi, and they really look more like little fingers. Look closer yet, and you'll see that each of the villi is made up of microvilli. The purpose of this design is to hugely increase the surface area to facilitate absorption of nutrients. Your colon is a tube about five feet long, but inside it has the same surface area as a tennis court.

Bacteria reside amid the microvilli. In return for free food and a warm place to live, they do good things for their host. That's the good news. The bad news is when fiberless, processed, fake food that doesn't belong there gets into the gut, bad bacteria grow, and these unwelcome party crashers cause problems.

First, the microvilli become blunted, shortened, and then start to slough off. Next, gaps develop between the protective cells that line the microvilli. These gaps leak material into the bloodstream that shouldn't get through—that's leaky gut syndrome. Also, when too many bad bacteria grow, too many good bacteria die, and when they die they release harmful chemical byproducts called lipopolysaccharides (LPSs). (Notice the root words for fat and sugar in there? Sounds like sticky stuff you don't want in your gut.) LPSs pass through the leaks in the damaged gut lining and into the bloodstream and trigger inflammation throughout the body.

It gets worse. The immune system identifies these LPSs as foreign invaders and starts fighting them, causing a metabolic mess we call inflammation in the intestinal lining.

Worse yet, because of these gaps, partly digested food molecules also leak into the bloodstream. The immune system misidentifies these, too, as foreign intruders, and mobilizes troops to fight them, leading to food allergies. For example, say some messed-up wheat particles get through and trigger the immune system to make antibodies against the wheat. Bingo, you're allergic to wheat. Leaky gut leads to food allergies. To help repair your leaky gut, eat the 5-S diet.

STRENGTH-BUILDING EXERCISES

S trength training benefits your transformation in many ways:

1. It increases strength, builds muscle mass, and protects bone health.
2. It maximizes your calorie burn through the afterburn effect.
3. It is the most efficient way to transform your body and maintain lasting results.

Be sure to listen to your body so you can push yourself to get better without pushing too hard and risking injury. These movements take practice—you will become stronger over time.

SAMPLE FULL-BODY RESISTANCE TRAINING CIRCUIT

Equipment needed: 1 pair of light to medium weights and one pair of medium to heavy weights.
Beginners/Intermediate: Light to medium weight = 5–10 pounds; Medium to heavy weight = 15–20 pounds
Intermediate/Advanced: Light to medium weight = 10–15 pounds; Medium to heavy weight = 20–25 pounds

Use the medium weight for the upper body and the heavy weight for the lower body. If you're a beginner, you can even eliminate the weights for the lower body. You will know what the right weight is for you if you're challenged by rep 12 in a 15-rep set.

- Warm up for 3–5 minutes (do any movement that gets your blood flowing).
- Complete combos 1 through 4.
- For each combo, complete 4 sets of 15 reps per move and a core exercise (1–2 minutes) between the combos.
- Alternate between lower-body and upper-body moves to allow the muscle groups to rest.

COMBO 1

Bicep Curls

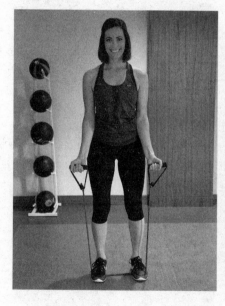 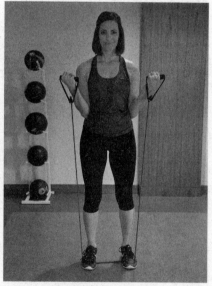

- Holding weights or a band (as pictured), stand with your legs shoulder distance apart and your arms extended.
- Curl your hands toward your shoulders by contracting your muscles. Return to starting position without overextending the elbow joint.

Squats

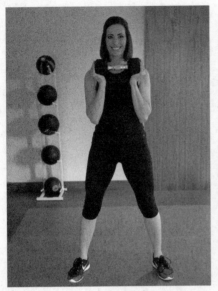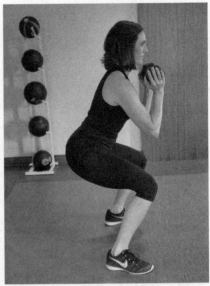

- Holding a weight with both hands in front of your chest, stand with your feet slightly wider apart than shoulder distance.
- Set your body weight in your heels, sit your bottom back, and squat while keeping your knees over your toes.

Core: Bicycle

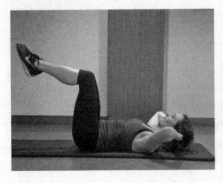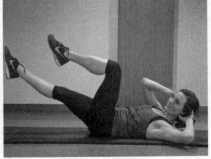

- Press your lower back to the floor, put your hands behind your neck, and bring your legs to a tabletop position.

- Rotate through your torso, bringing your left elbow to meet your right knee, and repeat on the other side.

COMBO 2

Shoulder Press (Single or Double)

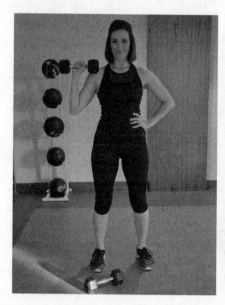 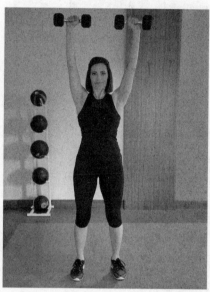

- Bend your knees slightly while holding the weight(s) at shoulder height.
- Extend your arm(s) toward the sky, keeping your arm(s) straight and your wrist(s) in line. (If you are doing the exercise with a single weight, repeat on the other side.)

Single-Leg Squats

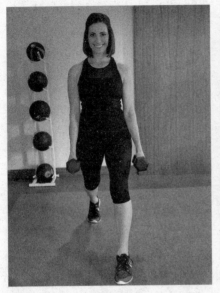 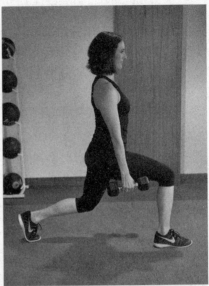

- Stand in split stance with weights hanging beside you.
- Bend both knees while keeping your front knee in line with your ankle.

Core: Plank

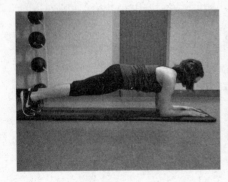 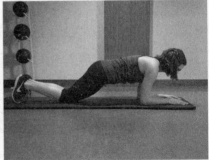

- Hold the Plank pose for 1 minute. (You may modify the pose by doing it with your knees on the ground, as pictured on the right.)

COMBO 3

Triceps Extension

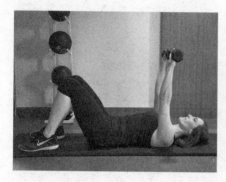 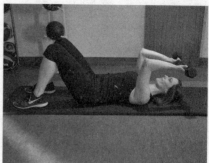

- Lie on your back and extend the weights in the air in line with your shoulders.
- Bend your elbows, bringing your wrists toward your forehead, and then return to the starting position (focus your strength on the back of your upper arms).

Core: Alternating Reach

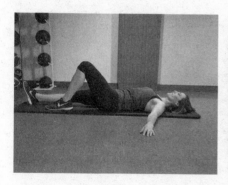 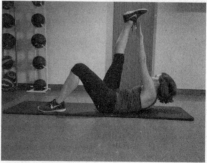

- Lie on your back with one knee bent. Extend both arms out to the side.
- Lift your leg and use the opposite arm to reach toward your ankle. Lower your leg/upper body and extend arm overhead.
- Repeat on the other side.

Bowler's Lunge

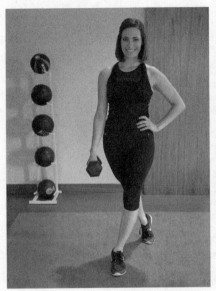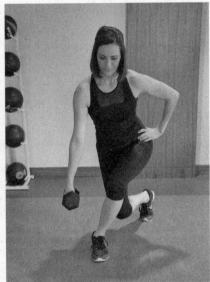

- Hold the weight in your right hand while extending your right leg back (as if you were bowling).
- Bend both legs while sticking your left hip out (bend forward slightly).
- Repeat on the other side.

COMBO 4

Upper-Back Row

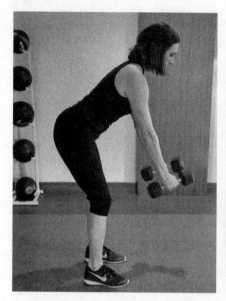 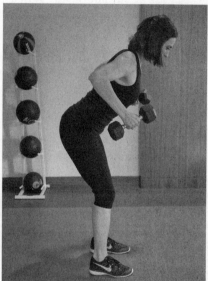

- Extend the weights in front of you at a slight angle while bending over.
- Pull back while squeezing your shoulder blades together.

Sumo Squat

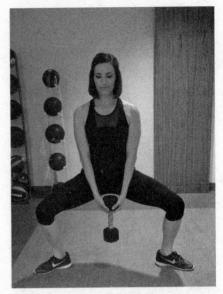

- Stand with your legs straight (not pictured) in a straddle position with your toes slightly turned out. Hold the weight between your legs.
- Bend and return to the starting position (keep your knees over your toes, your pelvis tucked, and your upper body straight).

Core: C-Crunch Extension

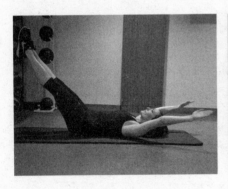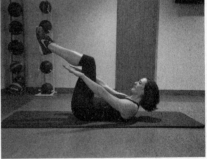

- Lie on your back and extend your arms and legs.
- Bring your knees to your chest while reaching your arms toward your feet, while keeping your lower back planted on the mat.

For more core ideas, see page 319.

APPENDIX B

YOGA AND PILATES

⊙ See Erin demonstrate and explain favorite yoga poses and Pilates movements at DrSearsWellness.org/T5/Yoga-Pilates.

YOGA

Yoga is not about touching your toes, it is
what you learn on the way down.
—JIGAR GOR

Practice the following moves by holding each pose for 5 deep breaths.

SOME STRENGTHENING POSES

Downward-Facing Dog: Strengthens and stretches the legs and shoulders. Calms the nervous system.

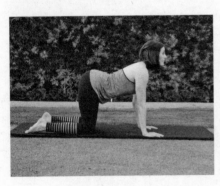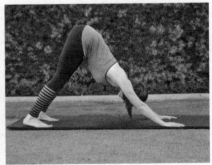

- Begin on all fours, with your feet a hip width apart and your wrists under your shoulders.

- Tuck your toes under and lift your tailbone to the sky. Extend your arms to lengthen your spine and spread your fingers wide.
- Relax your head between your biceps. Relax your shoulder blades down your back.

Plank: Strengthens and aligns the shoulders and core. (You may modify the pose by doing it with your knees on the ground, as pictured on the right.)

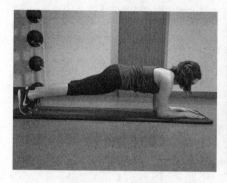
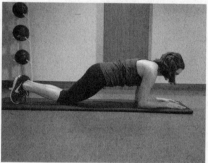

- Stack your shoulders over your elbows. Tuck your toes under and extend your legs.
- Energize and lengthen from your heels to your head.
- Keep your tailbone in line with your shoulders and engage your core.

Upward-Facing Dog: Lengthens the spine. Strengthens the core and triceps.

- Align your hands under the top of your ribs. Only your hands and the tops of your feet are on the mat.
- Lift your heart forward while relaxing your shoulders.

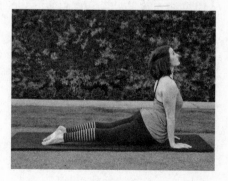

Warrior II: Strengthens and aligns the shoulders, legs, pelvis, and hips.

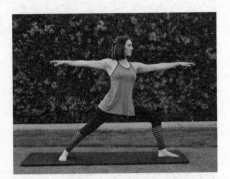

- Stack your front knee over your ankle, pointed in the same direction as your front toes. Align your front heel with the arch of your back foot.
- Energize your arms out to a T with your shoulders relaxed.
- Repeat on the other side.

Reversed Warrior II: Strengthens legs and tones/stretches the side body.

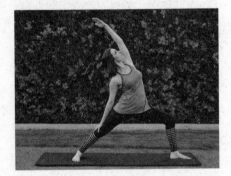

- Position your legs as in Warrior II. Extend your back arm down and reach your top arm over your head.
- Repeat on the other side.

Extended Side Angle: Strengthens the spine. Tones/stretches the side body.

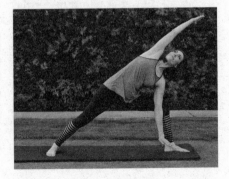

- Position your legs as in Warrior II. Bend your torso forward toward your front knee.
- Rest your front arm on your front thigh, or reach for your front ankle with your front arm.

- Extend your back arm overhead, creating a strong line of energy on the extended side.
- Repeat on the other side.

Low Crescent Lunge: Strengthens and aligns the legs. Opens the hip joints.

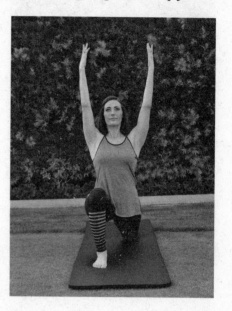

- Bend your front knee and stack it over your ankle. Keep the top of your back foot flat on the mat.
- Energize your arms toward the sky while relaxing your shoulders.
- Keep your core engaged to protect your lower back.
- Repeat on the other side.

Make this pose more challenging by tucking the toes of your back foot under and lifting your back knee off the mat.

Triangle: Strengthens and aligns the legs, hips, and arms. Gently rotates the spine.

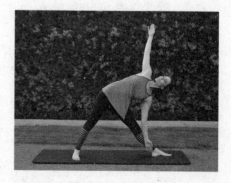

- Keep both your legs straight, with your front heel aligned with the arch of your back foot.
- Tilt your torso forward to stack your shoulders and open the chest. Energize your arms while relaxing your shoulder blades.
- Repeat on the other side.

Tree: Strengthens and stabilizes the legs. Promotes balance.

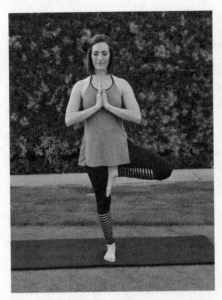
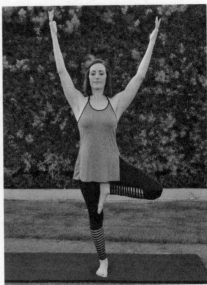

- Begin by balancing on both feet with your weight evenly distributed.
- Lift one foot and gently press it to the standing leg's calf or inner thigh.
- Lift out of the standing foot to the crown of your head.
- Keep your hips level. Put your hands in prayer position (pictured on the left) or extend them overhead (pictured on the right).
- Repeat on the other side.

Bridge: Strengthens the back, glutes, legs, hips, and ankles.

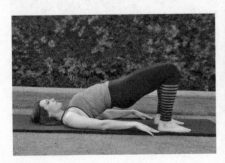
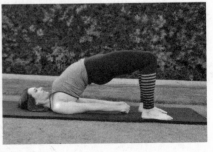

- Lie on your back and align your ankles under your knees.
- Keep your knees in line with your hips while engaging your inner thighs.
- Lift your pelvis toward the sky. Push away from the floor with your palms.
- Alternatively, interlace your fingers under your back and roll onto your shoulders.

STRETCH AND DETOXIFY

Revolved Low Crescent Lunge: Helps remove toxins from organs. Improves spinal flexibility.

- Assume the Low Crescent Lunge pose (see page 311).
- Plant the opposite palm next to the inside of your front foot and twist at mid-spine.
- Extend your top arm and try to stack your shoulders.
- Repeat on the other side.

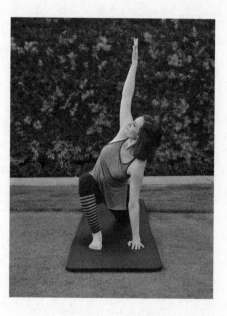

Twisted Wide-Legged Forward Fold: Helps remove toxins from organs. Improves spinal flexibility.

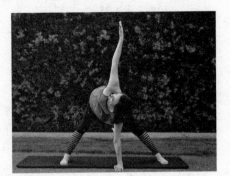

- Take a wide-legged stance with your feet facing forward.
- Find length in your spine and hinge forward. Lift your tailbone toward the sky.
- Lower one palm to the center and lift your other arm while twisting and stacking your shoulders.
- Repeat on the other side.

Seated Spinal Twist: Opens the rib cage and breath. Massages the digestive organs. Stimulates lymph flow and the immune system.

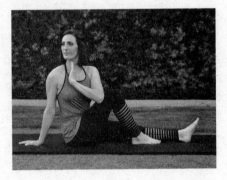

- Sit with both legs extended and a tall spine. Pull one knee toward your chest and plant the foot of that leg on the mat.
- Take the opposite elbow and cross the bent knee, reaching back with the other palm to lengthen your spine.
- Repeat on the other side.

Reclined Twist: Releases tension in the lower back.

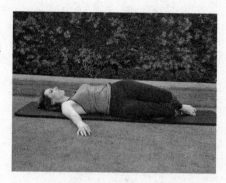

- Lie on your back with your knees bent and your feet on the mat.
- Extend your arms out to a T and lower your knees to one side. Keep your neck and shoulders relaxed.
- Repeat on the other side.

STRETCH AND RESTORE

Child's Pose: Gently flexes the spine, hips, knees, and shoulders. Massages the abdominal organs, kidneys, and adrenal glades.

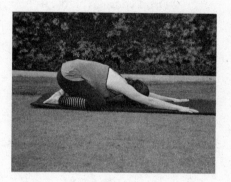

- Kneel on the mat with your knees spread wide (about mat width).
- Bow forward, lengthening through the spine.
- Alternatively, your palms can rest face up alongside your hips for a shoulder release.

Cat/Cow: Stretches the lower back and abdomen while stabilizing the wrists, shoulders, and knees.

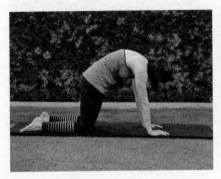 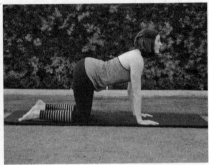

- Begin in a tabletop position, aligning your shoulders over your wrists and your hips over your knees. Spread your fingers wide.
- Press into the mat as your upper back rounds and your navel pulls toward your spine (Cat).
- Drop your navel toward the ground as you lift your sternum forward (Cow).
- Pull your shoulder blades down your back.

Forward Fold (Rag Doll): Promotes flexibility in the spine and hips. Stretches the hamstrings and lower back. Increases circulation to the brain.

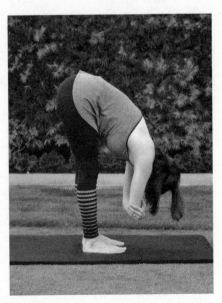

- Start standing. Fold from your hip joints while lengthening your spine (bend your knees as needed).
- Keep your head and neck relaxed as you grab your elbows.
- Add shoulder stretch or wide-legged variations (on next page).

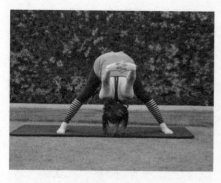
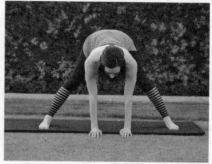

Supine Pigeon: Releases tension in the lower back, hips, and glutes.

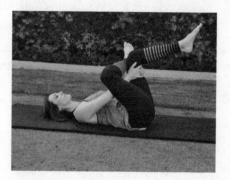

- Lie on your back with your knees bent. Cross one ankle over the opposite knee.
- Thread your hands around the uncrossed thigh and gentle pull it toward your chest.
- Keep your head and neck relaxed on the mat.
- Repeat on the other side.

Hamstring Extension: Promotes flexibility in the backs of the legs.

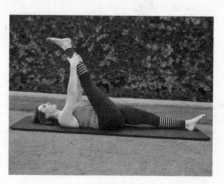

- Lie on your back and bring one knee to your chest. Extend the heel to the sky, working toward straightening the leg.
- Grab the leg wherever you can, except at the knee joint. If desired, you can use a strap or towel to assist you.
- Repeat on the other side.

Happy Baby: Releases the hips, inner thighs, and lower back.

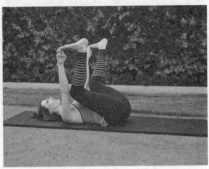

- Lie on your back and bend both knees toward your chest.
- Spread your knees wide apart, reaching toward your underarms.
- With your hands, grab your thighs, ankles, or feet, keeping your tailbone and shoulders on the mat as much as possible.

Supine Butterfly: Relieves stress. Stretches the hips, inner thigh, and groin. Promotes circulation.

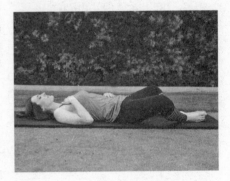

- Lie on your back. Place the soles of your feet together as your knees fly open.
- Place one hand on your navel and one on your heart.

PILATES/RESISTANCE BANDS

Keep your core engaged at all times and use your breath!

UPPER BODY

Biceps

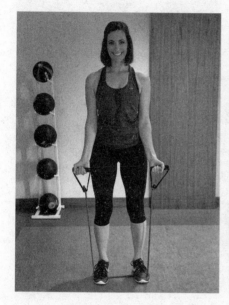 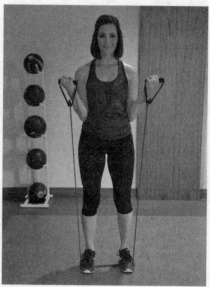

- Hold both handles of the band as pictured. Keep your knees bent slightly and your elbows hugging inward.
- Contract your biceps by bringing your wrists toward your shoulders and then slowly lower.

Shoulders

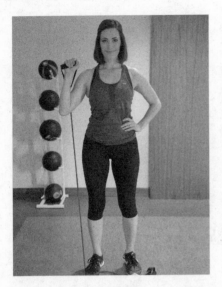
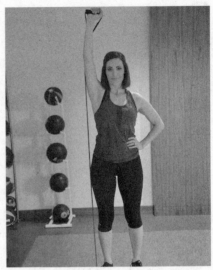

- Hold one handle of the band as pictured.
- Lift slowly until your arm is almost straight (avoid locking your elbow).
- Repeat on the other side.

Upper Back

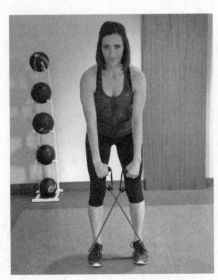
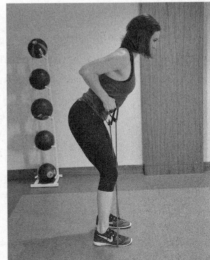

- Hold both handles of the band as pictured, with the bands crisscrossed.
- Hinge forward at the hips slightly and bend your knees.
- Contracting the upper back, try to pull your elbows together.

Triceps

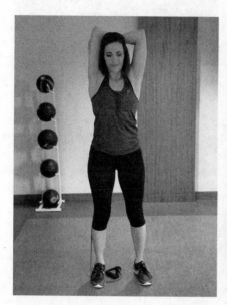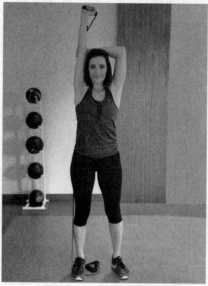

- Hold one handle of the band as pictured.
- With the palm of your empty hand, grab the opposite triceps.
- Leading with the pinky, extend the band toward the sky and return slowly.
- Repeat on the other side.

LOWER BODY

Glutes

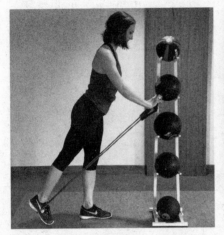 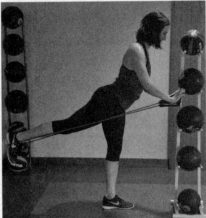

- Stand by a supportive surface (like a chair or couch) about hip or waist height and grab the handles of the band in each hand.
- Loop the band around one foot and lift and lower your foot, leading with the heel.
- Repeat on the other side.

For the floor version:

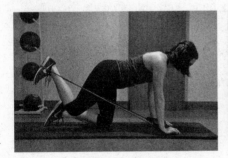 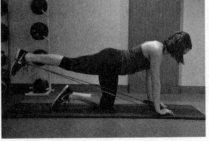

- Begin on all fours with a handle in each hand, and the band looped around one foot.
- Bend your knee in and extend your heel out.

Hamstrings

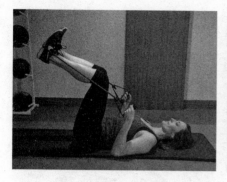 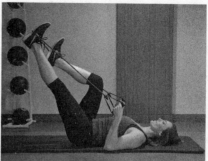

- Lay on your back and bring your knees to a table top position.
- Grab the handles of the band and loop the band itself around both feet.
- Extend your leg by pressing your heel away.
- Return to table top position and repeat on the other side
- Continue back and forth as if peddling a bike.

Quads and Core

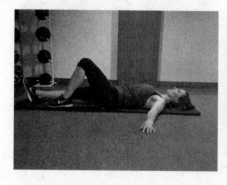 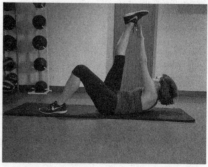

- Lie on your back with one knee bent. Extend both arms out to the side
- Lift your straight leg and use the opposite arm to reach toward your ankle. Lower your leg/upper body and extend arm overhead.
- Repeat on the other side.

MORE CORE

Side Plank

- Lie on your side.
- Align your lower elbow under your shoulder, extend your upper arm up to the sky, and lift your hips to the sky.
- Repeat on the other side.

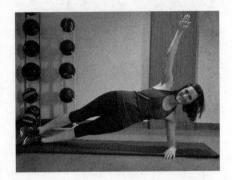

You may modify the exercise by lowering the bottom knee.

Plank with Extension

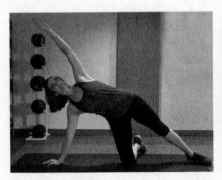
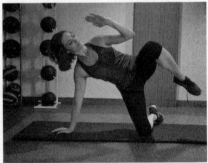

- Begin in a side plank with your shoulders stacked, one knee on the mat, and the other leg extended.
- Reach your top arm overhead and lengthen the side body from toe to fingertips.
- Engage your core and bend your upper knee and your upper elbow toward each other.
- Repeat on the other side.

Straddle

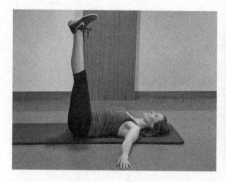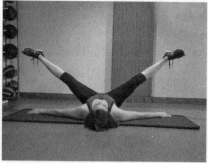

- Lie on your back with your legs straight up.
- Open your legs out to the sides.
- Activate your core and inner thigh to return your legs back up.

Oblique Twist

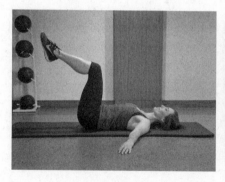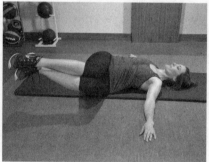

- Lie on the floor with your legs up and your knees bent at a 90-degree angle.
- Lower your knees to the side. Engage your core to draw the knees back to center.
- Repeat on the other side.

Toe Tap

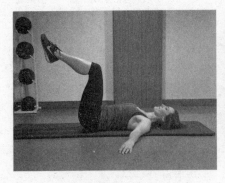 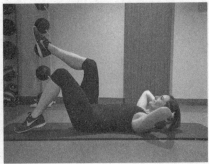

- Lie on the floor with your legs up and your knees bent at a 90-degree angle.
- Lower one foot or both feet to the floor.
- Return your leg(s) to 90 degrees.
- If you lowered only one foot, repeat on the other side.

For more support, put your arms out to the side (pictured on the left). For a more challenging exercise, put your arms behind your head and lift your chest (pictured on the right).

APPENDIX C

RECIPES

SALADS

SALAD IN A MASON JAR

By now you know that Dr. Bill and I are all about our salads! A couple years ago I was invited to a "salad in a jar" event that made me think, "Why didn't I think of that?" I left with five meals of yummy salads prepped. I have kept this in my T5 tool belt ever since because it is simple, fun, and convenient—the salads stay fresh for about five days!

Layer 1: The Dressing

The first layer of a Mason jar salad is always the dressing. You can use any type of dressing you like (that is T5 approved; see salad dressing recipes, page 330). I prefer an olive oil and balsamic vinegar dressing, which will come out of the Mason jar more easily. If you use a thicker dressing, you will have to give the jar a good shake and you will probably need to use your fork to scrape out the dressing. Use about 2 tablespoons of dressing.

Layer 2: Hearty Vegetables and Legumes

This layer is very important because it shields the dressing from the lettuce and other vulnerable ingredients. In this layer you should use vegetables that can hold up to being in dressing for up to a week. Choose raw vegetables like cherry or grape tomatoes, red onion, broccoli, cauliflower, asparagus, celery, carrots, peppers, beets, and any other hearty vegetable you like. Chop as desired.

Next sprinkle cooked legumes like black beans, kidney beans, lentils, or edamame, and less hearty raw vegetables like mushrooms, zucchini, sprouts, cucumber, and green beans. If you are using an avocado, then add it in this layer as well (sprinkle it with lime juice to keep it fresh). Basically, this layer acts as a second barrier between the dressing and the lettuce.

Layer 3: Pasta and Grains

This layer is for pasta and/or other healthy whole grains, such as couscous and/or quinoa.

Layer 4: Protein and Cheese

In this layer I put eggs and cheese. I like to keep these ingredients away from the dressing because they do not do well when they sit in dressing for a couple of days or more. If you are using shrimp or other seafood, add those ingredients to this layer. For cheese, I have used blue cheese, feta cheese, goat cheese, shredded parmesan or cheddar cheese, and various cubed cheeses in my Mason jar salad. Each of them has worked fine. Cheese tip: Generally, the harder, the healthier. For example, Parmesan is a good choice. However, remember to limit the amount of cheese or skip all together!

Layer 5: Lettuce, Nuts, Seeds, and Dried Fruit

In this last layer you want to put ingredients that would wilt or become too soft and soggy if exposed to dressing for too long. This definitely includes any type of lettuce or greens. I also include nuts in this layer because I have found that they sometimes lose their crunch if they are too close to the dressing layer. My favorite greens to use are arugula, baby spinach, kale, romaine, and mixed greens. Put nuts, seeds, and dried fruit in last.

After you fill the Mason jar with the different layers, just put the top on and close tightly. There's no rule for how much to put in each layer. You can even skip a layer or two. The layer you *always* want to include is layer 2, the hearty vegetables and legumes. Just make sure you have enough other ingredients to keep the dressing and lettuce away from each other until you're ready to enjoy your salad.

SALAD DRESSINGS

APPLE CIDER VINEGAR DRESSING

¼ cup apple cider vinegar
½ cup olive oil
2 teaspoons Dijon mustard
1 tablespoon minced garlic

1 teaspoon sea salt
1 teaspoon freshly ground black
   pepper + more if needed

Add all ingredients into a blender and blend until combined. Store in the refrigerator.

Serving size: 2 tablespoons

ZESTY TAHINI DRESSING

¼ cup tahini
¼ cup apple cider vinegar
¼ cup lemon juice

One teaspoon low-sodium tamari
   or soy sauce
½ cup nutritional yeast
1 tablespoon minced garlic

Add all ingredients into a blender and blend until combined. Store in the refrigerator.

Serving size: 2 tablespoons

CILANTRO LEMON VINAIGRETTE

⅓ cup olive oil or avocado oil
2 teaspoons water
2 handfuls cilantro
Juice of ½ lemon

2 teaspoons minced garlic
¼ teaspoon salt
1 teaspoon honey
2 tablespoons red wine vinegar

Add all of the ingredients to a blender and puree until smooth and emulsified. Store in the refrigerator.

Serving size: 2 tablespoons

DR. BILL'S ANTI-CANCER SALAD

The most motivated recipe designers are those fighting for their lives, or as described more aptly, eating for their lives. During my personal beat-cancer crusade, this is the science-based salad I came up with and continue to eat nearly nightly to this day. Here are the five "food groups" to choose from as you design your personal salad. You don't have to pick from all five to begin with, but eventually, as you shape your tastes and your gut feel, you'll choose the ones that work for you.

Greens
Kale
Spinach
Arugula
Red bell peppers
Jalapeño peppers
Leeks
Onions
Beet greens and roots
Broccoli
Red cabbage
Swiss chard
Collard greens
Asparagus
Mushrooms

Beans
Black beans (reduced sodium)
Lentils (my favorite legume)
Pinto beans

Hummus
Edamame (raw soybeans)

Seeds and Spices
Turmeric, with black pepper
Pumpkin seeds
Garlic

Dressing
Olive oil
Balsamic vinegar

Special additions
Cauliflower
Brussels sprouts
Berries
Nuts
1 (4-ounce) fillet wild salmon,
  baked

DR. BILL'S DELICIOUS, NUTRITIOUS MICROBIOME SALAD

1 (4–6-ounce) fillet wild salmon, baked

1 ounce goat cheese and/or cottage cheese

2 ounces organic, reduced-sodium black beans

1 cup spinach, kale, and arugula

¼ cup chopped tomato

4 spears asparagus

1 egg, hard-boiled and sliced

1 tablespoon extra-virgin olive oil

1 tablespoon diced onion

Juice of ½ lemon or lime

½ teaspoon ground turmeric

¼ teaspoon black pepper

1 teaspoon minced garlic

2 tablespoons T5-approved dressing of your choice

Optional additions

2 tablespoons cooked quinoa

Chili peppers

Preheat oven to 375 degrees and bake salmon in a baking dish for 10–15 minutes. Combine all the ingredients through diced onion in a large bowl. You may layer or mix everything together. Add the lemon/lime juice, turmeric, pepper, and garlic. Lastly, add the dressing. Enjoy a half portion to begin the meal, or a full portion as a salad entrée.

A hot tip: Put your salad in a steamer for a few minutes. You'll love the tangy cheese flavoring the warm vegetables. Use chopsticks so you savor it slowly. Enjoy!

DINNERS

LEMON DILL SALMON

This dish is great for those who are new to salmon.

Salmon
2 (6-ounce) fillets wild salmon
¼ teaspoon lemon pepper
¼ teaspoon dried or chopped fresh
   dill
Pinch of sea salt
Pinch of crushed red pepper
   (optional)
2 slices lemon

Sauce
1 tablespoon olive oil
1 tablespoon Dijon mustard
1 tablespoon fresh lemon juice
Pinch of black pepper

Preheat the oven to 375 degrees. Defrost the salmon if needed. Place the salmon fillets in a glass baking dish. In small bowl, mix the lemon pepper, dill, salt, and crushed red pepper, and sprinkle most of the mixture evenly over the fillets (save a little for the sauce). Place 1 lemon slice on each fillet. Bake the fillets for 10–15 minutes. While the fillets are baking, add all the sauce ingredients to the bowl with the reserved herb and spice mixture, and stir to combine. Serve the sauce either on top of the cooked fish or on the side.

Yield: 2 servings

Note: Always season to taste. If you like spicy food, use the red pepper. Also, instead of baking the salmon, you can sauté it. Cook the salmon in a teaspoon of olive oil in a skillet over medium heat for 4 minutes. Turn the fillets, top each fillet with 1 lemon slice, and cook for 4 more minutes.

HONEY BALSAMIC SALMON

2 (6-ounce) fillets wild salmon
1 tablespoon raw honey
1 tablespoon balsamic vinegar

1 teaspoon Dijon mustard
1 teaspoon olive oil

Preheat the oven to 375 degrees. Place the salmon in a baking dish. In a small bowl, mix together the honey, vinegar, mustard, and olive oil. Pour the mixture onto the fish and bake for 10–15 minutes.

Yield: 2 servings

Note: Alternatively, you can sauté the salmon in a little olive oil (about a teaspoon), with the sauce poured on top, in a skillet over medium heat for 4 minutes on each side.

SPAGHETTI SQUASH WITH SALMON

1 spaghetti squash (4–6 cups
    cooked)
Olive oil
1 teaspoon Italian seasoning
Sea salt
Black pepper
Crushed red pepper to taste

Fresh garlic or garlic powder
2 (6-ounce) wild salmon fillets
2 cups spinach
2 cups marinara sauce
Shredded aged Parmesan cheese
Fresh basil (optional)

Preheat the oven to 400 degrees. Use a fork to poke a few holes in the squash, place it on a microwave-safe plate, and microwave for 5 minutes to soften. Cut the squash in half lengthwise and place it in a baking dish. Scoop out the seeds with a spoon. Lightly drizzle with the olive oil and sprinkle with the Italian seasoning, salt, black pepper, crushed red pepper, and garlic. Place the squash face down and bake for about 30–45 minutes, depending on the size of the squash. If you can stick a fork in the cut side and can easily scrape it out, then it's done. Cool for about 10 minutes.

While the squash is cooling, bake the salmon for 10–12 minutes. While the salmon is baking, heat a little olive in a skillet over medium heat, add the spinach, and cook, stirring occasionally, until lightly wilted, 3–5 minutes. While the spinach is sautéing, heat up the marinara sauce in a small saucepan over medium heat, then simmer on low until needed. Once the squash has cooled, use a fork to scrape the flesh out of the shell. Cut the salmon into four pieces. For each serving, layer 1–1½ cups squash, ½ cup sauce, ½ cup spinach, and a piece of salmon. Lightly sprinkle with the Parmesan and basil if using. Enjoy.

Yield: 4 servings

LEMON GARLIC SHRIMP

3 teaspoons extra-virgin olive oil, divided

2 red bell peppers, diced

2 cups sliced asparagus (1-inch pieces)

2 teaspoons freshly grated lemon zest

½ teaspoon salt, divided

2 cloves garlic, minced

16 ounces raw shrimp, peeled and deveined

½ cup reduced-sodium chicken broth

1 tablespoon fresh lemon juice

Fresh or dried parsley to taste

Heat 1 teaspoon of the olive oil in a large nonstick skillet over medium-high heat. Add the bell peppers, asparagus, lemon zest, and ¼ teaspoon of the salt and cook, stirring occasionally, until just beginning to soften, about 6 minutes. Transfer the vegetables to a bowl; cover to keep warm.

Add the remaining 2 teaspoons olive oil and garlic to the pan and cook, stirring, for about 30 seconds. Add the shrimp and cook, stirring, for 1 minute. Add the broth to the pan along with the remaining ¼ teaspoon salt. Cook, stirring, until the sauce has thickened slightly and the shrimp are pink and just cooked through, about 2 minutes more. Remove from the heat. Stir in the lemon juice and parsley. Serve the shrimp and sauce over the vegetables.

Yield: 4 servings

ZUCCHINI AND TURKEY WITH BROWN RICE
PASTA OR WHOLE WHEAT PASTA

This is also great as a vegetarian meal—simply omit the turkey.

1 cup uncooked brown rice pasta
  or whole wheat pasta
4 medium zucchini
1 tablespoon olive oil
1 pound organic 90 percent lean
  ground turkey

½ teaspoon garlic powder
Salt to taste
Black pepper to taste
Crushed red pepper to taste
1 teaspoon Italian seasoning
2 cups marinara sauce

Prepare the pasta as directed on the package (be sure not to overcook the brown rice pasta). Use a vegetable peeler or spiralizer to cut the zucchini into strips/"noodles." Heat a large nonstick skillet with half the oil (½ tablespoon) over medium heat. Add the turkey, garlic, salt, black pepper, crushed red pepper, and Italian seasoning and cook, stirring occasionally, until there is no pink color. While the meat is browning, heat a separate skillet over medium heat using the remaining oil. Sauté the zucchini noodles for 3 minutes. Stir in the marinara sauce and cook for 2 more minutes. Combine the pasta, zucchini, and turkey into one skillet or a separate serving bowl.

Yield: 4 servings

TURKEY AND BLACK BEAN LETTUCE TACOS

The easy turkey and black bean filling in this recipe can serve as a base for many meals. Enjoy it as directed, add it to a salad, serve it on a corn tortilla, or mix it with quinoa and serve as a bowl.

1 tablespoon olive oil or spray
  olive oil

1 pound organic 90 percent lean
  ground turkey

¼ cup chopped onion
1 teaspoon cumin
2 teaspoons chili powder
¾ teaspoon garlic powder
¼ teaspoon sea salt
½ teaspoon black pepper
Crushed red pepper to taste

1 (15-ounce) can organic black beans
Romaine lettuce
½ cup low-fat plain Greek yogurt (optional)
Jalapeño peppers, chopped (optional)

Heat oil in a large nonstick skillet over medium-high heat. Cook the turkey until browned (a few minutes on each side), then break it up into a crumble. Mix in onion, cumin, chili powder, garlic powder, salt, pepper, and crushed red pepper, stirring occasionally. Add the beans and cook, stirring occasionally, until the turkey is fully cooked (no pink color). To serve, wrap the mixture in lettuce leaves, as if they were taco shells. Top with the yogurt and jalapeño peppers, if desired.

Yield: 4 servings

SLOW-COOKER CHICKEN VERDE TACO FILLING

You can add this tasty chicken filling to tacos, corn tortillas, salads, or burrito bowls.

1 pound organic free-range skinless, boneless chicken breasts

½ cup salsa verde
1 cup chopped green cabbage
¼ cup chopped white onion

Combine the chicken and salsa in a slow cooker. Cook on low for 6 hours or on high for 4 hours. Shred the chicken with a fork and sprinkle the cabbage and onion on top as desired. Use in tacos or other recipes, or for a salad or a rice bowl.

Yield: 4 servings

VEGGIE EDAMAME STIR-FRY

1–2 tablespoons olive oil

3 cups sliced mixed veggies (red bell pepper, onion, broccoli, snow peas, carrots, water chestnuts, and mushrooms)

½ teaspoon garlic powder

½ teaspoon ground ginger or finely chopped fresh ginger

Black pepper to taste

1½ cups shelled edamame

1 cup cooked brown rice

1 tablespoon sesame seeds

1 tablespoon reduced-sodium soy sauce

Add the olive oil to a wok and heat for 1 minute. Add the mixed veggies, garlic powder, ginger, pepper, and any of the additional ingredients (if using), and cook, stirring constantly, for 2 minutes. Mix in the edamame, rice, and sesame seeds. Sprinkle with the soy sauce. Cook, stirring constantly, until the veggies reach the desired tenderness.

Yield: 4 servings

Additional ingredients: Cubed tofu, bean sprouts, shrimp, any other veggies

VEGETARIAN BEAN CHILI

1 tablespoon olive oil

1 medium onion, chopped into ½-inch pieces (about 1 cup)

1 green bell pepper, chopped a little smaller than the onion

1 (16-ounce) can diced tomatoes (use the juice)

1 (15-ounce) can dark red kidney beans, rinsed and drained

1 (15-ounce) can white kidney beans, rinsed and drained

1 teaspoon salt

1 teaspoon black pepper

2–3 bay leaves

1–2 tablespoons chili powder

Pinch of crushed red pepper (optional)

Heat the olive oil in a small pan over medium heat, add the onion, and cook, stirring occasionally, for about 3 minutes. Add the cooked onion and the remaining ingredients to a slow cooker and heat on low for 6–7 hours or on high for 4–5 hours. Or use a large pot and cook on the stovetop for 1 hour.

Yield: 6 servings

VEGETABLE MINESTRONE SOUP

1 tablespoon olive oil
1 cup chopped onion
1–2 cloves garlic, minced
2 stalks celery, chopped
1 teaspoon dried or chopped fresh
  parsley
1 cup sliced zucchini
2 carrots, chopped
1 cup sliced green beans (1-inch
  pieces)

1 (15-ounce) can red kidney
  beans, rinsed and drained
1 (6-ounce) can tomato paste
1½ cups vegetable stock
6 cups water
1 teaspoon dried thyme
2 cups roughly chopped green
  cabbage
2 teaspoons Worcestershire sauce

Heat the olive oil in a large pot over medium-high heat. Add the onion, garlic, celery, and parsley and sauté for 5 minutes. Add the zucchini, carrots, green beans, kidney beans, tomato paste, stock, water, thyme, cabbage, and Worcestershire sauce. Cook over medium-low heat for 1½ hours.

Yield: 6–8 servings

SIDES

SAUTÉED SWISS CHARD

3 cups coarsely chopped Swiss
   chard (stems removed)
1–2 tablespoons olive oil
3 tablespoons walnut pieces
3 tablespoons organic raisins

1–2 cloves garlic, minced
Juice of ½ lemon
Salt to taste
Black pepper to taste

In a vegetable steamer over medium heat, steam the chard until it is lightly wilted or the desired tenderness. In a large skillet over medium-high heat, heat the olive oil. Add the walnuts and raisins and cook until the walnuts are lightly toasted, about 3 minutes. Add the garlic and cook for an additional 2 minutes. Add the chard, lemon juice, salt, and pepper and combine.

Yield: 2 servings

ZUCCHINI BITES

1 zucchini
Spray olive oil
Italian seasoning, to taste
Salt and pepper to taste

½ cup marinara sauce
¼ cup shredded low-fat
   mozzarella cheese

Slice the zucchini into ¼-inch slices. Spray a skillet with spray olive oil and heat over medium-high heat. Add the zucchini, and sprinkle with Italian seasoning, salt, and pepper. Sauté about 2 minutes, then flip. Top each slice with a spoonful of sauce, and a sprinkle of cheese. Reduce heat and cover for 2 more minutes.

Yield: 2 servings

SWEET POTATO FRIES

1 large sweet potato
2 tablespoons organic virgin
  coconut oil

Salt to taste
Black pepper to taste

Preheat the oven to 400 degrees. Cut the sweet potato into ¾-inch wedges. Place the wedges on a foil-lined baking sheet. Drizzle them with the coconut oil and sprinkle them with the salt and pepper. Bake for 30 minutes.

Yield: 2 servings

WILD RICE

2 cups wild rice
1 tablespoon Earth Balance vegan
  butter or Kerrygold Irish butter
¼ cup slivered almonds

2 tablespoons chopped green
  onions
Salt to taste
Black pepper to taste

Cook the wild rice as directed on the package. Heat the butter in a large skillet over medium-high heat. Add the almonds and green onions and cook, stirring occasionally, until the green onions are light brown, about 3 minutes. Add the rice, stir to combine, and cook for 2 minutes. Add the salt and pepper and mix.

Yield: 4 servings

SWEET TREATS

GLUTEN-FREE OATMEAL RAISIN COOKIES

¾ cup Earth Balance vegan butter or Kerrygold Irish butter

2 rounded tablespoons organic virgin coconut oil

¾ cup coconut palm sugar

¼ cup raw honey

1¼ teaspoons vanilla extract

2 eggs

1½ cups oat flour (or other gluten-free flour)

1 teaspoon baking soda

1½ teaspoons cinnamon

½ teaspoon sea salt

3 cups quick-cooking rolled oats

1 cup organic raisins

Preheat the oven to 350 degrees. In a large bowl, mix the butter, coconut oil, sugar, honey, and vanilla together using an electric mixer on medium speed until smooth. Mix in the eggs. In a smaller bowl, mix the flour, baking soda, cinnamon, and salt together. Add the flour mixture to the butter-sugar mixture in the large bowl, and mix together by hand. Stir in the oats and raisins. Scoop out rounded tablespoons of batter and place on an ungreased baking sheet. Bake for 8–10 minutes, until light brown. Cool for 1 minute and enjoy.

Serving size: 2 cookies   **Yield: 36 cookies**

BAKED PEAR WITH PISTACHIOS AND GREEK YOGURT

1 Bosc pear, halved and cored

1 tablespoon organic virgin coconut oil, melted

Cinnamon to taste

½ cup low-fat plain Greek yogurt

2 tablespoons chopped pistachios

Raw honey

Preheat the oven to 400 degrees. Place the pear halves in a glass baking dish. Drizzle with the melted coconut oil and sprinkle with the cinnamon.

Bake to the desired softness, 30–40 minutes. Top with the yogurt and pistachios and lightly drizzle with the honey.

Yield: 2 servings

CHOCOLATE AVOCADO PUDDING

1 ripe banana
1 small avocado, peeled and pitted
2 tablespoons almond or coconut
   milk, plus extra as needed

½ cup chocolate-flavored
   complete protein mix
2 teaspoons nut butter
Cinnamon to taste

Simply mash all the ingredients (except the cinnamon) together in a bowl or use a food processor. Start with the banana, then add the avocado, milk, complete protein mix, and nut butter. Add extra milk as needed to reach the desired consistency. Transfer the pudding to dessert bowls and sprinkle with the cinnamon.

Yield: 2 servings

SMOOTHIES

Invent your own delicious recipes from Dr. Bill's list of ingredients on page 9.

ENDNOTES

⊕ SEE MORE SCIENTIFIC REFERENCES

For a list of many scientific journal articles on the main T5 points in each chapter, see DrSearsWellness.org/T5/References.

Part I

CHAPTER 1

20. Science says salads are smart. In the Chicago Health and Aging Project (CHAP) and the Nurses' Health Study, high vegetable consumption is associated with a slower rate of cognitive decline. The researchers recommended that vegetables be consumed along with healthy fats, since fats increase the absorption of fat-soluble nutrients such as vitamin E, carotenoids, and flavonoids. Also, it has been proposed that flavonoids are neuroprotective in that they feed one of the most important types of brain cells, astrocytes, which provide energy for brain function. The famous Nun Study showed that high blood levels of folate, which is found in green, leafy vegetables, were associated with a decreased risk of Alzheimer's.

20. Love your legumes. Besides taming your tendency to overeat, legumes blunt after-meal insulin spikes. Brighenti F. et al., Colonic fermentation of indigestible carbohydrates contributes to the second-meal effect. *Am J Clin Nutr* (2006); 83:817–22.

22. Grow your own (tower) garden. Research shows that the shorter the distance between farm and fork, the more natural antioxidants fruits and vegetables retain. Our favorite is the Tower Garden, a vertical aeroponic growing system that requires no dirt, has no weeds, and requires less than 10 percent of the water and space of a traditional garden. See DrSearsWellness.orgT5/Tower-Garden for more about where to get this home garden device.

24. Spice up your transformation. For detailed information on how spices can improve brain and body health, see Aggarwal BB. *Healing Spices: How to Use 50 Everyday and Exotic Spices to Boost Health and Beat Disease.* New York: Sterling Publishing, 2011.

26. A six-ounce fillet of wild salmon. A six-ounce fillet of cooked wild sockeye salmon contains the following:

Average Nutrient Profile of 6 oz. (170 g) of Wild Alaskan Sockeye Salmon		
		Percent Daily Value[*]
Calories	287	—
Protein	43 g	86[**]
Carbohydrate	0 g	0
Total fat	11 g	17
Omega-3 DHA	1,200 mg[***]	—
Omega-3 EPA	900 mg	—
Cholesterol	100 mg	33
Minerals		
Calcium	20 mg	2
Iron	0.85 mg	5

		Percent Daily Value*
Magnesium	61 mg	15
Potassium	694 mg	20
Sodium	112 mg	5
Zinc	0.85 mg	6
Selenium	62 mcg	89
Vitamin C	0 mg	0
Thiamine	0.37 mg	25
Riboflavin	0.24 mg	14
Niacin	16.5 mg	83
Pantothenic acid	2.33 mg	23
Vitamin B_6	1.18 mg	59
Folate, total	15 mcg	4
Choline, total	191.6 mg	35
Vitamin B_{12}	9.64 mcg	161
Vitamin A	352 IU	7
Vitamin E	1.94 mg	10
Vitamin D	894 IU	224
Astaxanthin	8 mg	—

g = grams; mg = milligrams; mcg = micrograms; IU = international units.

* Percent Daily Values are based on a 2,000-calorie per day diet.

** This is the USDA Daily Value for protein, but I believe most adults need around 1 gram of protein per pound of their ideal body weight.

*** There is a wide range of omega-3 EPA/DHA content in seafood, depending on the species, time of year, and processing. While the USDA has yet to release an official Daily Value for omega-3 EPA/DHA, most authorities recommend 500–1,000 mg/day.

Source: USDA National Nutrient Database for Standard Reference, 2011.

For an informative and fun read about the scientifically referenced health effects of seafood, including my many fish stories and fishing trips with the top seafood scientists in the world, as well as the nutrient value of seafood and the safest seafood for all ages, see *The Omega-3 Effect* (Suggested Reading, page 381). Additional sources:

U.S. Department of Agriculture, Agricultural Research Service, Nutrient Data Laboratory website. USDA National Database for Standard Reference, Release 24. http://www.ars.usda.gov/ba/bhnrc/ndl. Accessed July 20, 2017.

U.S. Food and Drug Administration, "Mercury Levels in Commercial Fish and Shellfish (1990–2012)." https://www.fda.gov/food/foodborne illnesscontaminants/metals/ucm115644.htm. Updated January 18, 2017.

28. Seafood is healing food. Omega-3 fatty acids in fatty seafood, such as salmon, and in fish oil supplements can improve endothelial function, especially in people at risk for cardiovascular disease. The reason seems to be the natural biochemical anti-sticky-stuff action the omega-3 fatty acids exert on the components of the blood and the arterial walls. Nestel P, et al. The n-3 fatty acids eicosapentaenoic acid and docosahexaenoic acid increase systemic arterial compliance in humans. *American Journal of Clinical Nutrition.* 2002;76:326–330.

A seven-country study with a twenty-year follow-up of men who consumed an ounce per day of fish had a 50 percent lower chance of dying from cardiovascular disease than men who did not eat fish. Researchers concluded that the more omega-3s you eat, the longer you live. The mechanism seems to be, simply, omega-3s reduce the "sticky stuff" on the endothelial surface, or silver lining. Brown A, et al. Dietary modulation of endothelial function: Implications for cardiovascular disease. *American Journal of Clinical Nutrition.* 2001;73:673–686; Houston M. *Vascular Biology and Clinical Practice.* Philadelphia: Hanley & Belfus, 2002.

In my quest to learn more about why salmon is better than sirloin for keeping sticky stuff out of my blood, I went fishing for more knowledge in Norway with Dr. Jorn Dyerberg, who is credited with discovering much of the original fish oil science in the early seventies. Jorn loved my sticky-stuff explanation of illnesses. One night, as we sat down to enjoy the salmon we had caught, I asked Jorn, "What was your first clue that seafood didn't raise the blood level of sticky stuff?" He reinforced what I suspected. In the early seventies, when "fat is bad" was the weight-loss craze, he performed blood tests that revealed that people who ate more seafood (a high-fat and a right-fat diet) had lower levels of sticky stuff—that is, biochemicals that made the blood clot too quickly and get full of inflammatory biochemicals. Thirty years and over 22,000 journal articles later, the salmon-versus-sirloin theory has been proven. (See more of Dyerberg's studies and more research about this topic in *The Omega-3 Effect*.)

29. Suggested seafood sources. Our top pick is VitalChoice.com for the safest, most nutritious and delicious seafood, wild from Alaska and the Pacific coast. For a detailed list of traffic-light seafood eating (green light, yellow light, red light), see *The Omega-3 Effect*.

31. Eat more nuts, lose more weight. Weight-loss researchers found that the longer eaters chewed, especially on nuts, the more excess fat they lost. This is probably because chewing signals your appetite-control center not to overeat. Natoli S, et al. A review of the evidence: nuts and body weight. *Asia Pacific Journal of Clinical Nutrition.* 2007;16:588–597; Murakami K. Hardness (difficulty of chewing) of the habitual diet in relation to body mass index and waist circumference in free-living Japanese women aged 18–22y. *American Journal of Clinical Nutrition.* 2007;86:206–213.

32. Supplements fill the nutritional gaps. Most of us need supplements for these reasons:

Plant food and seafood supplements mute exercise-induced oxidative stress. Antioxidant supplements lower the wear and tear, called increased oxidative stress, following vigorous exercise. Colbert LH, et al. The Health, Aging, and Body Composition Study. *Journal of American Geriatrics Society.* 2004;52:1098.

Micronutrient deficiencies are huge. An analysis of our food sources reveals that modern produce does not offer the level of antioxidants it used to. Because of how plants and animals are fed and cared for, modern meat and produce, like modern humans, are becoming nutritionally deprived.

We eat out of the box. On its way from farm to fork, a lot of produce is packaged for longer shelf life. The longer food sits around, the more nutrients it may lose.

34. Fruit and vegetable supplements. Juice Plus+ is the most scientifically researched fruit and vegetable concentrate in the world. Right now, Juice Plus+ is the only nutritional supplement I eat daily. Over thirty university studies prove that Juice Plus+ lowers inflammatory biochemicals (sticky stuff) and raises blood levels of antioxidants—the two health effects you want from plant-based foods. Canas JA, et al. Insulin resistance and adiposity in relation to serum beta-carotene levels. *Journal of Pediatrics.* 2012;161(1):58–64; Lamprecht M, et al. Supplementation with a juice powder concentrate and exercise decreases oxidation and inflammation, and improves the microcirculation in obese women: randomized controlled trial data. *British Journal of Nutrition.* 2013;110(9):1685–1695. Kiefer I, et al. Supplementation with mixed fruit and vegetable juice concentrated increased serum antioxidants and folate in healthy adults. *Journal of the American College of Nutrition.* 2004;23:205–211; Nantz M, et al. Immunity and antioxidant capacity in humans is enhanced by consumption of a dried, encapsulated fruit and vegetable juice concentrate. *Journal of Nutrition.* 2006;136:2606–2610; Bellavia A, et al. Fruit and vegetable consumption and all-cause mortality: a dose-response analysis. *American Journal of Clinical Nutrition.* 2013;98:454–459; Plotnick GD, et al. Effect of supplemental phytonutrients on impairment of the flow-mediated brachial artery vasoactivity after a single high-fat meal. *Journal of the American College of Cardiology.* 2003;41(10):1744–1749; Kawashima A, et al. Four week supplementation with mixed fruit and vegetable juice concentrates increased protective serum antioxidants and folate and decreased plasma homocysteine in Japanese subjects. *Asia Pacific Journal of Clinical Nutrition.* 2007;16(3):411–421.

For a detailed summary of the research behind Juice Plus+, mainly for immune and vascular health (which translates to brain health), see AskDrSears.com/Juice-Plus.

35. Know your omega numbers. In 2012, I had the honor of hosting at our home a two-day roundtable discussion on omega balance. Attending were six of the top omega scientists in the world, who among them have authored more than 1,500 scientific articles. From these brilliant researchers I learned that omega balance is an often-overlooked key to overall health.

Omega balance is one of the newest and most important concepts in modern nutrition. It requires eating foods that are high enough in both omega-3 and omega-6 oils, yet in the proper balance. The T5 real-food diet has an optimal omega-6:omega-3 ratio of between 2:1 and 3:1. Yet in the standard American diet (SAD) that ratio can be as out of balance as 10:1 or 20:1. Here is the problem with the SAD. Omega-3 oils are found mainly in seafood. They are the most expensive oils, and they spoil quickly. Food companies purposely put more omega-6 oils into their foods for two reasons: they cost less and last longer on the shelf.

Here's the science made simple: our cell membranes, especially in our brain tissues, need both omega-3s and omega-6s in a healthy balance. Think of these two omegas as personal friends who play nicely together and don't try to overwhelm each other. When they are in balance, you have wellness. Yet, when we eat too many 6s and not enough 3s, the excess 6s use up all the enzymes for their own selfish metabolism, so there is not enough left over to metabolize the omega 3s. The body then is left with an omega-6 excess and an omega-3 deficiency, which can lead to illness. We also call this the "bully effect." The excess omega-6s overpower the omega-3s. In a nutshell, the T5 eating plan provides the optimal balance of both of these essential fatty acids.

Brenna JT, et al. ISSFAL official statement Number 5, alpha-linolenic acid conversion to n-3 long-chain polyunsaturated fatty acids in humans. (Personal communication with Dr. Tom Brenna, Chairman of the International Society for the Study of Fatty Acids and Lipids.) For more detailed information about omega balance, see *The Omega-3 Effect* in the reference list; also Simopoulos AP. The importance of the ratio of omega-6/omega-3 essential fatty acids. *Biomedicine and Pharmacotherapy.* 2002;56:365–379.

A simple test to measure your omega numbers is available at www .VitalChoice.com.

YOUR OIL TRANSFORMATION

Enjoy in moderation	Eat less	Eat none
• Fish oil (supplements)	• Corn oil	• Hydrogenated oil
• Algae oil (supplements)	• Soy oil	• Cottonseed oil***
• Olive oil*	• Sunflower oil	• Canola oil****
• Flax oil, hemp oil	• Safflower oil	
• Coconut oil, virgin**		
• Avocado oil		

*One tablespoon a day is our recommended serving.

**The MCTs (medium-chain triglycerides) in coconut oil may improve cognitive function in patients with dementia, and are healthy fats for intestinal health. Coconut oil was unscientifically maligned as a "saturated fat." Yet, because of its healthy biochemical properties, it doesn't increase the sticky stuff in the blood vessels like the saturated fats in meats. Besides, new nutritional insights reveal that some saturated fat is healthful after all.

***A cheap oil most likely to be contaminated with pesticides and containing one of the highest pro-inflammatory omega-6:omega-3 ratios of greater than 200:1.

**** Too highly processed and chemicalized.

36. Astaxanthin. To paraphrase what Dr. Oz said on his TV show: astaxanthin is one of the most important nutrients you need but have heard the least about. It is one of Mother Nature's most powerful antioxidants and anti-inflammatories. Since new insights reveal that most brain diseases have their roots in inflammation, it makes sense to add this anti-inflammatory to your brain-health diet.

READ MORE ABOUT IT

Natural Astaxanthin: Hawaii's Supernutrient, William Sears, MD, 2015. Download a free e-copy at Nutrex-hawaii.com.

39. T5 lowers sticky-stuff spikes. The following article supports the health effects of lowering sticky stuff: Blaak EE, et al. Impact of postprandial glycemia on health and prevention of disease. *Obesity Reviews.* 2012;13:923–984.

A group of twenty authors from top university nutritional departments around the world reviewed the top medical studies on postprandial glycemia (sticky stuff.) Their review revealed the challenges of interpreting these studies. (If experts have a tough time interpreting the studies, no wonder the general public is confused!) Yet they did conclude that the more consistently you lower sticky-stuff spikes, the better your health.

Among the important findings of this review article is the matter of *intra-meal satiety*, the point at which you become satisfied during a meal and follow your prompts to stop eating. Foods with low glycemic index reduce hunger and promote satiety better than those with high glycemic index. Translation: As we've said throughout the book, real foods show the least sticky-stuff spikes—mainly those that are high in protein, moderate in healthy fats, and slow-release, fiber-rich carbs.

Even though many of the authors disclosed that they are advisors to some of the top food makers, I was impressed with their ability to stay scientifically unbiased.

Eating the T5 way showed a lower insulin peak and a slower rise of the hunger hormone, ghrelin—again, just what you want in order to prolong your satiety, the time before you get hungry again.

Note to savvy readers: Not all the studies listed by these authors came to the conclusion that real foods promote more satiety. *But the majority of the studies concluded that the higher the protein, fiber, and healthy fat content of the food, and the less processed the food, the faster you get comfortably full and the longer you stay that way.*

Another important point these authors made that support our "real foods" concept is that specific soluble fibers could increase the viscosity of the food-goo, slow down digestion, and stimulate the release of satiety hormones as another mechanism of feeling more comfortably full faster. Fiber coats the lining of the intestine like a gooey paint, which slows digestion. Further, certain fibers ferment in the large intestine, producing short-chain fatty acids that also promote satiety.

Another part of this article we like is the authors' use of the word "glucolipotoxicity," chemistry-speak for high blood levels of sticky-stuff molecules composed of unhealthy sugars and unhealthy fats.

Yet another important finding in the article was the higher the sugar spikes, the higher the spikes of HbA1c, the most common marker doctors use to measure sticky stuff. Other markers associated with high sugar spikes were lumped into what are called "adhesion factors." Also, the sticky-stuff spikes that follow a high-glycemic meal increase oxidative stress and reduce oxidative defenses—more reason to get plenty of antioxidants in your diet and via supplements.

All this boils down to common sense: eat mostly real foods at a meal. And if you *do* eat processed foods, chase them with a salad, so that the antioxidants blunt the effect of the oxidants you ate.

Another highly referenced article supporting our sticky stuff explanation: Downey, M. Controlling after-meal blood sugar spikes. *Life Extension Magazine*, October 2016, pages 59–65.

NO sticky stuff response. These authors also gave scientific support to what we mention in chapter three that sticky-stuff spikes reduce NO release in the silver lining of the arteries. In other words, the higher the sticky stuff, the stiffer the arteries; the lower the sticky stuff, the more relaxed they are. More relaxed arteries give more blood flow. And, as you also learned throughout the book, the richer the blood flow to each organ, the healthier it is.

39. "Sticky stuff" made simple. The higher the level of the sticky biochemicals, the higher the chances of your getting a neurodegenerative disease such as Alzheimer's. Feng C, et al. Hyperhomocysteinemia associates with small vessel disease more closely than large vessel disease. *International Journal Medical Science.* 2013;10:408–412. Also, a higher level of sticky stuff such as hemoglobin A1c is associated with an increased incidence of neurodegenerative diseases, especially Alzheimer's; Kimattila SM, et al. Chronic hyperglycemia impairs endothelial function and insulin sensitivity via different mechanisms in insulin-dependent diabetes mellitus. *Circulation* 1996;94:11276–11282.

40. You put sticky stuff in your mouth. Researchers at the University of Maryland School of Medicine studied hospital-employee volunteers to see if feeding them a sticky-stuff breakfast caused sticky stuff in their blood, or what they called *endothelial dysfunction*. Sure enough, endothelial function started dropping quickly after the sticky-stuff breakfast. Within three hours endothelial function was only half of what it had been before the meal. Yet endothelial function was not changed in the group that ate a no-sticky-stuff breakfast. (Plotnick GD, et al. Effect of antioxidant vitamins on the transient impairment of endothelium-dependent brachial artery vasoactivity following a single high-fat meal. *Journal of the American Medical Association.* 1997;278(20):1682–1686.

45. How carbs make you fat. What happens to the extra sugar we eat? Suppose you ignore your body's biochemical prompts to slow your eating. Your body has three kinds of fuel tanks: liver, muscle, and fat cells. After a meal your storage hormone, insulin, decides which one of these tanks to fill. Suppose you're stuffed. You've overeaten and filled your liver, and now you're lying around, not moving, so that your liver or muscles don't have to burn those stored calories. The excess sugar goes to the third tank, fat cells, mainly belly fat. Sugar is packaged as triglycerides, a fuel-efficient way to transport them. Triglycerides circulate in the blood to provide an immediate energy source. The rest of the unused sugar is stored in fat cells. Lasting weight loss means releasing more, storing less.

It's all about insulin, the master sugar wrapper. Insulin packages sugar for deposit and rapid withdrawal. The biochemical key to lasting weight or fat control is your blood insulin level. Too high and you store more fat and get sick; too low and you can't withdraw sugar from your bank for fuel, and you get tired. Just right and you stay *lean and energetic.*

T5 works because it teaches insulin to behave right. The biochemical cause of obesity and related illnesses is that insulin is too high for too long. When someone compliments you, "You look so good. What are you doing?" respond, "I'm teaching my insulin to behave." This is more fun and biochemically correct than "I'm on a diet."

50. A gram of protein per pound. The T5 eating plan is naturally protein-rich. Here is a short list of protein numbers: wild salmon, 6 oz., 40 grams; Greek yogurt, 1 cup, 20 grams; tofu, firm, 3 oz., 13 grams; nut butter, 2 tbsp, 8 grams; egg, 6 grams; beans, ½ cup, 7 grams; cheese, 1 oz., 8 grams; protein powder supplement in smoothie, 13 grams.

53. A big, fat, sweet lie. Researchers at the University of California, San Francisco (UCSF), examined internal documents from the Sugar Research Foundation (SRF), which had sponsored research beginning in 1965 that touted fat and cholesterol as the dietary causes of cardiovascular disease and covered up evidence that sugar consumption was also a risk factor. According to the UCSF authors, the SRF's funding and role in the study had not been disclosed. This fascinating article reports the detective work revealing that substituting healthy fats for added sugars caused a large *improvement* in serum triglyceride levels in healthy persons. Further, it showed that substituting legumes for added sugar caused a large improvement in cholesterol levels. So it was "added sugar," sucrose, that raised cholesterol and could lead to coronary heart disease, not the dietary fats found in real foods. Kearns CE, et al. Sugar industry and coronary heart disease research. A historical analysis of internal industry documents. *JAMA: Internal Medicine.* 2016;176(11):1680–1685. doi:10.1001/jamainternmed.2016.5394.

In his masterpiece of detective research, *The Case Against Sugar*, journalist Gary Taubes exposes that Big Food, Big Pharma, big government, and big universities were in cahoots in perpetrating the big, fat, sweet lie.

More on the big, fat, sweet lie. The sickest nutritional advice in America is this: "Eat a low-fat diet."

For fifty years or more, news media and even the U.S. government preached an unhealthy and absurd message: "Eating fat makes you fat." As our diets got lower and lower in fat, and as food marketers convinced us to eat more and more fat-free, carb-laden, processed foods, Americans just got fatter—and worse yet, sicker. We got fewer and fewer calories from slowly digested fats, and more from spike-inducing factory-made carbs—what we now call "junk carbs."

In the seventies, carbs got junkier still with the introduction of high-fructose corn syrup and chemical sweeteners. Before long, the average American dinner plate was full of brain-busting "dumb" carbs. Factory-food makers saw that replacing the natural fats in foods (which spoil faster) with cheaper, longer-lasting chemical carbs could fatten their profits. This also made Americans fatter.

The bought have been caught. Once upon a time, nearly all trusted medical research was funded by grants from the National Institutes of Health, where I had the privilege of spending two years of my career. Research protocols were examined by wise scientists who were not under the influence of Big Food, Big Pharma, or other outside profiteers.

Over the last forty years, however, more and more researchers have received funding from companies who are more interested in results that support their profits than in valid, objective results.

This isn't to say that all research funded by for-profit corporations is suspect. Far from it. Many valuable drugs and therapies are developed with private funding in hope of profit. Yet there has been a great deal of bad science issued on behalf of the diet industry.

However, the bought have been caught. In the last few years, honest scientists have publicly exposed the fallacy that high-fat diets are the cause of many diseases: for example, Dr. Walter Willett, professor and chairman of the Department of Nutrition, Harvard Medical School; and Dr. Robert Lustig, Director of the Weight Assessment for Teen and Child Health Program, University of California, San Francisco. They have had both the wisdom and the courage to teach that you don't get fat by eating fat, but by eating junk carbs.

A double fault. In the early 1980s, as the low-fat diet craze hit its peak, artificial sweeteners and flavor enhancers also entered Americans' diets—and their brains. A double whammy. Not only were people not eating the right fats to protect their brains, they were eating more artificial and chemical foods that harmed their health. A close look at our misreading of science and misfeeding of Americans shows that the increase in neurodegenerative diseases seems to parallel the junking-up of the standard American diet (SAD).

You don't get fat by eating fat. Over the past two decades there has been a steady decline in the percentage of fat in the American diet, yet a huge increase in the rate of obesity. The general conclusion of people who have studied this, especially Dr. Willet, is that you don't get fat by eating fat, and high-fat diets are not to blame for the high prevalence of obesity in Western countries. Willett WC. Dietary fat plays a major role on obesity: No. *Obesity Reviews.* 2002;3:59–68.

Yet while refined carbs are the chief culprits, new insights are proposing that the type of fats and the change in fatty acid composition of our foods may be contributing to the obesity epidemic, especially in the increasing ratio of omega-6 to omega 3-fatty acids. This is especially important in the role of excess omega-6s in promoting obesity. Ailhaud G, et al. Fatty acid composition of fats is an early determinant of childhood obesity: a short review and an opinion. *Obesity Reviews.* 2004;5:21–26; Ailhaud G, et al. Temporal changes in dietary fats: Role of n-6 polyunsaturated fatty acids and excessive adipose tissue development in relationship to obesity. *Progress in Lipid Research.* 2006;45:203–236; Ailhaud G, et al. Fatty acid composition as an early determinant of childhood obesity. *Genes Nutrition.* 2007;2:39–40.

CHAPTER 2

56. Chew-chew, times two. For more scientific evidence for the rule of twos, see Robinson E, et al. A systematic review and meta-analysis examining the effect of eating right on energy intake and hunger. *American Journal of Clinical Nutrition.* 2014;100:123–151.

These authors did a literature survey and concluded that a slower eating rate was associated with a lower volume of eating compared to fast eaters. Again, common sense tells us that if we take time to chew longer, rest between bites, and eat more slowly, we're going to be fuller faster, simply because you give the head brain and the gut brain more time to say "slow down, you've eaten enough, stop!" As we've said, fast eaters eat right through these signals.

Researchers also found that slower eating results in slower gastric emptying, so the stomach feels fuller longer. Further, the more slowly you eat, the longer these enjoyment-taste nerves are exposed to the food, and the faster you feel full. The authors mentioned that slower eating is related to the number of sips, bites, or chews per volume of food.

Two studies reviewed in this article showed that increasing the number of chews, bites, or sips while keeping the eating rate constant leads to being satisfied sooner with a smaller amount, as did increasing the number of chews per unit volume of food. *Smaller bites and more chews lead to greater satiety.*

57. Grazers Are Healthier Than Gorgers. One of the most often quoted studies showing the health benefits of grazing was done by Dr. David Jenkins and his team at the University of Toronto. They divided eaters into two groups. Both ate the same amount of the same foods, yet one group ate the three standard meals a day, whereas the other group, called nibblers, ate mini-meals throughout the day. After two weeks the nibblers showed 15 percent lower cholesterol, 17 percent lower cortisol (the stress hormone), and 28 percent lower insulin. Jenkins JA, et al. Nibbling versus gorging: metabolic advantages of increased meal frequency. *New England Journal of Medicine.* 1989;321:92–934. Another trusted reference on the benefits of grazing is Dr. Dean Ornish in his book *Eat More, Weigh Less* (New York: HarperCollins, 2001).

58. But the point is that by eating less ... To learn more about the latest research on caloric restriction, read the excellent article in *Life Extension Magazine,* October 2016. Remember, "caloric restriction" means cutting down on calories without cutting down on healthy nutrients.

60. This is your brain on broccoli. In the June 2017 issue of *Scientific American Mind,* food scientists at Tufts University studied how a change in food habits can change cravings. They had volunteers eat mainly foods such as those recommended in our T5 real-food diet: low sugar, high protein and fiber, and moderate in healthy fats. The researchers did brain scans on fifteen of these volunteers, which revealed that the pleasure centers in the subjects' brains lit up more when they viewed pictures of the healthy foods than when they viewed pictures of junk foods.

65. *Umami*: Enjoying Healthful Food. A delicious read on the subject of how blending certain ingredients creates biochemical synergy, or *umami*, is the book *Umami, Unlocking the Secrets of the Fifth Taste* by Ole Mouritsen and Klavs Styrbaek (New York: Columbia University Press, 2014). There's an unsurprising story in this book about the taste-enhancing natural biochemicals that are found in human breast milk (far more than in cow's milk) that enhance its flavor. After fifty years of watching babies breastfeed, I am still touched by that sweet little face that conveys the feeling "This is delicious."

72. Eat Early. Early eaters are more likely to stay lean. Dr. Robert Lustig, in his book *Fat Chance*, postulates that the reason seems to be the level of your appetite-regulating hormone, leptin (the "eat less, you're satisfied" biochemical prompt.) Levels are naturally higher in the early evening hours.

73. Snacks are *good* for you. Nutrition experts wisely caution that snacking can actually be harmful for your health in two ways: snacking on unreal foods and snacking on too much, too frequently, especially when you're not hungry. Cameron JD, et al. Increased meal frequency does not promote greater weight loss in subjects who were prescribed an 8-week equi-energenic, energy-restricted diet. *British Journal of Nutrition.* 2010;103:1098–1101.

The grazing and rule of twos parts of our T5 program do go to pot, as it were, if you snack or graze too much and on unreal foods. Fung, J. *The Obesity Code.* Vancouver, BC: Greystone Books, 2016; Ohkuna T, et al. Association between eating right and obesity: a systematic review and meta-analysis. *International Journal of Obesity.* 2015;39(11):1589–1596. Also, *The DNA Restart* by Sharon Moalem (New York: Rodale, 2016), p. 256.

There also can be confusion between the terms "snacking" and "grazing." Grazing implies small, frequent mini-meals, or the rule of twos, as opposed to eating snacks. Again, *it's the type of snacks that is important*, which is why we don't use the term "snacking." Grazing is a more healthful term.

For more on grazing, see:

- Li J, et al. Improvement in chewing activity reduces energy intake in one meal and modulates plasma gut hormone concentrations in obese and lean Chinese men. *American Journal of Clinical Nutrition.* 2011;94(3):709–716.
- Bellisle F, et al. Meal frequency and energy balance. *British Journal of Nutrition.* 1997;77:Suppl 1:S57–S70.
- Cameron JD, et al. Increased meal frequency does not promote greater weight loss in subjects who were prescribed an 8-week equi-energetic energy-restricted diet. *British Journal of Nutrition.* 2010;103(8):1098–1101.
- Holmstrup ME, et al. Effects of meal frequency on metabolic profiles and substrate partitioning in lean healthy males. *European Society for Clinical Nutrition and Metabolism.* 2010;5(6):e277–e280.
- Jenkins DJ, et al. Nibbling versus gorging: metabolic advantages of increased meal frequency. *New England Journal of Medicine.* 1989;321(14):929–934.
- Wang YQ, et al. Increased eating frequency is associated with lower obesity risk, but higher energy intake in adults: a meta-analysis. *International Journal of Environmental Research and Public Health.* 2016;13(6):E603.
- Dashti HS, et al. Recommending small, frequent meals in the clinical care of adults: a review of the evidence and important considerations. *Nutrition in Clinical Practice.* 2016;32(3):365–377.

82. "Added sugar" leads to added weight. Yang Q. Gain weight by "going diet?" Artificial sweeteners and the neurobiology of sugar cravings. *Yale*

Journal of Biology and Medicine. 2010;83(2):101–108; Suez J, et al. Artificial sweeteners induce glucose intolerance by altering the gut microbiota. *Nature.* 2014;514(7521):181–186.

Are fakies a health food? Absolutely not! Do they help a person lose weight? Rarely. Large studies have shown that people of all ages who eat the most fakies tend to gain the most weight (see Yang article, note to page 82). One of the suggested reasons is that people who lessen their calories by substituting artificial sweeteners for sugar tend to take this as a license to eat more.

Fakies mess with your microbiome. Studies in humans and mice show that artificial sweeteners such as sucralose, aspartame, and saccharin mess with the gut bacteria (the microbiome) and blood sugar balance, and can lead to obesity.

In the past few years, an increasing number of scientific articles have concluded that artificial sweeteners change the microbiome, resulting in metabolic upheavals such as glucose intolerance and leaky gut (see Suez article, note to page 82). Basically, the gut brain reacts to fakies the same way the head brain does: "This is chemical food, not real food. It doesn't belong here, so we're going to react to it with inflammation, which causes leaky gut."

How fakies fool the brain. Let's follow what happens in the nervous system as you swallow a fakie. The taste receptors on your tongue (which contains an especially rich supply of nerves) send a biochemical signal to the happy center in the brain, which rewards the fakie-eater by releasing the pleasure hormone dopamine. We are creatures of habit. The more the tongue tells your brain's happy center, "I like it, let's eat more," the greater your craving for these fakie-polluted foods. Neuroimaging techniques let us watch how people's brains respond to what they eat. Suppose we look at the brain of a person consuming a fakie such as a "diet" soda. You'll see that fakies confuse the pleasure centers of the brain and actually *increase appetite and decrease satiety*, prompting the person to crave more food, especially more of the fakie and the junk food it came in. Good for the junk food business, bad for the brain. Neuroscientists generally conclude that unsweetening the world's diet is a key to reversing the obesity epidemic.

CHAPTER 3

91. Think of NO as the pharmacist. *Endotheliologists* (yes, I made that word up) say, "The endothelium passes gas." Nitric oxide (NO) is really a gas that is squirted out of the 1.2 trillion cells in the endothelial wall as prompted by enzymes. Because it's a gas, NO works its way into the blood and blood cells more easily than would liquid biochemical messengers. What a smart design! While the endothelial pharmacy makes many medicines, the big ones are antioxidants, anticoagulants (which keep the blood from getting too sticky), and vasodilators (which keep the arteries relaxed and make them open wider when needed). Vascular biologists have another name for NO: endothelium-derived relaxing factor. The categories of "medicines" that have been isolated from the endothelium so far are:

1. Biochemicals that relax and constrict vessels as needed
2. Maintenance medicines that keep the endothelium, the "silver lining," healthy
3. Anti–sticky stuff that regulates blood clotting
4. Anti-inflammatories that keep inflammation out of the blood and off the vascular lining
5. Antioxidants and natural medicines that decrease wear and tear on tissues

Houston M. *Vascular Biology and Clinical Practice.* Philadelphia: Hanley & Belfus, 2002.

The erectile dysfunction drug Viagra works similarly to NO by relaxing, opening up, and prolonging the widening of the blood vessels in the penis.

92. Sam suffers from "sitting disease." Let's look at the biochemistry of a sitter. When you don't move your muscles, they wither. You don't want that at any age, and when you're older it can be disabling. So move more, all your life. According to researcher Wolf Dröge, author of the excellent book, *Avoiding the First Cause of Death*, when we sit too much, our muscle-building mechanism, protein synthesis, dials down. Amino acids, the building blocks of proteins, travel around our bodies waiting to be incorporated into proteins that are made into muscle. In sitters, because their muscles are withering, not growing, amino acids get sidetracked onto two other roads: body fat, especially belly fat, and sticky stuff in the blood vessels. In people who move a lot, those building blocks are made into stronger muscles and bones, which helps us stay in motion all our lives and reduces the chances of falls and fractures—all while burning more fat and storing less of it.

93. This can contribute to coronary artery clogging. Researchers showed that smokers tend to have high concentrations of sticky stuff in their blood, sticky molecules called ICAM-1, VCAM-1, and selectin. Brown A, et al. Dietary modulation of endothelial function: Implications for cardiovascular disease. *American Journal of Clinical Nutrition.* 2001;73:673–686.

94. The brain gets bigger. Researchers at the University of Illinois studied nine- and ten-year-olds to show that exercise can alter brain structure and improve cognitive abilities. MRIs showed that fitter children scored better on tests of attention. They have significantly larger basal ganglia, which are a part of the brain that aids and maintains attention and the executive control needed to coordinate actions and plans. Also, the hippocampus, a brain structure important to memory, was found to be larger in the fitter children. Chaddock L, et al. A neuroimaging investigation of the association between aerobic fitness, hippocampal volume, and memory performance in pre-adolescent children. *Brain Research.* 2010;1358:172–183; Erickson KI, et al. Aerobic fitness is associated with hippocampal volume in elderly humans. *Hippocampus.* 2009;19:1030–1039.

95. The gut feels good. Move more, eat healthier. A must-read article in the October 2015 issue of *Scientific American Mind* titled "Don't Diet" discusses research showing that movers who consistently did a six-month exercise regimen dialed down their cravings for unhealthy treats.

95. Cells are more insulin-sensitive. Researchers studied the blood sugar effects of an after-meal walk and found that a 15-minute walk after a meal improved blood sugar regulation. DiPietro L, et al. Three 15-minute bouts of moderate postmeal walking significantly improves 24-hour glycemic control in older people at risk for impaired glucose tolerance. *Diabetes Care.* 2013;36:3262–3268.

107. Gotta dance! Those were the headlines in an August 2016 *Harvard Health Letter* article. A study of 48,000 people over forty years of age in the United Kingdom, reported in the June 2016 *American Journal of Preventive Medicine,* found that dancers had healthier hearts. Researchers theorized that dancing is such good exercise for the brain and heart because there are bouts of higher-intensity exercises, dancers make social connections, and dancing dials down stress.

116. That's why I love that studying the neuroscience of nature . . . The delights of nature help you learn. Studies by Roger Ulrich using EEG measurements showed that viewing scenes of nature produced higher alpha wave amplitudes, which are associated with increased production of serotonin, the "happy chemical." Higher alpha wave activity dials down the arousal and anxiety centers and dials up the calm center just as meditation does. Anxiety, on the other hand, is associated with lower alpha wave amplitude and higher beta waves. Ulrich's studies also showed that subjects whose anxiety had been raised by watching a tragic video recovered more rapidly if they then watched scenes of nature. This is why scientists call natural scenes "visual Valium." The study also revealed lowered aggression and angry thoughts in those who watched nature videos. Schoolteachers and therapists could use this knowledge in dealing with aggressive children. (See references to chapter three, DrSearsWellness.org/T5/References.)

116. Healing effects of nature. Does the brain work more peacefully in the presence of nature and, if so, how? What's going on when people report feeling more tranquil and peaceful when viewing pictures of nature and being in scenes of nature? MRI studies give us the answer: viewing nature stimulates an area of the brain (the parahippocampal gyrus) that is rich in opiate receptors, natural pain-relieving cells that stimulate release of dopamine into the system in response to nature. The conclusion is that experiencing nature relaxes the brain. The research showed that the delights of nature dial down and calm the arousal centers in the brain, while scenes such as crowds, malls, markets, traffic, and rush hour rev up the brain and eventually tire it out. I have personally experienced this mental fatigue during long commutes in busy traffic, crowds, and malls. Moreover, neuroimaging studies show that the fear center of the brain is more active in urban dwellers.

118. Lessons from Leaves. Researchers from Kansas State University found that flowering plants can stimulate calming waves as shown by EEG. Researchers from Taiwan and Ulrich's research (see note to page 116) also showed EKG and electromyogram effects that were more therapeutic, in addition to decreased heart rate, when people watched scenes of nature and forests versus hectic urban scenes. A 2004 study of mentally ill patients in Japan revealed lower heart rates when viewing scenes of nature versus urban scenes. The presence of green plants lowered blood pressure and heart rate, in addition to amplifying alpha wave activity.

119. Don't Worry, Go Outside and Play. Studies from the Japanese Society of Forest Medicine revealed some interesting findings about *shinrin-yoku*, which translates literally as "forest bathing." The agency's Dr. Miyazaki showed that 40 minutes of walking in a forest improved mood and vitality and lowered blood levels of the stress hormone cortisol, proving what anthropologists have long suspected: we are wired to walk. The Japanese researchers also showed that 20 minutes of *shinrin-yoku*, compared with 20 minutes of "city bathing," showed an increased state of relaxation in the forest bathers.

A few years ago Martha and I were invited speakers at a medical and parenting conference in Osaka, Japan. After a long and mentally exhausting day, our host, Mr. Sakinishi, announced, "We are going to take you and Mrs. Sears out for some *shinrin-yoku*." I thought this was a Japanese drink. As he drove us up a mountain road that weaved through a pine forest, I realized that he was taking us not to a bar but to his special "happy place" to enjoy the scenery, sounds, and fresh air on his mountain. After an hour of "forest bathing," our minds were reset to a calmer level.

Forest bathing and the immune system. Researchers at Nippon Medical School showed that forest bathing can boost the circulating number of the immune cells called natural killer cells. Evergreens also have been shown to secrete into the air natural, immune-boosting phytochemicals called *phytoncides.* Forest air seems to trap moisture, which traps the secretions from the evergreen. This suggests a scientific basis for the healing benefits ancient healers ascribed to taking a deep breath in the middle of the forest. Selhub EM, Logan AC. *Your Brain on Nature.* Hoboken, NJ: Wiley, 2012.

Many other studies have replicated findings of lower levels of cortisol, lower blood pressure and pulse, and increased variability in heart rate, a measure of cardiac health that cardiologists interpret as turning up the calming pathway from the brain to the heart (parasympathetic nervous system, PNS) and turning down the pump-faster branch of the nervous system (sympathetic nervous system, SNS). These researchers concluded that what calms the brain also calms the heart.

121. My early nature therapy. Here is my speculation as to why ADD, ADHD, and many other brain "Ds" are now epidemic among teens and even young adults. Once upon a time humans celebrated the big brain D—*differences.* There was probably a time when it was easier for adolescents to be whoever they are and still find useful roles and fit in with the tribe. Joe is rather impulsive, restless, can't sit still, but he can really hyperfocus when he's out in the woods. So he becomes a hunter. And because he's so sensitive, the tribe makes him the chief lookout for predators and warriors. When it comes to, say, making tools or building huts, Joe can't seem to stay on task. Fine. The tribe has plenty of other people who can.

Fast-forward into today's classroom. Joe doesn't fit into the standardized forms and norms of modern education. There is a mismatch between how Joe's brain works and how the teacher wants him to work, learn, and behave.

The system could educate Joe according to his needs and abilities, to help him find his own individual path, but in most schools, that would be too time consuming and too costly, not to mention that most educators don't really know how to do it. So they and Joe's parents take the easy way out. Instead of "drugging" our school system, they drug Joe to help him fit. The more uniquely Joe thinks, the more drugs he gets. After they took recess out of schools, Ritalin prescriptions went up. Any correlation? We think so.

CHAPTER 4

124. You Can Rewire Your Worry Circuit. Schwartz, JM, et al. Systematic changes in cerebral glucose metabolic rate after successful behavior modification treatment of obsessive-compulsive disorder. *Archives of General Psychiatry*, 1996 53;109–113. See also: Schwartz J, Begley S. *The Mind and the Brain: Neuroplasticity and the Power of Mental Force.* New York: Harper Collins, 2002.

125. Mind over medicines. Why not just pop a pill? Some medications are touted to help manage stress, for example, by dialing down stress hormone levels in people who are manic or anxious, or by elevating the mood of people who are depressed. The problem with pills is that, unlike the internal, natural medicines you can make for your own brain (which T5 promotes), synthetic medications seldom get it right. They either turn the dials down too low for too long, so that the person becomes "flat," or they turn them up too high for too long, so that the depressed person becomes "hyper." This imbalance of the medication's effect is called *cerebral disharmony.* There is also the *cocktail effect* in people who are on two, three, even five psychoactive medicines. Unlike the players in the body's natural symphony orchestra, these medications don't communicate with one another. Each does its own thing—playing too loud, too soft, or too long. On the other hand, your own natural mood-mellowing neurochemicals are all interconnected and orchestrated. When one plays too loud, the others say "cool it, dial down," like a conductor gesturing to the drummer to play more softly.

The belief effect. A landmark 2002 study published in the most respected medical journal at that time, *The New England Journal of Medicine,* strongly suggests that doctors and patients should give more respect to the "mind healing" of the placebo effect, also called the belief effect. A study on patients who were undergoing surgery for knee pain found that those who had a "fake surgery" (had wound prep and incisions performed, etc., but nothing done inside the knee) improved as well as those who had actually undergone some surgical manipulation on the inside of the knee. The placebo patients didn't find out that they belonged to that group for a couple years after their "surgery," but they continued to heal as well. Moseley JB, et al. A controlled trial of arthroscopic surgery for osteoarthritis of the knee. *New England Journal of Medicine.* 2002;347:81–88; Niemi M. Placebo effect: a cure in the mind. *Scientific American Mind.* 2009;20:42–49.

126. Think-changing skills better than pills. Studies at the University of Toronto found that cognitive behavioral therapy (CBT, which we prefer to call TCB, or think-changing the brain) dialed down the firings of sad-center nerves and dialed up the happy center. The scientists went on to conclude that relapse rates with TCB are much lower than with medication, which, they found, "in many cases seems to be no more effective than a placebo for anything but the most severe depression." Goldapple Z, et al. Modulation of cortical-limbic pathways in major depression: treatment-specific effects of cognitive behavior therapy. *Archives of General Psychiatry.* 2004;61:34–41.

132. Breathe deeply through your NO-rich nose. Nasal deep breathing is even better since it increases the release of nitric oxide, which may assist in lowering anxiety. Increased nasal NO also leads to decreased pulmonary vascular resistance, a benefit for people with asthma or pulmonary disease.

133. Why cats purr. Exhaling while pursing your lips or placing the tip of your tongue against the inside of your upper teeth is called *resistance breathing*. In their excellent book, *The Healing Power of the Breath* (Shambhala Publications, Boulder, CO), medical doctors Richard Brown and Patricia Gerbarg describe how partially obstructing the airflow during exhalation stimulates the calming nerves in a cat's brain. When you hear a cat purr, they are actually self-medicating and self-calming.

133. Breathe better to think better. When you deeply inhale you activate stretch receptors in the lungs, like pulling a cord that signals the brain to "relax, cool it." Deep breathing dials down the SNS, the busy stressor center that says "move fast!" SNS is often associated with increased heart rate, because it's a quick-reaction survival mechanism. Deep breathing dials up the PNS—the quiet center—which decreases heart rate, blood pressure, and metabolic rate; decreases the wear and tear of oxidative stress; and increases melatonin, the sleep hormone, which is why deep breathing is good before bedtime.

ANOTHER T5 EFFECT: BREATHE FIVE TIMES A MINUTE

After breathing more from the belly, more slowly, and nearly always through the nose, besides feeling self-calming "medicine," I noticed an unexpected T5 effect: I was naturally breathing more slowly, averaging five breaths per minute. I was curious what science says about breathing techniques. Compared with fast upper-chest mouth-breathing, slow, nasal, rhythmic belly breathing:

- Provides more oxygen delivery to tissues because the lower parts of the lungs are larger, contain more blood supply and air sacs, and are more easily inflated with belly breathing.
- Maintains just the right body chemistry (levels of oxygen and carbon dioxide and acid-base balance) to increase oxygen delivery to better energize tissues.
- Improves self-detoxing by increasing lymphatic drainage of the waste products of metabolism.

Take slow, deep belly breaths while reading an informative book: McKeown, Patrick, *The Oxygen Advantage,* New York, Harper Collins, 2015.

136. Tread water to shed worries. Warm-water bathing improves the balance between the two branches of the nervous system that trigger stress: dialing down the rev-up neurochemicals (the SNS), and dialing up the rest-and-relax PNS branch. (See SNS and PNS balance, page 151.)

137. Have an Attitude of Gratitude. Neuroscientists, using new brain-imaging technology, revealed that we can grow the gratitude center in our brains. When we focus on what we have to be thankful for, the good things in our lives, we light up an area of the brain called the anterior cingulate, which is connected to our happy center, the hippocampus. The gratitude center is also connected to the amygdala, the fear center, helping us dial down stress. Kini P, et al. The effects of gratitude expression on neural activity. *NeuroImage.* 2016;128:1–10.

139. Dr. Bill's meditation story. There are approximately twenty references to meditation in the Bible, which should serve as an answer to some modernists who downplay meditation as "too Buddhist." In fact, Christianity has a rich historical tradition of "contemplative prayer," which we now call meditation. In Genesis, "Isaac went out to meditate in the field." In Joshua, "Followers are commanded by law to meditate day and night." In the twelfth century there were four levels of monastic practice: *lectio* (read it), *meditatio* (ponder the deeper meaning of what you read), *oratio* (pray about it), and *contemplatio* (listen to what God tells you about it).

139. Meditate like a monk. In this famous monk study, researchers did functional MRIs on Buddhist monks, revealing that years of daily meditation had literally changed their brains, especially improving brain centers associated with the ability to sustain concentration and focus. Their conclusion was that long-term meditation might help to reduce what the researchers called "neural noise," or what we would call annoying "brain chatter" or "brain clutter." Davidson RJ, et al. Buddha's brain: neuroplasticity and meditation. *IEEE Signal Process Magazine.* January 1, 2008;25:176.

140. Windows into your brain. For fascinating neuroimaging studies on how nature affects the brain, see *Your Brain on Nature* by Harvard neurologist Dr. Eva Selhub.

153. Unresolved stress. According to *The Lancet Interheart Study*, stress is responsible for nearly 40 percent of heart attacks. During the stress response, epinephrine makes circulating platelets more likely to clump together. If there are some tears in the lining of the vessel, these clumps of sticky stuff are more likely to collect there, clogging the artery. Furthermore, the lower the heart rate, the longer we tend to live. An insightful and scientific explanation of the stress response in various animals and how it applies to humans during cardiovascular, immunological, and cerebral illnesses is found in Robert Sapolsky, *Why Zebras Don't Get Ulcers: An Updated Guide to Stress-Related Diseases and Coping,* 3rd ed., New York: Holt Paperbacks, 2004.

155. A waist size greater than 40 inches. Since waist size is now the most accepted predictor of health, your doctor may measure your waist-to-height ratio (WHR) during checkups. Your waist size should be less than half your height. If you have a waist size of 36 inches and you're 68 inches tall, you need to lose two inches off your waist. While this ratio is an easier measurement, another WHR—waist-to-hip ratio—may be more meaningful. A waist-to-hip ratio of less than 1.0 for men and less than 0.85 for women is considered a healthy goal.

Part II

CHAPTER 6

190. The "second brain." One of the brainiest books I have ever read is *The Second Brain*, by Michael Gershon, MD (Quill, 2003).

191. These gut bugs manage your intestinal health. Meet a few of your "pharmacy staff," the good bacteria that are in probiotics:

- *Lactobacillus bulgaricus*
- *Lactobacillus rhamnosus*
- *Lactobacillus casei*

- *Lactobacillus acidophilus*
- *Bifidobacterium lactis*
- *Bifidobacterium breve*

There are actually over a thousand species of gut bugs. These are six of the most common ones seen on probiotic labels.

196. Fermenting fats. Three SCFAs made by your microbiome are acetate, butyrate, and propionate. The intestinal cells rapidly absorb these SCFAs and use them as energy sources to keep the gut lining growing. They also regulate how much extra food energy is stored as fat, especially around the waist.

199. Your gut bacteria can produce neurohormones. Brain medicines your microbiome makes include serotonin, dopamine, acetylcholine, histamine, catecholamines, melatonin, GABA (the mood-balancing neurotransmitter), NGF (nerve growth factor, fertilizer for your brain garden), Vitamin B_{12}, and many more.

203. SAD from top to bottom. How does fast food harm gut-bug health? Here's the inside scoop on why fast food is bad for your microbiome. An interesting experiment was done in 2015 by Tim Spector, professor of genetic epidemiology at King's College in London. Tim set out to test the effects of junk food on the microbiome. For his guinea pig, he chose his son, Tom, a student of genetics.

The experiment: Tom ate all his meals at the local fast-food burger joint for ten days. His diet consisted of greasy cheeseburgers, chicken nuggets, fries, and cola. Dad collected his son's fecal samples before, during, and after to see what was happening to his son's gut bugs in response to this drastic change in diet. Not surprisingly, Tom was bothered by this change of diet even more than his gut bugs. He became literally sick and tired and emotionally down, as well. His friends told him he even looked sick, with a "strange grey color." Tom was suffering from inflammation of the gut lining, where most of the serotonin, the happy hormone, is made, which accounted for his moodiness.

His gut bugs also became sick. The good guys, called *Firmicutes,* were replaced by bad guys, *Bacteroides.* And the really good guys, the bifida bacteria, on which we rely to keep our inflammation balanced, were reduced by half. The biggest change was in diversity: Tom lost nearly 40 percent of the 1,400 species of gut bugs that he had when the experiment began. Two weeks after the experiment was over, his microbes still had not recovered.

Parents and grandparents, read Tom's sad story to your young. Millennials, do you really want that SAD stuff in your body?

Stetka B. In search of the optimal brain diet. *Scientific American Mind.* 2016;27:26–33.

203. More SAD effects. Pediatricians and neurologists are becoming increasingly concerned about the increasing number of younger children who are being drugged for a variety of "disorders." As of 2014, it is reported that over 10,000 American *two- and three-year-olds* are now being medicated for ADHD. Renowned neurologist David Perlmutter in his insightful book *Brain Maker* raises a red flag that we are giving too many children brain-changing drugs at this vulnerable time in brain development without much scientific knowledge of what they actually do to the brain. He has written widely about how the SAD diet, low in plant fiber and high in processed and artificial chemical foods, contributes to ADD and Alzheimer's. (See related section, "The Brain Accumulates Sticky Stuff," page 217.)

209. Artificial sweeteners. There's a revealing read about how artificial sweeteners harm the health of your microbiome in the July 2015 *Life Extension Magazine* on page 67, entitled "Artificial Sweeteners Promotes Weight Gain."

209. Sugar-sweetened carbonated beverages. Carbonated beverages mess with the microbiome. Carbonation interferes with taste and intestinal satiety-hormone balance, triggering you to crave more sweets and eat and drink more. An interesting neuroimaging study showed that carbonation reduced the perception of sweetness, which may prompt the drinker to drink more sweet stuff to become satisfied—just what the beverage industry loves. Di Salle F, et. al. Effect of carbonation on brain processing of sweet stimuli in humans. *Gastroenterology.* 2013;145:537–539.

A new study from John Hopkins School of Public Health reveals that overweight people who drink diet sodas tend to consume more calories. MRI studies showed that carbonation decreased the neuroprocessing of sweetness-related signals, prompting researchers to speculate that artificial sweeteners increase appetite and stimulate the reward centers of the brain, which leads the person to eat more by triggering hunger via the same mechanism as sugar.

CHAPTER 7

225. Exercise Goes to Your Head. After reviewing over 1,600 scientific papers, scientists at the Mayo Clinic concluded that exercise:

- Helps prevent cognitive decline
- Lessens Alzheimer's disease
- Improves performance test scores at any age
- Improves moods
- Facilitates motivation
- Improves energy

Ahlskog JE, et al. Physical exercise as a preventive or disease-modifying treatment of dementia and brain aging. *Mayo Clinic Proceedings.* 2011;86:876–884.

226. Movement makes more blood vessels. Since aerobic exercise gets blood flowing faster, it builds more blood channels in the brain. This finding parallels research in animals that showed that chronic aerobic exercise can lead to growth of new capillaries in the brain, increase the length and number of dendritic interconnections between neurons, and even increase cell growth in the hippocampus. The increase in brain volume is most likely due to an increase in brain-growth fertilizers (BDNF and IGF-1), which grow more small blood vessels and more interconnections between brain cells.

226. Movement makes healthier blood vessels. You've read herein how, when you move, your internal endothelial pharmacy makes more nitric oxide (NO), which is really a multipurpose medicine. NO dilates, or widens, blood vessels during exercise, but it's also a neurotransmitter, one of those vital messengers that relay chemical signals from one nerve fiber to another and are needed for thought processes and moods. NO is also a natural antioxidant, or anti-rust, neurochemical, and brains need more NO, because they are more prone to rust. A new discovery shows that the brain, like the endothelium, makes a lot of NO, a revelation that is prompting neurologists to wonder if Alzheimer's could be a NO deficiency.

226. A visit to Veggieland. Researchers in the United Kingdom advised people with high blood pressure to make one simple change: eat more fruits and vegetables, even if it's just one extra serving a day of each. After two months, those who increased their daily fruit and vegetable eating the most showed the best improvement in endothelial function. McCall DO, et al. Dietary intake of fruits and vegetables improves microvascular function in hypertensive subjects in a dose-dependent manner. *Circulation.* 2009;119(16):2153–2160.

229. Science says: Movement makes brain medicines. Here are the main brainy neurochemicals that increase with movement: dopamine, testosterone, norepinephrine, acetylcholine, vascular endothelial growth factor, opiates (which are natural analgesics, sedatives, and anxiolytics), endorphins (only if intense exercise), and adiponectin. Deslandes, A, et al. Exercise and mental health: many reasons to move. *Neuropsychobiology.* 2009;59:191–198.

Chapter 8

244. Alzheimer's Begins in Young Adults. The higher the level of the sticky biochemicals, the higher the chances of your getting a neurodegenerative disease such as Alzheimer's. Feng C, et al. Hyperhomocysteinemia associates with small vessel disease more closely than large vessel disease. *International Journal Medical Science.* 2013;10:408–412.

Also, a higher level of sticky stuff such as hemoglobin A1c is associated with an increased incidence of neurodegenerative diseases, especially Alzheimer's. Kimattila SM, et al. Chronic hyperglycemia impairs endothelial function and insulin sensitivity via different mechanisms in insulin-dependent diabetes mellitus. *Circulation.* 1996;94:11276–11282.

245. The omega-3 effect on blood vessels. Like the antioxidants in fruits and vegetables, omega-3s help endothelial function in two ways: decreasing sticky stuff and relaxing the blood vessels, which promotes greater blood flow. Omega-3 molecules work their way into the membranes of the red blood cells, making them less likely to sludge together, resulting in smoother blood flow, what scientists call *cellular fluidity*. Researchers suggest that omega-3s either increase the production of nitric oxide (NO) or make the arterial wall more responsive to it. Either way, they do help relax the arteries. Researchers found a clue to the vasodilating effects of omega-3s when they studied coastal villagers in Japan, who tend to eat more fish compared with those who live inland, and found that the arteries of the fish eaters relaxed more. This article also showed research that omega-3s given to diabetics increased arterial NO production. Brown A, et al. Dietary modulation of endothelial function: implications for cardiovascular disease. *American Journal of Clinical Nutrition.* 2001;73:673–686.

259. Why smoothing out sugar spikes with a plant-based diet helps fight cancer. The number one finding on which all studies and all scientists agree: a predominantly plant-based diet is the best cancer-prevention medicine. Moreover, convincing science says that people who eat more red meat are more likely to get cancer. Further, a November 2008 study in the *American Journal of Clinical Nutrition* showed that men who ate fish at least five times a week had an almost 50 percent lower prostate cancer death rate than those who didn't. Chavarro J, et al. A 22-y prospective study of fish intake in relation to prostate cancer incidence and mortality. *American Journal of Clinical Nutrition.* 2008;88:1297–1303.

The SAD diet promotes cancer, as shown by the *Journal of American Medical Association*, August 15, 2007. Patients with the highest intake of a Western diet (high in red meat, sugary desserts, fat, and refined grains) had a threefold increase in colon cancer. Meyerhardt J, et al. Association of dietary patterns with cancer recurrence and survival in patients with stage III colon cancer. *Journal of American Medical Association.* 2007;298(7):754–764.

Dr. Dean Ornish, a friend and one of my most trusted scientists, showed that a plant-based diet can suppress cancer growth. Ornish D, et al. Intensive lifestyle changes may affect the progress of prostate cancer. *Journal of Urology.* 2005;174:1065–1070.

259. Cancer Causes . . . sedentary lifestyle. Movement reduces risk of colon cancer, possibly because moving the body moves the food and stools through the intestine faster, so that any cancer-causing chemicals in this stuff have less contact with the cells lining the intestines. However, the main reason movement reduces cancer is that movers have more effective immune systems than sitters do. Lee, IM. Physical activity and cancer prevention—data from epidemiological studies. *Medicine and Science in Sports and Exercise.* 2003;35:1823–1827. Rockhill B. A prospective study of recreational physical activity and breast cancer risk. *Archives of Internal Medicine.* 1999;159:2290–2296. Pedersen L, et al. Voluntary running suppresses tumor growth through epinephrine and IL-6 dependent NK cell mobilization and redistribution. *Cell Metabolism.* 2016;23:554–562. Friedenreich C. Physical activity and cancer prevention: from observational to intervention research. *Cancer Epidemiology, Biomarkers & Prevention.* 2001;10:287–301.

One of the proposed mechanisms is that exercise increases insulin sensitivity, thereby lowering the blood level of insulin growth factor (IGF/1), a potent cancer cell fertilizer. Westerlind K. Physical activity and cancer prevention—mechanisms. *Medicine and Science in Sports and Exercise.* 2003;35:1834–1840.

CHAPTER 9

281. Cheating on eating. You spike after a binge. Science suggests that even one big sticky-stuff meal can harm your heart. The most noticeable effect of a big, fat "pig-out" is that dreaded term *endothelial dysfunction.* When healthy volunteers had their arterial function measured after a sticky-stuff eating binge, it showed their blood vessels got stiffer within two hours after the binge. This seems to be the explanation for the *steakhouse syndrome* in which cardiologists have noticed a higher incidence of heart attacks after eating big, sticky steaks. Vogel RA, et al. Effect of a single high-fat meal on endothelial function in healthy subjects. *American Journal of Cardiology*. 1997;79:350–354.

283. Mother Nature does it for you. In the June issue of *Scientific American,* scientists at Tufts University Human Nutrition Research Center wrote an insightful article on the relationship between the daily calories you consume and the weight you gain or maintain. This was one of the most insightful and well-researched articles on clearing up calorie confusion that I have ever read. The conclusions of these researchers:

- Different people control their weight differently with different foods. One person may eat 100 calories of nuts and store or burn a different number of those calories than another person. Two persons eating the same diet might burn or store energy differently by as many as 500 calories a day. There are genetic burners and genetic storers.
- How a food is processed affects the calories it yields. For example, because raw almonds are digested more slowly, we extract fewer calories from them than if the same number of calories were obtained from almond butter.
- The higher the fiber content of a food, the fewer calories extracted from the food and the more calories the body burns or excretes. A person eating a high-fiber cereal would store fewer calories and burn more than if she had eaten a cereal with less fiber, even if the calories listed on the package label are the same. (That's one of the main points of T5: fiber feeds weight control.)
- Because metabolism—calorie burning—slows down with age, the older we get, the fewer calories we need.

- Because metabolic rate drops during weight loss, the body protects itself by becoming more fuel efficient. This is how increased exercise compensates for the reduced metabolic rate (decreased calorie burning) and helps maintain the weight loss.
- The higher the carb spike of a meal, the more a person tends to eat and the hungrier they are after the meal. For example, a bowl of boxed cereal (low in protein, fat, and fiber) leaves the eater hungrier than if she consumed the same number of calories in a breakfast of eggs and oatmeal.

287. Move more, drug less. Mood specialists have long known that the more you move, the better you feel. Studies showed that many people can get just as good an antidepressant effect from exercise as they could from drugs, but without the unpleasant side effects. Schuch FB, et al. Exercise as a treatment for depression: a meta-analysis adjusting for publication bias. *Journal Psychiatric Research.* 2016;77:42–51; Cooney GM, et al. Exercise for depression. *Cochrane Database of Systematic Review.* 2013;12(9):CD0043GG; Ratey JJ. *Spark: The Revolutionary New Science of Exercise and the Brain.* New York: Little, Brown, 2008.

287. T5 for Depression. While antidepressant medications have been health-savers, even life-savers, for some people, when you mess with your neurotransmitters, either with thoughts or medications, you can also change your personality—for better or worse. Psychiatrists notice that while some persons treated with medications are less depressed and less anxious, others may become less creative, less interesting, and "flat." As one of my friends said to his medicated wife, "You are no longer you." A ten-year-old patient of mine told his parents that he wanted to stop his "focus pills" during the school-free summer months, saying, "I just want to be me!"

SUGGESTED READING

Other related books by Dr. William Sears:

Sears, William. *The Inflammation Solution.* Denver: Dr. Sears' Wellness Institute, 2015.

Sears, William, and James Sears. *The Omega-3 Effect.* New York: Little, Brown, 2012.

Sears, William, and Martha Sears. *Prime-Time Health: A Scientifically Proven Plan for Feeling Younger and Living Longer.* New York: Little, Brown, 2010.

More suggested reading:

Asprey, Dave. *The Bulletproof Diet.* New York: Rodale, 2014.

Borysenko, Joan. *The Plant Plus Diet Solution.* Carlsbad, CA: Hay House, 2014.

Davidson, Richard J., and Sharon Begley. *The Emotional Life of Your Brain.* New York: Plume, 2013.

Fortanasce, Vincent. *The Anti-Alzheimer's Prescription: The Science-Proven Prevention Plan to Start at Any Age.* New York: Gotham Books, 2008.

Ludwig, David. *Always Hungry*. New York: Grand Central Publishing, 2016.

Lustig, Robert H. *Fat Chance: Beating the Odds Against Sugar, Processed Food, Obesity, and Disease*. New York: Plume, 2012.

Newberg, Andrew, and Mark Robert Waldman. *How God Changes Your Brain: Breakthrough Findings from a Leading Neuroscientist*. New York: Harper Wave, 2016.

Ornish, Dean. *Love and Survival: 8 Pathways to Intimacy and Health*. New York: HarperCollins, 1998.

Ornish, Dean. *The Spectrum: A Scientifically Proven Program to Feel Better, Live Longer, Lose Weight, Gain Health*. New York: Ballantine Books, 2007.

Ratey, John J., with Eric Hagerman. *Spark: The Revolutionary New Science of Exercise and the Brain*. .New York: Little, Brown, 2008.

Servan-Schreiber, David. *Anti-Cancer: A New Way of Life*. New York: Viking, 2008.

⊕ SCIENTIFIC JOURNAL REFERENCES

For our list of over 100 references supporting our T5 plan, visit DrSearsWellness.org/T5/References.

SUBJECT INDEX

RECIPE INDEX

GRATITUDES

FROM DR. BILL:

A huge thanks to my mentors, who taught me the tools to use in my own health transformation: *Richard Van Praagh, MD*, professor of pediatrics at Harvard Medical School, who instilled in me the show-me-the-science mindset. *Louis Ignarro, PhD*. Thank you, Dr. Lou, for teaching me about your Nobel Prize–winning research revealing where in the world of our body is our own personal pharmacy and what medicines it makes. *Dean Ornish, MD*, one of the original pioneers in preventive medicine, founder and president of the Preventive Medicine Research Institute, and clinical professor of medicine at the University of California, San Francisco. Dr. Dean's books and personal guidance taught me to appreciate the concept of "doctor" first as preventer of disease and second as prescriber of medicines. *Randy Hartnell,* owner of Vital Choice Seafood Company, whom I call "my favorite fisherman." Thank you, Randy, for the privilege of fishing with you while you taught me to appreciate seafood as one of the top nutrients in mind and body transformation. *Vincent Fortanasce, MD*, author of *The Anti-Alzheimer's Prescription* and clinical professor of neurology at the University of Southern California School of Medicine. Thank you, Dr. Vince, for teaching me that prevention of brain illnesses, especially Alzheimer's, must begin in young adults. *Gerry Cysewski, PhD,* who taught me about an important nutrient that is left out of most wellness plans—astaxanthin. *David Katz, MD,* founding director of Yale University's Preventive Research Center, for his continued writings on preventive medicine. *Tom Aarts,* founder of the NBJ Summit, for introducing me to the leaders in the field of preventive medicine, many of whom are referenced throughout this book.

FROM ERIN:

My deepest gratitude goes out to so many people who have supported me along this journey. First and foremost, I thank God for the beautiful gift of life. To my sweet John, you have been there every step of the way as my biggest cheerleader; I love you. To my parents for your unconditional love and belief in me. Dad, a special thanks to you for your guidance and encouragement through this process. My friends and mentors Pam Lasich, Joy Bess, and Kyczy Hawk, your presence in my life helps keep me grounded and soaring at the same time. Thank you to Amber D'Anna and East West Yoga for guiding me through the transformational world of yoga. I would also like to acknowledge Linda Carlberg, graphic designer extraordinaire. Matt Sears, you are a lifesaver; major thanks for your hard work. Lastly, I am so grateful for all the clients I've been blessed with throughout the years. You teach me every day how to thrive in this life, and I am so honored to walk through it together.

FROM THE BOTH OF US:

A special thanks to our team of "co-workers": *Martha Sears, R.N.,* Dr. Bill's wife of 51 years, Erin's mother, patient proofreader, and untiring cheerleader; *Tracee Zeni,* Dr. Bill's diligent editorial assistant for over 25 years; *Matthew Sears,* our research assistant, for his untiring search for the best science behind our transformation tools; *Jonathan Sears*, our online medical journal detective. Special hugs to Dominique Hodgin, director of the Dr. Sears Wellness Institute. Thank you for having many of our wellness coaches read the manuscript and, together with your own comments, provide valuable material for this book. Big smiles to our graphic artist, *Debbie Maze,* who makes readers smile as they read. We deeply thank our literary agents, Denise Marcil and Anne Marie O'Farrell, at the Denise Marcil Literary Agency, for making the perfect match with BenBella

Books. A special thanks to the diligent staff at BenBella Books for their untiring patience and insightful suggestions: Leah Wilson, Editor-in-Chief; Dave Bessmer, Chief Grammar Detective, otherwise known as "editor"; Heather Butterfield, Senior Marketing Manager; Jessika Rieck, Deputy Production Manager; Adrienne Lang, Deputy Publisher; and Glenn Yeffeth, Publisher and CEO.

We wish you all a big dose of the helper's high for your contributions to this book!

—WILLIAM SEARS AND ERIN SEARS BASILE